Orthodontic-Surgical Treatment of Dentofacial Anomalies: An Integrated Esthetic-Functional Approach

First published in Italian as *Dismorfie dento-facciali: Trattamento ortodontico-chirugico, Approccio integrato estetico-funzionale* by Quintessenza Edizioni Srl. Translation by Frances Cooper.

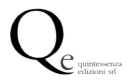

Quintessenza Edizioni Srl
20017 Passirana di Rho (MI)
via Ciro Menotti, 65
Italy
www.quintessenzaedizioni.it

Printed in Italy

Orthodontic-Surgical Treatment of Dentofacial Anomalies

An Integrated Esthetic-Functional Approach

Paolo Ronchi, DMD

Head of Oral and Maxillofacial Surgery
Sant'Anna Hospital
Como, Italy

With a DVD Presenting a Live Surgery

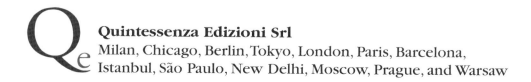

Quintessenza Edizioni Srl
Milan, Chicago, Berlin, Tokyo, London, Paris, Barcelona,
Istanbul, São Paulo, New Delhi, Moscow, Prague, and Warsaw

To Prof Paolo Gotte, with recognition and gratitude

To Patrizia, Stefano, and Silvia, for their support and patience

TABLE OF CONTENTS

INTRODUCTION

CHAPTER 1

CHAPTER 2

CHAPTER 3

CHAPTER 4

CONTRIBUTORS

Dr Luigi Colombo
Specialist in Oral and Maxillofacial Surgery
Level I Medical Director
Maxillofacial Surgery
Sant'Anna Hospital
Como, Italy

Dr Alberto Guariglia
Specialist in Orthodontics
Private Practice
Milan, Italy

Dr Andrea Di Francesco
Specialist in Oral and Maxillofacial Surgery
Level I Medical Director
Maxillofacial Surgery
Sant'Anna Hospital
Como, Italy

Dr Giorgio Novelli
Specialist in Oral and Maxillofacial Surgery
Level I Medical Director
Maxillofacial Surgery
Sant'Anna Hospital
Como, Italy

Dr Stefano Panigatti
Specialist in Oral and Maxillofacial Surgery
Level I Medical Director
Maxillofacial Surgery
Sant'Anna Hospital
Como, Italy

FOREWORD

Almost at the close of my university career, it gives me great satisfaction to present the book *Orthodontic-Surgical Treatment of Dentofacial Anomalies* by Paolo Ronchi.

Life brings events that are predictable and others that are not, the latter perhaps being more frequent and often the cause of regret that we did not predict their possible occurrence. Those belonging to the first category, however, are the natural consequences expected from a series of events, and Paolo Ronchi's career clearly fits into this category.

I first met Paolo Ronchi in November 1976 when he entered the Oral and Maxillofacial Surgery Clinic at the University of Verona. His studies at our school culminated in a diploma in oral and maxillofacial surgery (1989). During this period of development, he became interested in orthodontic treatment for dysgnathic anomalies and subsequently in the surgical techniques available to resolve maxillary and mandibular anomalies.

In 1986 Dr Ronchi was made head of the Oral and Maxillofacial Surgery Department at Sant'Anna Hospital in Como, Italy, a position he still holds. Over the next 13 years, he amassed expansive experience in dentofacial anomalies, and he has chosen to pass on this experience by publishing this book.

The success of this book lies in its great clarity in expressing the essence of surgery for dentofacial anomalies. This essence stems from Dr Ronchi's experience as a surgeon and from his ability to cleverly integrate functional requirements and esthetic rules. These are the goals and the guidelines of every rehabilitation. The style is easy to read and elegant, simple and understandable, and the case descriptions, supplemented with numerous illustrations, make this text highly practical and clinically relevant.

Paolo Gotte
Professor and Director
Oral and Maxillofacial Surgery Clinic
University of Verona
Verona, Italy

FOREWORD

When we write a book, we transmit the ideas of our experience gained through years of application and dedication to our work. For a book to be successful, though, something more is needed, some feature that represents a fresh contribution. With this book, I believe there are two innovative features: The first is the special consideration given to function and esthetics, and the second is the accompanying DVD, which presents video of the surgeries described in the text.

Mandibular and maxillary surgery must inevitably and particularly take into account functional aspects. Experience has proven to me, time and again, that it is impossible to change the inclination and dimension of the maxilla or mandible without also producing a significant, even a determinant change at the muscular level. Relapses, patient discomfort, and tension-related muscular pain after surgery, in my experience, tend to originate from excessive concentration on the structural bony components while neglecting the muscular situation. In the same way, it is important to consider esthetic aspects; much space in the literature has been dedicated to this aspect, and Paolo Ronchi, in this book, has succeeded in giving this issue the proper focus and, above all, the possibility of practical clinical application.

The ability to observe on the DVD what is explained in the text is important for rapid and effective learning. University teaching is now moving in this same direction, using direct observation as a form of instruction to improve learning and understanding. The author has succeeded in implementing this approach to more effectively impart his knowledge to the reader.

In light of these considerations, I believe that the work of Paolo Ronchi is an innovative contribution to university teaching, as well as a worthwhile update for those who wish to perfect their skills in the field of maxillofacial surgery.

Giorgio Nidoli
Professor
Faculty of Medicine and Surgery
Department of Orthodontics
University of Insubria
Varese, Italy

PREFACE

Orthodontic-surgical treatment of dentofacial deformities is a continually evolving discipline whose practice is becoming more widespread. This book was written for orthodontists and maxillofacial surgeons who are already working in this fascinating field, as well as for those who are preparing to do so. Drawing on more than 30 years of clinical experience, I have illustrated in this text the essential aspects of treatment of dentofacial anomalies while avoiding long theoretical explanations. My primary aim is to achieve clarity and simplicity so that orthodontists can more easily understand the surgical problems involved in such treatment, and likewise surgeons can become more familiar with the orthodontic aspects.

The philosophy that must guide us in treating dentofacial deformities is that of integrating function and esthetics. Technologic progress gives us increasingly sophisticated instruments, but nevertheless, underlying a good result and a good relationship between doctor and patient must always be a large dose of clinical common sense. For this purpose, I have provided practical information related to the various therapeutic phases—from the initial planning through the orthodontic and surgical phases and finally to the postoperative reeducation. I have also given particular importance to some aspects that have recently emerged in the literature: relationships with temporomandibular joint dysfunction, problems surrounding rigid fixation and condylar position, aspects of postoperative rehabilitation, and the possibilities that may be offered by new surgical techniques such as distraction osteogenesis. There is also an important chapter concerning how to prevent and manage errors and complications. The final chapter is devoted to presenting and discussing 33 clinical cases that exemplify the different types of anomalies as well as different therapeutic solutions. The DVD accompanying the book illustrates a complete case from start to finish with particular emphasis on surgery. The entire procedure is presented, including footage of all the principal stages.

I hope that this work will be a simple and practical tool for study and consultation for anyone who treats patients with dentofacial anomalies, whether it is to review a single aspect in greater depth or to learn how to avoid some of the most frequent errors. Indeed, if this work helps only one colleague to better understand one aspect of treatment or avoid a mistake, then I can say that I have truly achieved my most important goal.

ACKNOWLEDGMENTS

My thanks to all my co-authors and collaborators who have helped in the writing of this book, as well as to those who have worked with me in past years. Very heartfelt thanks to all the postgraduates of Milan University who have attended my department over these years, as well as to the nursing staff, who amid continual difficulties have succeeded in working alongside me successfully and unceasingly all these years; without them this book could never have been written.

Particular thanks to my friends Dr Aurelio Levrini and Prof Luca Levrini for their valuable advice in the orthodontic and publishing fields.

The most important and most sincere thanks naturally go to Prof Paolo Gotte, who taught me surgery, and to Prof Giorgio Nidoli. They have accompanied and presented my work with words that are both moving and stimulating. I hope someday to be able to live up to them.

Lastly, I cannot forget my patients. It is thanks not least to their willingness to agree to publication that the documentation, which I feel is essential to any book of this type, is so rich and I hope so demonstrative.

Indications for Orthodontic-Surgical Treatment

The correction of dental malocclusions has always had a dual goal: function and esthetics. Normal stomatognathic functioning associated with satisfactory facial esthetics must inevitably have significant repercussions on a patient's general state of health. The physical health of patients with severe malocclusion may be altered or compromised in various ways; if the problem is such as to significantly reduce masticatory capability, there may be repercussions on the digestive tract or, in some cases, impossibility of ingesting certain types of food. Marked dentoskeletal malposition may cause problems with speech or induce respiratory deficiency in the upper airways. It is also known that some dentoskeletal anomalies are closely linked with obstructive sleep apnea syndrome, with all its repercussions on the cardiorespiratory apparatus. If teeth are irregular, protruded, or crowded, it is more difficult to maintain good oral hygiene, with a consequent increased predisposition to caries, and periodontal problems may become severe. Some conditions also predispose to an increased probability of temporomandibular joint pain and/or dysfunction.

Nevertheless, we believe that the esthetic aspect of severe malocclusion with its related psychosocial impact is more important than the correlated physical problems, particularly in modern society, which assigns increasing importance to appearance. Both self-image and images of others are closely influenced by facial and dental appearance. Suffice it to recall the stereotype of the mentally challenged person with long face, open bite, and labial incompetence, which contemporary society frequently proposes: This type of alteration may thus become a particularly severe disability for our patients. The positive effect of an attractive face on an individual's mind-set is clear in terms of self-confidence and self-respect. On the other hand, it is quite probable that a subject with a severe dentoskeletal alteration may develop a lack of self-confidence, or even depression of varying severity, that might lead to suicidal feelings in some cases. Thus the cornerstone for valid treatment must be to combine acceptable functionality with satisfactory esthetics.

In recent years, increasing numbers of patients have elected to undergo orthodontic-surgical treatment to correct severe malocclusion not responsive to simple orthodontic solutions. Currently this type of alteration is defined as *dentofacial anomaly* or *dentofacial deformity*. Treatment of these types of anomaly, as of less severe cases of malocclusion, is clearly elective; in other words, it is not vital in the true meaning of the word as, for example, surgical treatment is vital for heart disease or to remove a tumor. Nevertheless, it may be extremely important to improve the quality of life for our patients, from both the physical and the mental standpoints, which is why treatment may be justified and necessary.

But who should be given orthodontic-surgical treatment? The most immediate and the simplest reply to this question is that orthodontic-surgical treatment is necessary whenever orthodontics alone is insufficient to resolve the problem. In reality, this response is both inexact and insufficient, and furthermore it conceals a severe risk: that of beginning exclusively orthodontic treatment only to realize, after treatment is underway, the impossibility of achieving an acceptable final result. This may leave the patient with a dramatic, irreversible situation. Thus the response must be both more complete and more complex, and this is what is provided in this book.

In cases of severe malocclusion with dentoskeletal discrepancy, there are generally only three possible therapeutic options: modification of growth, camouflage through dental compensation, and surgical repositioning of the bony bases. Proffit's well-known discrepancy diagram (Proffit and Ackerman 1994)

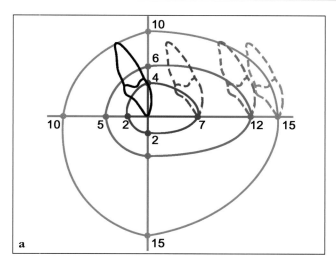 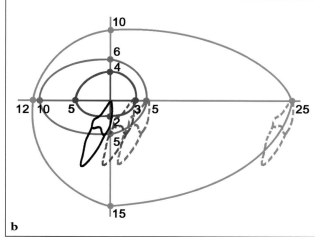

Fig 1 *(a and b)* Proffit's discrepancy diagram: displacements on the sagittal and vertical planes. (Reprinted from Proffit and Ackerman 1994 with permission.)

demonstrates these concepts in detail (Fig 1). The inner circle indicates the limits of orthodontic treatment alone (camouflage); the middle circle indicates tooth movement associated with growth modification; and the outer circle indicates surgical correction. However, the precise extension of these circles and thus the true possibilities for orthodontic and/or orthopedic treatment may be debatable, since not all data are supported by scientifically impeccable research; some are only based on subjective clinical evaluation. The precise dimensions of the diagram, however, are less important than the philosophical concept they express, which must be applied individually to each case.

First and foremost, an overriding rule is that vertical problems, in general, are more difficult to correct from the orthodontic and growth standpoints than are purely sagittal problems; thus a vertical problem in a subject who has completed growth is unlikely to be resolved through orthodontics alone. This concept holds for anomalies of both vertical excess and vertical deficiency. Furthermore, again from the general standpoint, the diagram provides no transverse references, whereas in some malocclusions transverse problems may require surgical solutions. This principle is virtually absolute for all types of dentofacial asymmetry.

With regard to growth, it is obvious that the fundamental parameters we must consider are age, gender, type of malocclusion, and skeletal involvement in the defect. Clearly, age and gender impose precise limits with regard to the timing of any orthopedic-functional treatment. Furthermore, at present there is reasonable consensus on two fundamental points. First, growth may be modified favorably only in some types of pa-

tients, which limits this approach; the maxilla or the mandible may be stimulated to grow by a few additional millimeters (it is much more difficult to limit growth by the same amount) than would have occurred naturally. Thus it is not possible to obtain significant transformations. Second, during all orthopedic-functional treatment the teeth inevitably also move in the direction of the correct occlusal relation. This tooth movement, which may be called *dental compensation for skeletal discrepancies* hinders complete orthopedic-skeletal correction and introduces some elements of dental camouflage.

It can be deduced from these considerations, for example, that in Class III situations, orthopedic treatment only plays a role in cases of slight isolated maxillary hypodevelopment with no mandibular protrusion and without significant vertical alteration (Fig 2). In all other cases treatment should be postponed until the end of growth, when surgical correction will be applied (Fig 3). In Class II cases, almost all of which are characterized by mandibular retrusion or hypodevelopment, dentofacial orthopedics during growth may in some cases play a determinant role. Nevertheless, some distinctions must also be made in these cases, since not all Class II patients may be treated in this way with satisfactory and stable results. An article by Proffit et al (1992) provides detailed indications for the therapeutic choice of orthodontic, orthopedic, or orthodontic-surgical treatment for subjects during growth (Fig 4). Important considerations may also be gained from this study for malocclusion characterized by open bite and vertical excess. As was said above, in general, vertical problems are much more difficult to correct without the help of surgery.

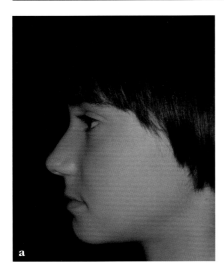

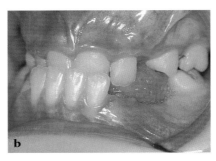

Fig 2 *(a and b)* Example of skeletal Class III malocclusion with growth pattern favorable for an early gnatho-orthopedic correction with the Delaire mask.

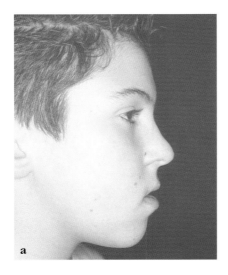

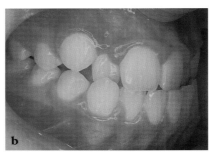

Fig 3 *(a and b)* Example of skeletal Class III malocclusion with growth pattern unfavorable for gnatho-orthopedic correction.

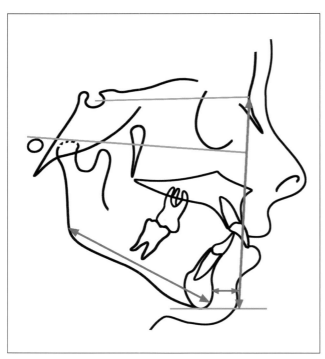

Fig 4 Indications for surgical treatment in adolescent subjects with severe Class II malocclusion: anterior overjet more than 10 mm, anterior vertical height more than 125 mm, distance from pogonion to nasion–Frankfort perpendicular more than 18 mm, length of mandibular body less than 70 mm. (Reprinted from Proffit et al 1992 with permission.)

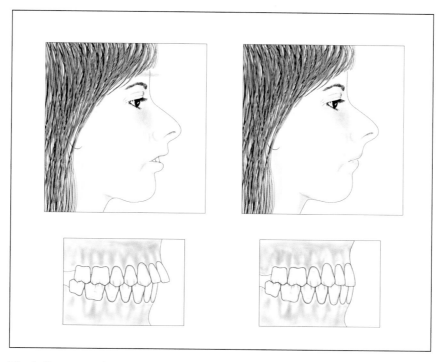

Fig 5 Changes in the profile after correction of Class II malocclusion by repositioning the maxillary incisors alone (whether orthodontically or surgically).

If we look now at the inner circle, relating to purely orthodontic treatment, with regard to subjects in whom growth is complete, it is clear that the limits of the diagram are purely theoretical and do not take into account any contingent difficulties relating to tooth movement: periodontal conditions, bone support, morphologic and structural characteristics of the alveolar bone in which the teeth must move, patient collaboration, and compliance. Furthermore, these camouflage corrections, even if possible from the theoretical and technical standpoints, are not always associated with improvement in facial esthetics. In reality dental camouflage leads to an effective improvement of esthetics only in a few situations. More frequently it has no significant influence on facial esthetics, as occurs, for example, with purely orthodontic correction of Class III cases, or when it is used to attempt correction of a Class II malocclusion at the end of growth simply by lingualizing the maxillary incisors (Fig 5). Obviously, all these implications relating to facial esthetics must be interpreted from both the sagittal and the vertical standpoints.

We are now in a position to give a more complete reply to the question, who should be given orthodontic-surgical treatment? In a subject still undergoing growth, malocclusion may be considered too severe to be corrected without the help of surgery when the changes to growth that can be achieved with dentofacial orthopedics for that type of condition are not sufficient to ensure an optimal functional and esthetic result. In an adult with dentoskeletal discrepancy, surgery is the only sure treatment option if the dental defect cannot be corrected by orthodontics alone or if dental camouflage would involve technical or periodontal contraindications, or would not produce a marked esthetic improvement.

We may therefore reasonably say that vertical dentoskeletal problems and dentofacial asymmetry are unlikely to be treatable without the help of surgery. The great majority of adult Class III patients require orthodontic-surgical treatment, chiefly in order to provide an optimal solution to their esthetic problems. In Class II cases the choice of orthodontics versus surgery may in some cases be subtle and difficult to make, requiring careful clinical and esthetic evaluation by both the surgeon and orthodontist that takes into account the patient's expectations. The diagrams and the considerations in this introduction may help the clinician in this decision.

Finally, we must consider that the improvement that has come about in surgical techniques over recent years has undoubtedly helped to decrease surgery-related complications and to improve patients' postoperative progress. We may therefore assume that indications for orthodontic-surgical treatment of dentoskeletal discrepancies will continue to increase, above all in the interest of patients. However, we must not forget that such treatment is always elective, though it is also in part therapeutic and in part preventive; that it involves at the same time and with equal importance both esthetics and functionality; and that fundamentally it must contribute to improving the quality of life for our patients from both the psychologic and physical standpoints. This is the approach and the philosophy that must always guide the physician in his or her work and treatment choices.

Bibliography

Athanasiou AE, Melsen B, Mavreas D, Kimmel F. Stomatognathic function of patients who seek orthognathic surgery to correct dentofacial deformities. Int J Adult Orthodon Orthognath Surg 1989;4:239-253.

Bell R, Kiyak HA, Joondeph DR, Johnston LE Jr. Perceptions of facial profile and their influence on decision to undergo orthognathic surgery. Am J Orthod 1985;88:323-335.

Cassidy DW Jr, Herbosa EG, Rotskoff KS, et al. A comparison of surgery and orthodontics in borderline adults with Class II, division 1 malocclusions. Am J Orthod Dentofacial Orthop 1993;104:455-470.

Cunningham SJ, Hunt NP, Feinmann C. Psychological aspects of orthognathic surgery: A review of literature. Int J Adult Orthodon Orthognath Surg 1995;10:159-172.

De Clercq CAS, Neyt LF, Mommaerts MY, Abeloos JSV. Orthognathic surgery: Patients' subjective findings with focus on the temporomandibular joint. J Craniomaxillofac Surg 1998;26:29-34.

Heldt L, Hafflker EA, Davis F. The psychological and social aspects of orthognathic treatment. Am J Orthod 1982;82: 318-328.

Kiyak HA, Hohl T, Sherrik P, et al. Sex differences and motives for outcomes of orthognathic surgery. J Oral Surg 1981; 39:757-763.

Laskin BM, Ryan WA, Greene CS. Incidence of temporomandibular symptoms in patients with major skeletal malocclusions: A survey of oral and maxillofacial surgery training programs. Oral Surg Oral Med Oral Pathol 1986;61: 537-541.

Proffit WR, White RP Jr. Who needs surgical-orthodontic treatment? Int J Adult Orthodon Orthognath Surg 1990;5: 81-89.

Proffit WR, Phillips C, Dann C 4th. Who seeks surgical-orthodontic treatment? Int J Adult Orthodon Orthognath Surg 1990;5:153-160.

Proffit WR, Phillips C, Tulloch JFC, et al. Surgical versus orthodontic correction of skeletal Class II malocclusion in adolescents: Effects and indications. Int J Adult Orthodon Orthognath Surg 1992;7:209-220.

Proffit WR, Ackerman JL. Diagnosis and treatment planning. In: Graber M, Vanarsdall RL Jr (eds). Orthodontics: Current Principles and Treatment. St Louis: Mosby, 1994.

Snow MD, Turvey TA, Walker D, et al. Surgical mandibular advancement in adolescents: Postsurgical growth related to stability. Int J Adult Orthodon Orthognath Surg 1991;6: 143-154.

Thomas PM. Orthodontic camouflage versus orthognathic surgery in the treatment of mandibular deficiency. J Oral Maxillofac Surg 1995;53:579-587.

Tucker MR. Orthognathic surgery versus orthodontic camouflage in the treatment of mandibular deficiency. J Oral Maxillofac Surg 1995;53:572-578.

White CS, Dolwick F. Prevalence and variance of temporomandibular dysfunction in orthognathic surgery patients. Int J Adult Orthodon Orthognath Surg 1992;7:7-14.

Recommended Reading

Proffit WR, White RP Jr. Surgical-Orthodontic Treatment. St Louis: Mosby, 1991.

1

Clinical and Diagnostic Considerations

- Class III malocclusion
- Class II malocclusion
- Dentofacial asymmetry
- Open bite
- Functional evaluation and the clinical record

The introduction showed that some dentomaxillofacial skeletal anomalies exist that, with greater frequency and incidence, require orthodontic-surgical treatment. Based on clinical experience gained over a number of years, it seems that, from the numeric and statistical standpoints, the dentofacial anomalies of most interest for clinician, surgeon, and orthodontist are Class III, skeletal Class II, dentofacial asymmetry, and skeletal open bite. Therefore, without intending to make any type of classification, the organization of this book will take the various aspects of these malocclusions—esthetic, orthodontic, and surgical—into consideration.

There are, however, many other, rarer situations associated with Class I dental malocclusions, or even normal occlusion, in which surgical correction is the only possibility available to achieve a stable and esthetically satisfactory solution to the problem. These are essentially lateral crossbite, skeletal deep bite, and pure long face syndrome. These anomalies are discussed, in all their clinical and therapeutic aspects, in chapter 12.

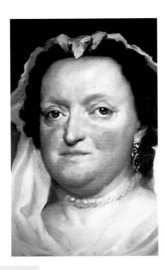

Fig 1-1 Portrait of Mary Josephine of Hapsburg (Mengs, 1750, State Museum of Dresden, Germany).

Class III Malocclusion

Incidence and etiology

Not only in the Italian population, but also in that of the rest of Europe and Asia, the incidence of Class III malocclusion shows some significant geographic variations that are undoubtedly due to a familial or hereditary predisposition. It is known that this anomaly, characteristic of some Prussian and Austrian dynasties and families, is most frequently found in central Europe (Austria and Germany in particular), and it is not by chance that orthognathic surgery was mainly developed in those countries (Fig 1-1). As an inevitable consequence of this situation, the incidence of Class III cases is higher in northern Italy than in the rest of the country, due to the influx of populations originating from central Europe. In eastern Asia, likewise, there are certain areas, such as Japan, in which Class III malocclusion is widespread. Thus, although no specific genetic responsibility for this alteration has yet been found, there is undoubtedly some phenotypic heredity responsible for the high incidence of Class III cases in some family groups and in certain geographic areas, not only in Italy but also in other nations and continents. On the other hand, the national and international migration that has occurred over the last several decades has increased the diffusion of this dentoskeletal anomaly throughout Italy, including in some areas where the incidence was initially low.

Alongside an etiopathogenesis of a hereditary or familial type, there are some intrinsic and extrinsic factors that, during the various phases of development and growth, contribute to the onset of Class III malocclusion: stenosis, or inadequacy of the upper airways, primarily the nose, with consequent hypodevelopment of the palate and maxilla; severe hypertrophy of the

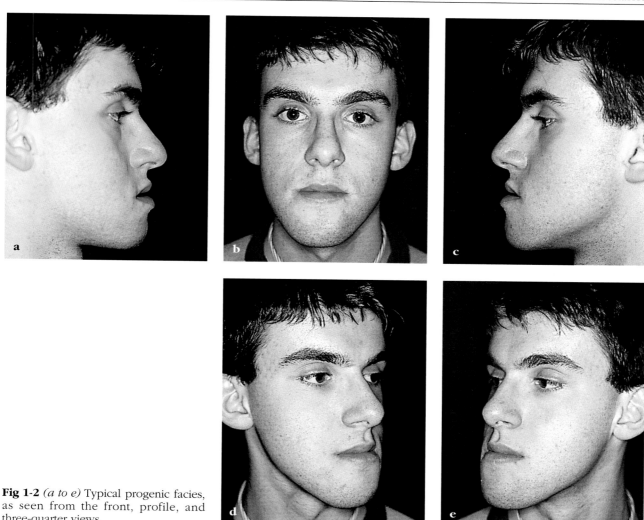

Fig 1-2 *(a to e)* Typical progenic facies, as seen from the front, profile, and three-quarter views.

tonsils with reduction of the air space in the mouth and pharynx and tendency for positional or structural mandibular protrusion; tooth agenesis or traumatic tooth loss in the maxilla (particularly the lateral incisors and premolars); prolonged retention or complete impaction of the maxillary canines; early loss of mandibular molars with absence of posterior contacts and anterior sliding of the mandible; and positional anomalies of the tongue or undesirable habits such as atypical swallowing. Changes in tongue volume, once held to be responsible for many Class III malocclusions, are only the consequence of excessive mandibular growth; it has been shown that in reality the tongue adapts to the space available.

Clinical characteristics

Clinical examination of a patient with Class III malocclusion, as indeed with all types of dentofacial anomaly, must be extremely thorough; it must analyze oc-

clusion and, above all, carefully evaluate the morphologic characteristics of the face. This type of anomaly cannot and must not be examined only in the sagittal direction because transverse or vertical alterations that are so significant as to influence the treatment plan frequently exist. Thus the term *progenic syndrome*, coined by the school of Gotte, appears particularly apt and comprehensive to define this dentoskeletal anomaly, within which, in a general way, mandibular, maxillary, and mixed forms can be determined.

Clinical examination of the face takes time and is of particular importance. The face should be evaluated from the front, in profile, and in three-quarter profile (Fig 1-2). For simplicity, data may be transcribed onto the medical record only for the frontal and profile views, but the evaluation must always be as complete as possible. (We must remember that the patient always sees himself or herself from the front or in three-quarter profile, almost never in profile.) The clinical examination should begin at the top, proceeding from

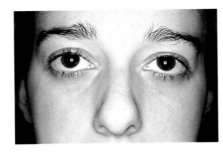

Fig 1-3 Evident scleral exposure.

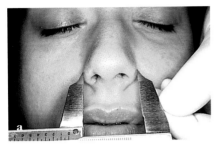

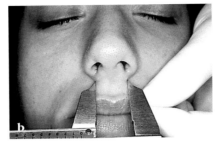

Fig 1-4 Measurement of the width of the alar base: *(a)* maximum; *(b)* minimum.

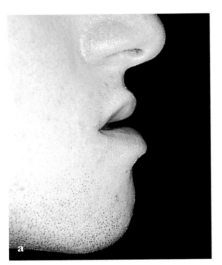

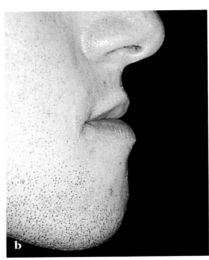

Fig 1-5 Incompetent lips *(a)*; contraction of the mentalis muscles during lip closure is evident *(b)*.

forehead to neck. The following features should be considered: hairline, frontal eminences, palpebral fissures, intercanthal distance, prominence of the cheekbones, and thickness of the cheeks and of the soft tissues in general. Particular attention must be paid in these patients to the suborbital area, also evaluating the characteristics of the infraorbital rim and determining the presence of scleral exposure when looking forward (Fig 1-3).

The nose, the central structure of the face, is of great importance in the clinical examination; glabella, dorsum, hump (if present), tip, columella, and opening of the nares should all be carefully examined. The width of the alar base should be measured, both the maximum distance and that at the point of insertion on the upper lip (Fig 1-4); the mobility of the nares during speech and smiling should also be observed. Anterior rhinoscopy can reveal any deviation of the septum and the presence of endonasal synechia. The lips must also

be examined both at rest and in movement, evaluating shape, thickness, and muscle tone, as well as the shape and characteristics of the prolabium and of the Cupid's bow; any hypertrophism of the frenulae; and labial competence or incompetence (evaluated with the lips completely relaxed with no contraction; Fig 1-5). Particular attention should be paid to the relationship between lips and teeth and between lips and gingiva, both at rest and during smiling, with consideration given to tooth exposure and gummy smile, if any (Fig 1-6). Last, the nasolabial angle and the paranasal areas must be examined for depressions (Fig 1-7), as should the nasogenial fold, which in some cases may be highly accentuated (Fig 1-8).

With regard to the clinical examination of the lower third of the face, the overall shape of the mandible should be evaluated, considering the characteristics and position of angles of the mandible (Fig 1-9), the shape and symmetry of the chin, and the presence and

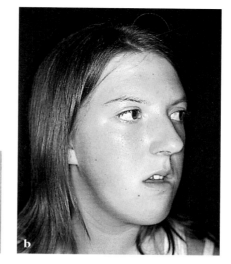

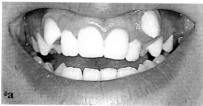

Fig 1-6 Typical gummy smile *(a)* due to an increased skeletal vertical dimension *(b)*.

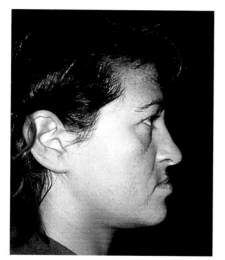

Fig 1-7 Nasolabial angle and depression in paranasal areas.

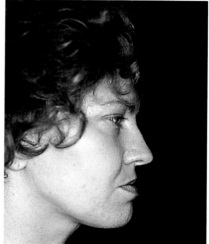

Fig 1-8 Accentuation of the nasogenial fold.

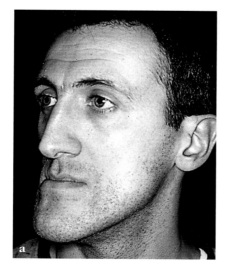

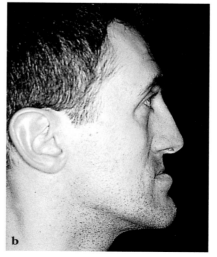

Fig 1-9 Open and receding mandibular angle *(a)* and increased angle between chin and neck *(b)*.

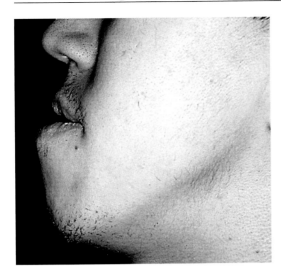

Fig 1-10 Disappearance of the labiomental angle in a Class III patient.

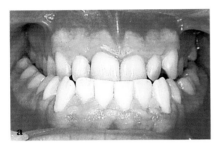 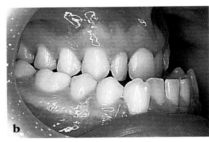 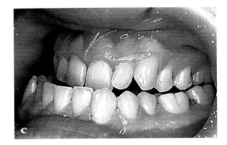

Fig 1-11 *(a to c)* General intraoral examination.

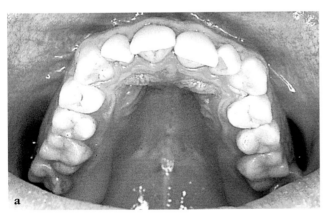 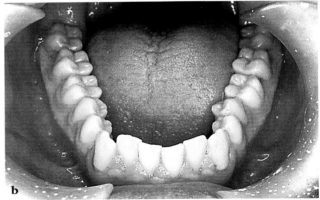

Fig 1-12 *(a and b)* The two dental arches are evaluated separately.

extent of the labiomental angle (Fig 1-10). It is also important to evaluate the shape and characteristics of the angle between the neck and chin and of the soft tissues beneath the chin (thickness, tone, hypertrophy, excess of soft or adipose tissue) (see Fig 1-9). The intraoral examination must only be dedicated in part to the maxillomandibular relationship (Fig 1-11). In practice the most significant aspect of this relationship consists in quantifying the negative overjet evaluated at the incisal level; any anterior open bite also should be evaluated. From the first examination, it is necessary to become accustomed to seeing the two arches independently, since this is the way they will be treated and prepared for definitive surgical correction (Fig 1-12).

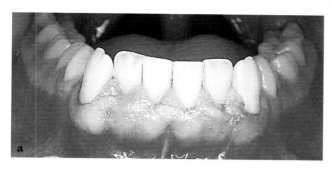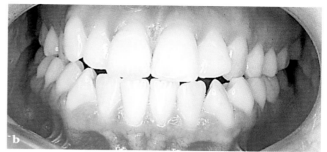

Fig 1-13 Periodontal evaluation of mandibular incisors: sufficient quantity of adherent gingiva *(a)*; adherent gingiva is almost entirely lacking *(b)*.

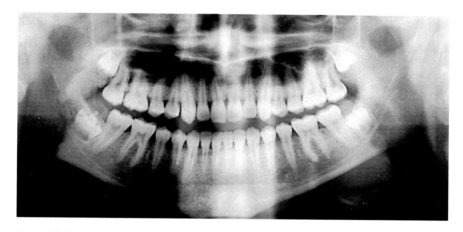

Fig 1-14 Panoramic radiograph of a Class III patient.

The presence and number of teeth must be evaluated, along with any agenesis, tooth rotation, and crowding. The periodontal condition of the maxillary incisors and especially the mandibular incisors must be carefully evaluated (Fig 1-13); these are the critical points in the treatment plan for these patients. Simple clinical examination can reveal the presence and extent of dental compensation at this level. The quality and quantity of adherent gingiva must be evaluated, as must any pockets and the characteristics of the frenu-

lum linguae and of the frenulum labii inferioris. Lastly, true macroglossia (a very rare condition) must be determined, along with the presence of undesirable habits and/or swallowing abnormalities.

Radiologic examination, including full panoramic radiography, completes the clinical examination of the arches, providing useful elements concerning the presence of impacted teeth and the inclination and direction of tooth roots (Fig 1-14). Lateral radiography completes the diagnostic classification (see chapter 2).

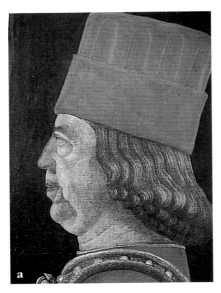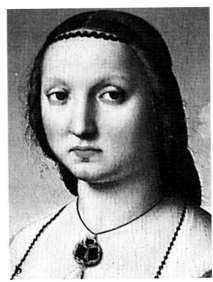

Fig 1-15 *(a)* Portrait of Borso d'Este (Baldassarre d'Este, 1470, Castello Sforzesco Art Gallery, Milan, Italy). *(b)* Portrait of Maddalena Doni (Raphael, 1506, Palatine Gallery, Florence, Italy).

Class II Malocclusion

Incidence and etiology

The incidence of Class II malocclusion in the Italian population is, in general, lower than what has been recorded in the United States or in northern European countries (United Kingdom, the Netherlands, Scandinavia), for example. As for Class III malocclusions, for this type of anomaly there are undoubtedly genetic and/or familial components, as well as environmental ones, and we may speak of phenotypic heredity and predisposing factors. A geographic distribution may also be determined for Class II cases, although to a lesser extent than for Class III cases, with greater incidence in central Italy than in the remainder of the country. This may be seen in some paintings of the Italian Renaissance, such as the family portraits of the Estenses and some of the Florentine nobility painted by Raffaello (Fig 1-15).

With regard to intrinsic factors linked to development and growth, oral respiration certainly plays an important part, whether it is due to a reduction of nasal patency, to hypertrophy of the adenoids or tonsils, or simply to a bad habit. Agenesis of the mandibular premolars or traumatic loss of some teeth in the mandibular arch, as well as condylar trauma during growth, must not be underestimated in the onset of this type of anomaly.

Clinical characteristics

Clinical examination of a patient with Class II malocclusion, again from the front, profile, and three-quarter profile, must evaluate some fundamental aspects and characteristics. First and foremost, we can say with reasonable certainty that a characteristic common to the great majority of Class II malocclusions is mandibular retrusion, both structural and positional; the shape of maxilla in skeletal terms is exceptional; dental protrusion must not be confused with skeletal position. These concepts will be further developed in chapters 2 and 9. Furthermore, in addition to the sagittal dimension, the transverse and vertical dimensions must be taken into particular consideration from the start; this enables clinicians to immediately distinguish cases of excessive vertical dimension, classified as Class II, division 1 (Fig 1-16) and cases of reduced vertical dimension, Class II, division 2 (Fig 1-17).

In the middle third of the face the clinician must carefully evaluate the nose, the central structure of the face (in Class II situations it is often prominent); however, this may be accentuated by concomitant mandibular retrusion, and in some cases only prominence of the nose may be apparent (Fig 1-18). Glabella, dorsum, tip, and hump (if present) must be carefully considered. Measurement of the internostril distance is also very important, both at rest and during smiling and speaking; narrow and wide noses can

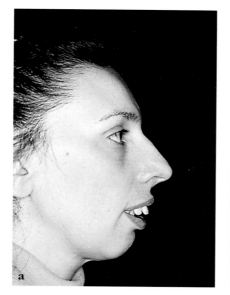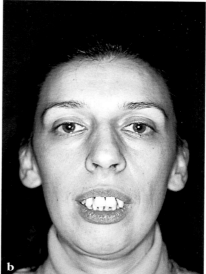

Fig 1-16 *(a and b)* Typical example of Class II, division 1 malocclusion, with increased vertical dimension.

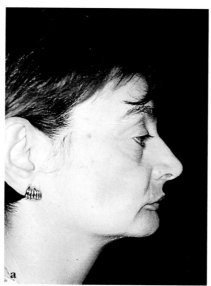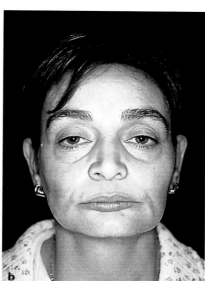

Fig 1-17 *(a and b)* Typical example of Class II, division 2 malocclusion, with reduced vertical dimension.

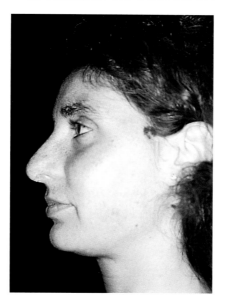

Fig 1-18 The nose is visually more prominent in a Class II patient because of mandibular retrusion.

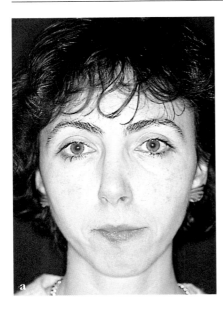

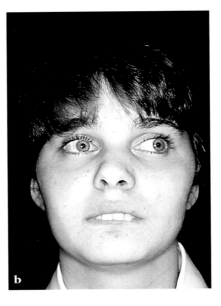

Fig 1-19 Typical examples of a narrow nose *(a)* and a wide nose *(b)*.

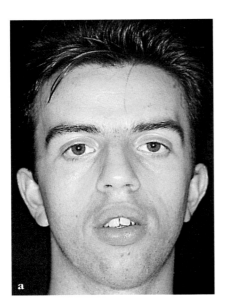

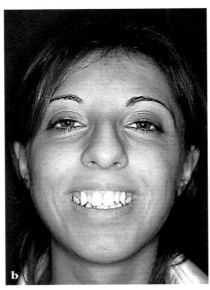

Fig 1-20 Short upper lip with excessive dental exposure *(a)* and gummy smile due to maxillary vertical excess *(b)*.

be generically distinguished (Fig 1-19). Obviously a careful functional evaluation is also necessary, possibly with an anterior rhinoscope.

With regard to the labiodental relationship and tooth or gingival exposure, it is important to remember that the upper lip in these patients is frequently short, sometimes "curled" upward, contributing to a gummy smile. This is frequently associated with atypical swallowing and biting of the lower lip, which in this case is often hypertonic. Naturally the gummy smile may also be due to an excessive skeletal vertical dimension, so that clinicians must carefully evaluate the extent to which each of the two components

is responsible for the clinical situation (Fig 1-20). Lastly, we must evaluate and measure the nasolabial angle (right, acute, or obtuse angle) and the labial competence or incompetence when the lips are perfectly relaxed (Fig 1-21).

Clinical examination of the lower third of the face in almost all cases shows true mandibular retrusion, of both the structural and the positional types; structural hypodevelopment of the mandible may be revealed, at the level of both the ramus and the body of the mandible, and frequently coexists with true structural hypodevelopment of the chin (Fig 1-22). In general, clinicians can distinguish a mandibular form with nor-

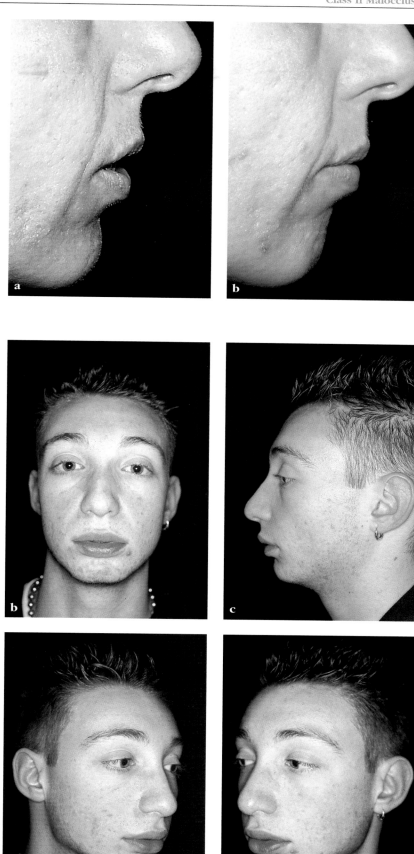

Fig 1-21 Labial incompetence with relaxed lips *(a)* and contraction of mentalis muscles during closure *(b)*.

Fig 1-22 *(a to e)* Typical hypodevelopment of the lower third of the face in a Class II patient, as seen from the front, profile, and three-quarter views.

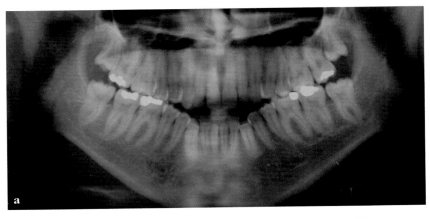

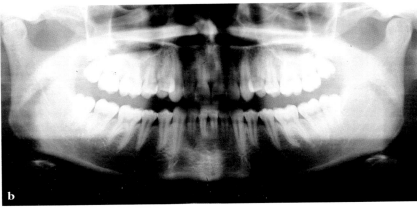

Fig 1-23 Panoramic radiograph of a Class II patient with increased vertical dimension *(a)* and one with reduced vertical dimension *(b)*.

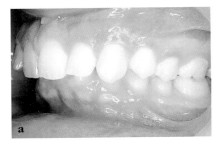

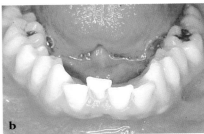

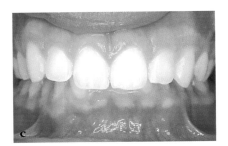

Fig 1-24 *(a to c)* Intraoral photographs showing evident crowding of mandibular incisors.

mal or open angle (Class II, division 1) in which the vertical dimension is normal or increased, and a mandibular form with closed angle (Class II, division 2) with reduced vertical dimension (Fig 1-23). In these patients there is often also muscular hypertrophy, especially of the masseter muscles.

The occlusal examination must first of all evaluate the presence of any posterior premature contacts with anterior sliding of the mandible and thus a double occlusion, frequently found in skeletal Class II patients; sometimes this double occlusion is deliberately though unconsciously sought by the patient in an attempt to compensate for the skeletal defect.

The intraoral examination must evaluate crowding, tooth rotation, agenesis, and impacted or embedded teeth (Fig 1-24). Periodontal evaluation is very important, especially for the mandibular incisors, in view of preoperative orthodontic treatment; periodontal problems at the mandibular incisors are frequent in both division 1 and division 2 cases, though with different pathogenetic mechanisms (Fig 1-25). With regard to the maxillary incisors, flaring of these teeth may be accompanied by gingival recession and severe periodontal problems (Fig 1-26).

Panoramic radiographic examination, in addition to the intraoral clinical examination and better classification of the mandibular forms with open or closed

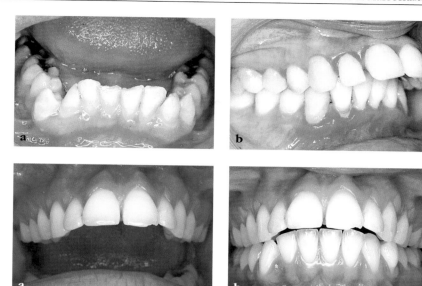

Fig 1-25 Severe periodontal problems at the mandibular incisors in a Class II, division 2 case *(a)* and in a Class II, division 1 case *(b)*.

Fig 1-26 *(a and b)* Severe periodontal problems at the maxillary incisors in a Class II, division 1 case.

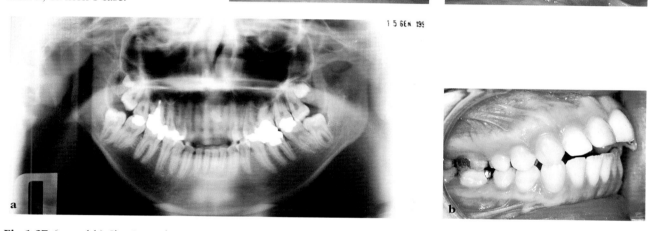

Fig 1-27 *(a and b)* Classic, and severe, condylar resorption in a young woman with Class II, division 1 malocclusion and open bite.

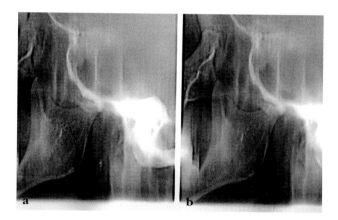

Fig 1-28 *(a and b)* Stratigraphy of the TMJ of the patient in Fig 1-27.

angle, may provide essential information on the morphology of the mandibular condyles. In underweight young women with a tendency for open bite, condylar resorption of varying degrees of severity may exist (Fig 1-27). The radiologic examination should be integrated in such cases with stratigraphy of the temporomandibular joint (TMJ) to enable the morphology and structure of the condyles to be monitored over time (Fig 1-28). In these subjects particular care also must be taken during the various phases of treatment to avoid any manipulation that might produce compression of the joint structures, particularly of the condyles, which would further aggravate the resorption. Lateral radiography completes the clinical evaluation (see chapter 2).

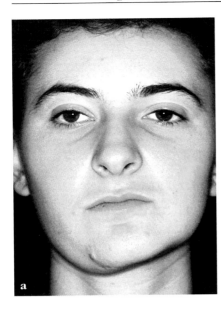
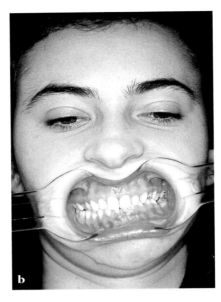

Fig 1-29 Classic case of hemimandibular hyperplasia *(a)* with canting of the occlusal plane *(b)*.

Dentofacial Asymmetry

Incidence and etiology

In the field of dentofacial asymmetries, hereditary, familial, geographic, and/or racial factors are less important than they are for Class III or Class II malocclusion. In these anomalies, the determinant phase of the etiopathogenesis is asymmetric growth of the mandibular condyles, which causes an altered development not only of the mandible, but also of the entire maxillomandibular complex. A number of hypotheses have been put forward to explain the genesis of this anomaly; undoubtedly trauma in early childhood can play an important role, as can temporomandibular ankylosis, which can cause unilateral condylar hypodevelopment and thus may generate significant dentofacial asymmetry. In most cases, however, the developmental anomaly is flanked by persistent precartilaginous cell activity at the level of the condylar growth center. There may be a number of different causes for this hyperactivity (neurotrophic disorders, alteration of local circulation, hormonal disorders, partial hypertrophy); however, the causes originating this asymmetric growth are not yet clearly understood.

In their milestone publication in 1986, Obwegeser and Makek distinguished two forms of asymmetric growth: hemimandibular hyperplasia and hemimandibular elongation. Hemimandibular hyperplasia is characterized by the three-dimensional enlargement of one side of the mandible, which may be limited to the condyle alone or may also involve the ramus and body of the mandible; in this case, the hypertrophy stops exactly on the median line. Growth of the maxilla is affected by the asymmetric mandibular growth, creating a situation in which the occlusal plane is inclined to a greater or lesser extent (Fig 1-29).

Hemimandibular elongation is characterized by deviation of the mandible and chin horizontally toward the healthy side, generally with no repercussions on the occlusal plane. There is a slender form with a thin and extended neck of the condyle, and a nonslender form with an apparently normal neck of the condyle at radiologic investigation; in this case we may suppose the growth anomaly to be limited to the cellular level (Robiony et al 1997) (Fig 1-30). Naturally there are also incomplete or mixed forms with unilateral or bilateral involvement or in which hemimandibular hyperplasia is associated with hemimandibular lengthening.

Within the immense field of dentofacial asymmetries, congenital malformations also exist that relate to different situations of hemifacial microsomia. These abnormalities, however, require a multidisciplinary therapeutic approach during the various phases of growth. We therefore believe that treatment of these specific forms lies largely outside the contents and scope of this book; the reader is referred to specific works for further information.

Clinical characteristics

In the clinical examination of patients with dentofacial asymmetry, it is of utmost importance to examine the patient from the front and from below, although evaluation in profile and in three-quarter profile should, of course, not be neglected (Fig 1-31). It should be remembered that some degree of asymmetry between the two halves of the face is present in every individual;

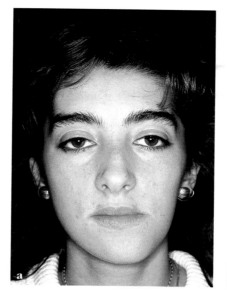

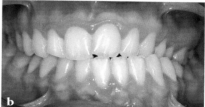

Fig 1-30 Classic example of hemimandibular elongation *(a)* with no canting of the occlusal plane *(b)*.

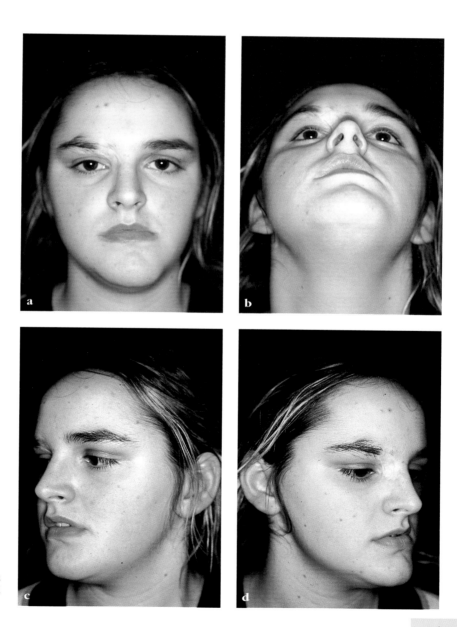

Fig 1-31 *(a to d)* Clinical examination of the face of a patient with dentofacial asymmetry.

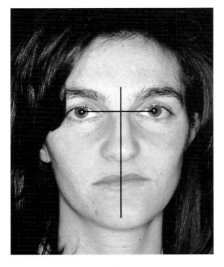

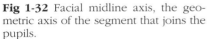

Fig 1-32 Facial midline axis, the geometric axis of the segment that joins the pupils.

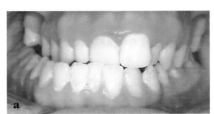

Fig 1-33 *(a and b)* Evaluation of the inclination of the occlusal plane.

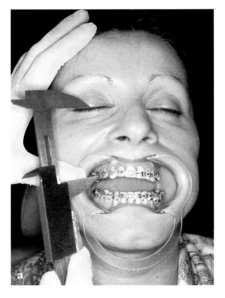

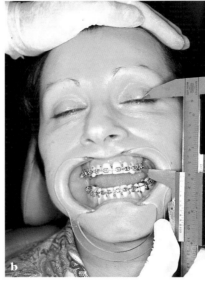

Fig 1-34 *(a and b)* Evaluation of the inclination of the occlusal plane during orthodontic treatment.

only in a small percentage of cases is the difference so evident as to be considered true dentofacial asymmetry.

For an exact clinical classification of these patients, the fundamental points and planes of reference are the bipupillar plane, the inner canthi, and the palpebral fissures with eyes closed. To be evaluated with regard to these planes of reference are the occlusal plane (and more precisely that relating to the maxilla); the dental midlines, maxillary and mandibular; and the point characterizing the mental symphysis. It is important upon starting the examination to define and determine the facial midline axis; this is the axis of the segment that unites the center of the pupils, the center of the palpebral fissures with eyes closed, or the two inner canthi, depending on the reference points used. The facial

midline axis may be determined more accurately on a photograph of the patient, which in this respect becomes a vital diagnostic aid (Fig 1-32).

Evaluation of the cant of the occlusal plane may be facilitated by the use of a wooden tongue depressor (Fig 1-33); measurement becomes both more precise and simple during therapeutic phases if an orthodontic arch is present because it constitutes an optimal point of reference with regard to the inner canthi (structures that are relatively fixed but not sufficiently far apart) or with respect to the center of the pupils or of the palpebral fissures when the patient is completely relaxed (Fig 1-34). The latter anatomic points are less fixed than the inner canthi with the patient vigilant, and for this reason the patient must be carefully instructed on how to

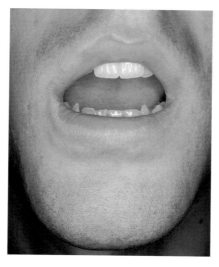

Fig 1-35 Evident deviation of the maxillary dental midline with respect to the center of the upper lip.

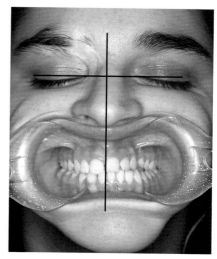

Fig 1-36 Evaluation of the maxillary dental midline with respect to the facial midline axis.

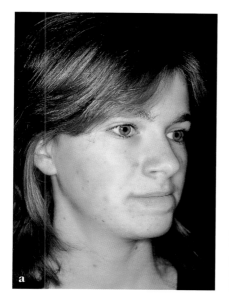

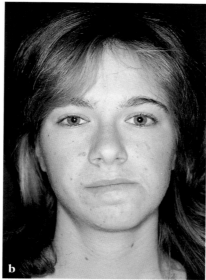

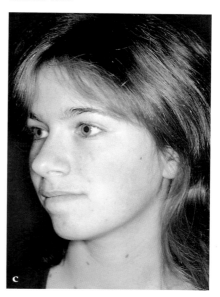

Fig 1-37 *(a to c)* Evaluation of different morphology of the angle of the mandible on the two sides.

keep his or her eyes closed and relaxed, or how to look at a fixed point straight ahead if the pupils are used as reference points. In any case, it is advised to repeat the procedure several times to be certain that a sufficiently reliable measurement has been obtained. With some experience, and if patient collaboration is good, these measurements are highly indicative and do not require the use of dedicated spectacles or masks that, if not perfectly positioned and stabilized, can lead to error.

With regard to the dental midlines and their relationship with the facial midline axis, the central point of the Cupid's bow is more useful as a clinical reference point than are the structures of the nose (tip and columella), which may be deviated (Fig 1-35). How-

ever, for a more precise evaluation, a photograph of the patient taken with cheek retractors, on which the facial midline axis is carefully traced, may also be used (Fig 1-36).

The point that characterizes the mental symphysis and its relationship with the facial midline axis should be determined through palpation and clinical examination of the patient from the front, from below, and from above; here, too, study of a photograph enables precise evaluation of the degree of deviation of the prominence of the chin (see Fig 1-32). Lastly, the shape, position, and characteristics of the angles of the mandible should be carefully evaluated from the front and in three-quarter profile (Fig 1-37).

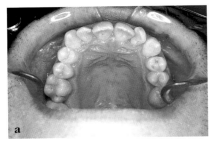
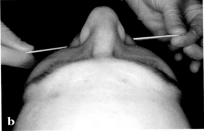
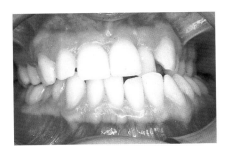

Fig 1-38 *(a and b)* Evaluation of the symmetry of the maxillary canines.

Fig 1-39 Evident inclination of the mandibular incisors as dental compensation for malocclusion.

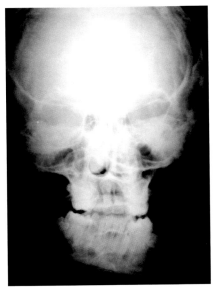
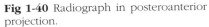
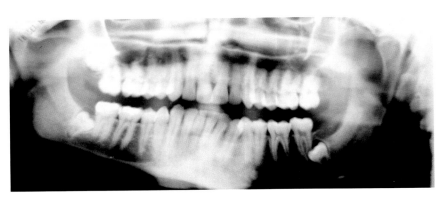

Fig 1-40 Radiograph in posteroanterior projection.

Fig 1-41 Evident structural asymmetry of the mandibular condyles, visible in a panoramic radiograph, which requires further diagnostic investigation via computerized tomography and/or scintigraphy.

With regard to the intraoral examination, as well as the observations and evaluations that are common to all cases of dentofacial anomaly and that have already been discussed for Class III and Class II malocclusions, the presence of any deviating premature contacts and the position of the maxillary canines are of particular importance. In some patients with dentofacial asymmetry there may be a precontact at the level of the canines or premolars, which alters and aggravates the mandibular lateral deviation; it is obvious that clinical evaluation must always be performed in centric relation and not at maximum intercuspation. With regard to the position of the maxillary canines, this should be evaluated both by examining the maxillary arch from below and by observing the patient from above with the help of a wooden tongue depressor or a rigid metallic wire to unite the cusps of the canines; in this way the position of the canines within the arch may be determined precisely and any asymmetry revealed (Fig 1-38). Lastly, mesiodistal inclination of the mandibular incisors must be carefully examined; this is frequently present as a natural attempt to compensate for the skeletal lateral deviation (Fig 1-39).

In these patients the diagnostic classification is completed with radiography in lateral and posteroanterior projection (see chapter 2) as well as with panoramic radiography, if necessary accompanied by stratigraphy of the TMJs to evaluate condylar asymmetry (Figs 1-40 and 1-41). An indispensable examination to verify whether condylar growth is still active and to better differentiate condylar asymmetry from the functional and growth standpoints is technetium-99 scintigraphy (see chapter 9). Use of single-photon emission computed tomography (SPECT) is reserved for select cases.

Open Bite

Incidence and etiology

Although open bite may occur in any type of dentofacial anomaly (Class III, Class II, or dentofacial asymmetry), the classic open bite with long-face syndrome is found in patients whose skeletal relationship is generally Class I, with increased anterior vertical dimension and/or decreased posterior vertical dimension and transverse contraction of the maxilla. From the etiopathogenetic standpoint, for open bite, as for dentofacial asymmetries, environmental and growth factors appear to be more important than hereditary, racial, or geographic factors. Among environmental factors recognized as potentially causing a predisposition to open bite are oral respiration, lingual interposition, masticatory forces, and posture of the mandibular muscles, both at rest and during movement.

Two different types of tests have shown a relationship between oral respiration and open bite: the first is based on animal experiments, the second on observation in man. The animal experiments entailed completely obstructing nasal patency. Because in man complete nasal obstruction never occurs, the relationship between nasal and oral respiration—that is to say the percentage of airflow that passes through the nose versus that through the mouth—during development and growth is more important. It would appear reasonable to suppose that the transverse contraction of the maxilla (often where there is a narrow triangular maxillary arch) and/or the presence of hypertrophic tonsils or abundant adenoidal tissue might constitute an important etiologic factor in predisposition to oral respiration and thus to open bite.

Lingual interposition has also been implicated in the onset of open bite. In reality, the lingual interposition that occurs during atypical swallowing appears to be more responsible for dental flaring and dentoalveolar problems than for severe skeletal problems. In this respect alteration of the tongue posture downward would seem important, as it would condition the growth of the mandible clockwise, causing an increase of the anterior vertical dimension and a tendency to open bite. Atypical swallowing can also contribute to postoperative relapse and must therefore be carefully evaluated and corrected, if possible, through appropriate physiotherapy.

With regard to the posture of muscles with mandibular insertion, both elevator and depressor muscles, it may be hypothesized that they could influence the direction of growth of the mandible through a dual mechanism. On one hand, an imbalance might come about between the two groups of muscles, with preva-

lence of the depressor muscles and thus a tendency toward increased vertical dimension and open bite. On the other hand, weaker muscular force and weaker masticatory force might favor dentoalveolar eruption in the posterior sectors, with development of open bite and increased vertical dimension. Greater tooth eruption in the posterior sectors is commonly found in patients with this anomaly.

Clinical characteristics

Clinical examination of a patient with open bite must take into account all the etiopathogenetic implications mentioned above and must therefore place more emphasis on the functional and dynamic aspects than on the strictly morphologic one. In any case the facies of subjects with open bite and long face is very characteristic, and diagnosis is obvious (Fig 1-42).

Particular attention should be paid to medical history in order to determine any problems of nasal respiration and/or those relating to adenoids or tonsils. The characteristics of the nose and upper airways and the type of respiration should be carefully evaluated: The nose is frequently narrow and may have a bony or cartilaginous hump and reduced nostril opening (Fig 1-43). Respiration is almost always prevalently oral, even where there is no evident deviation of the nasal septum. The turbinates are often hypertrophic to an extent that the patency of the nasal fossae is sometimes compromised (Fig 1-44).

Lingual interposition should be looked for both in the active phase, during swallowing or speech, and at rest; in this case it may be due to an altered posture of the tongue and its musculature. True macroglossia is very rarely found. Some pathognomonic clinical signs help to ascertain whether there is an actual increase in the size of the tongue. If at maximum protrusion the tongue extends beyond the labiomental fold to reach the tip of the chin, then there is a prevalently longitudinal increase. On the contrary, if the tongue, again at maximum protrusion, extends in width to reach the corners of the mouth, then there is a prevalently transverse increase (Fig 1-45).

Lastly, both the depressor and the elevator muscles should be palpated to determine the degree of hypotonia of the mandibular musculature. Muscle hypotonia is frequently found in the orbicularis oris muscles, and this certainly aggravates labial incompetence and contributes to the disappearance of the labiomental fold (Fig 1-46).

Intraoral examination will readily reveal a higher incidence of caries in patients with open bite, including in the anterior teeth, caused by oral respiration and labial incompetence (Fig 1-47). In almost all cases there

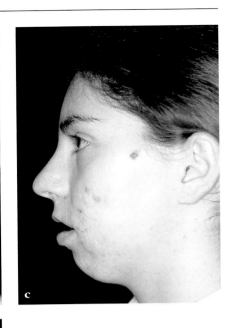

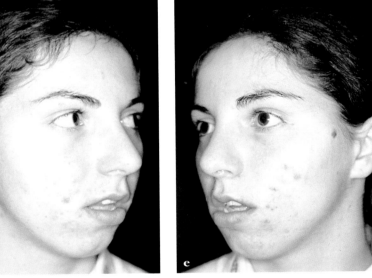

Fig 1-42 *(a to e)* Typical facies of a patient with open bite.

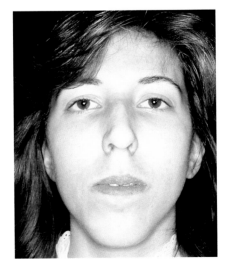

Fig 1-43 Typical narrow, humped nose in a patient with open bite.

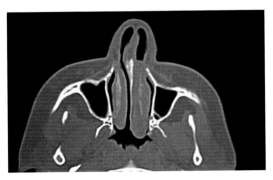

Fig 1-44 Marked hypertrophy of the turbinates in a patient with open bite.

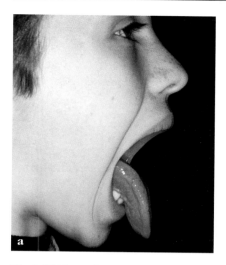
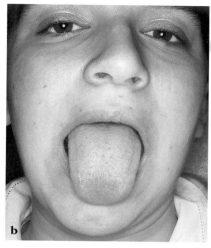
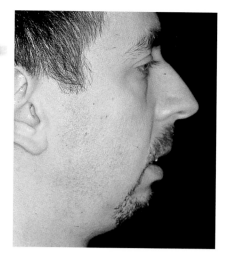

Fig 1-45 Macroglossia with chiefly longitudinal increase *(a)* and with chiefly transverse increase *(b)*.

Fig 1-46 Labial incompetence and disappearance of the labiomental fold.

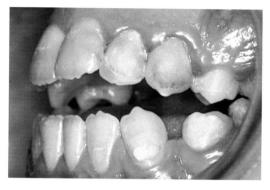
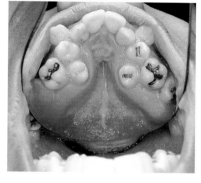

Fig 1-47 Widespread caries and periodontal problems linked to open bite.

Fig 1-48 Severe transverse contraction of the maxilla with narrow triangular palate and marked crowding.

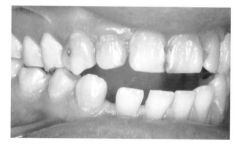
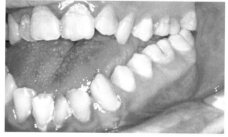

Fig 1-49 Flaring of maxillary and mandibular incisors in open bite.

Fig 1-50 Evident inversion of the curve of Spee with the reverse situation in the maxilla. Severe periodontal problems are partly due to oral respiration.

is transverse contraction of the maxilla, and the maxillary arch is narrow and triangular, sometimes with severe crowding (Fig 1-48). The anterior teeth, in both the maxillary and mandibular arch, are frequently flared (Fig 1-49). Any signs of abrasion or wear should also be determined; these are frequently present in the posterior sector at the molars, where the only tooth contacts occur. The curve of Spee is often inverted, with the reverse effect in the curve formed by the cusps and incisal edges of the maxillary teeth (Fig 1-50).

Standard radiologic examination for these patients also includes panoramic and lateral radiography; the latter examination in this type of anomaly is of particular importance, undoubtedly more so than in cases of Class III or Class II malocclusion, as will be clarified in chapter 2.

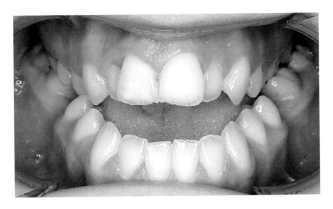

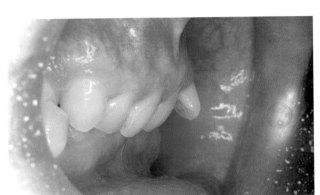

Fig 1-51 Tooth contact is almost nonexistent in a severe case of Class III malocclusion, which produces evident masticatory functional problems.

Fig 1-52 Severe periodontal problems in a patient with Class II, division 2 malocclusion that can only be resolved through an orthodontic-surgical approach.

Functional Evaluation and the Clinical Record

The incidence of TMJ disorders in subjects with dentofacial anomalies is practically the same as that found in subjects without dentomaxillofacial skeletal alterations, including among the latter group both subjects with normal occlusion and subjects with occlusal alterations that do not require surgical treatment. The existence of a direct relationship between dentofacial anomalies and joint disorders is thus extremely debatable; there is no scientific evidence of a direct relationship between skeletal anomalies in the widest sense and TMJ disorders. Nevertheless, a number of studies have shown a clear correlation between type of malocclusion and dysfunction or pain at the TMJ. This chiefly occurs with Class II, division 2 and Class III malocclusions or dentofacial asymmetry with anterior interference and/or anterior deep bite. Another type of malocclusion in which there is some increase in TMJ disorders is open bite, primarily in Class II cases. How-

ever, it remains to be demonstrated whether the correlation is actually due to the skeletal model or to the parafunction that is associated with or triggered by these types of malocclusion. In any case, in this type of patient, orthodontic-surgical treatment obviously brings about an improvement in the clinical situation as a whole. In all other situations, at least from the theoretical standpoint, the dentofacial anomaly may at most be considered a predisposing factor, in the long term, for dental, periodontal, muscular, or joint problems. However, there are other functional aspects, in the widest sense, that should not be neglected. For example, individuals with open bite and severe Class III malocclusion may have such little tooth contact that the masticatory capability is seriously compromised, from both subjective and objective standpoints (Fig 1-51). The same may be said for the periodontal aspect; there are some situations (typically Class II, division 2) in which orthodontic-surgical treatment is the only possible way to solve serious dental and periodontal problems, especially at the incisors (Fig 1-52).

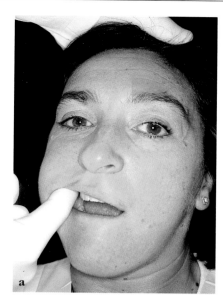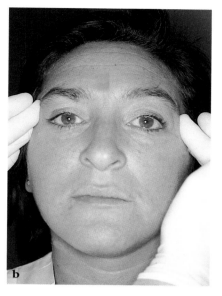

Fig 1-53 Palpation of the external pterygoid *(a)* and temporal muscles *(b)*.

There are therefore three different possible situations influencing our approach to a patient: the patient is subjectively asymptomatic and seeks medical assistance only for his or her occlusal and morphologic problem, with requirements that are almost exclusively esthetic; the patient has no subjective symptoms of TMJ disorder and requests treatment for objective difficulty in mastication, or has severe dental and/or periodontal problems that can be related to malocclusion and that cannot be solved without an orthodontic-surgical approach (in both these situations there may also be initial clinical signs of TMJ disorders, not yet noticed by the patient); or the occlusion is clearly dysfunctional, both from subjective and objective standpoints, and the patient requests treatment to solve all of his or her problems.

In any case, functional evaluation in patients suffering from dentofacial anomalies must include kinematic study of the mandible, including measurement of the degree of mouth opening, opening and closing pathways, and protrusive and lateral movements; palpation and auscultation of the TMJ (palpation may also indicate the degree of translation of the condyles and any pain at pressure); and palpation of the mas-

ticatory muscles, especially the external pterygoid and temporal muscles (Fig 1-53), as well as the cervical musculature, especially the suprahyoid and sternocleidomastoid muscles. In subjectively asymptomatic patients, a thorough clinical examination is sufficient upon beginning therapy and during all the various phases to monitor and control joint and muscle functionality, avoiding any risk of iatrogenic problems. The clinical examination may be supplemented in these patients by an oblique transcranial radiograph of the TMJ (see chapter 3), which is especially useful in the preoperative and postoperative phases for checkup and monitoring.

In patients with occlusal dysfunction, the clinical examination must be completed with instrumental investigations that, depending on clinical indications, may include transcranial radiography or stratigraphy of the TMJ; computerized tomography or nuclear magnetic resonance imaging of the TMJ; and electromyography of the masticatory muscles with kinesiographic examination. These problems will be dealt with in more detail in chapter 3.

Clinical data must be completed with cephalometric evaluation, as discussed in the next chapter, and must be entered into the clinical record. An example of such a clinical record is provided on the following pages.

DENTOFACIAL ANOMALIES

NAME: _____

DIAGNOSIS: _____

FRONTAL VIEW OF FACE

FOREHEAD

    HAIRLINE _____

    FRONTAL EMINENCES _____

    ORBITAL RIM _____

EYES

    INTERCANTHAL DISTANCE _____

    ORBITAL RIMS _____

    BIPUPILLARY LINE _____

    SCLERAL EXPOSURE _____

NOSE

    GLABELLA _____

    DORSUM _____

    TIP _____

    WIDTH OF ALAR BASE _____

    COLUMELLA _____

    SEPTUM _____

EARS

    MEATUS ACUSTICUS (LEVEL) _____

ZYGOMAS AND CHEEKS

    CHEEKBONES _____

    THICKNESS OF CHEEKS _____

    NASOGENIAL FOLD _____

LIPS

　　CUPID'S BOW _____

　　PROLABIUM _____ UPPER _____ LOWER _____

　　TONE _____ UPPER _____ LOWER _____

　　CLEFT LIP SEQUELAE _____

　　COMPETENT ☐　　　　INCOMPETENT ☐　_____ mm

CHIN

　　SHAPE _____

　　SYMMETRY _____

MANDIBLE

　　BORDER _____

　　ANGLES _____

FACE IN PROFILE

FOREHEAD

　　VAULT _____

NOSE

　　GLABELLA _____

　　DORSUM _____

　　TIP _____

　　NASOLABIAL ANGLE _____

ZYGOMAS AND CHEEKS

　　ORBITAL RIMS _____

　　CHEEKBONE _____

　　PARANASAL AREAS _____

LOWER THIRD

　　PROJECTION OF UPPER LIP _____

　　PROJECTION OF LOWER LIP _____

　　LABIOMENTAL FOLD _____

　　ANGLE BETWEEN CHIN AND NECK _____

31

INTRAORAL EXAMINATION

DENTAL FORMULA _____

UPPER DENTOLABIAL RELATIONSHIP AT REST _____

LABIAL RELATIONSHIP WHEN SMILING _____

GUMMY SMILE _____

CURVE OF SPEE _____

MAXILLARY DENTAL MIDLINE (versus facial midline axis) _____

MANDIBULAR DENTAL MIDLINE (versus facial midline axis) _____

MAXILLARY OCCLUSAL PLANE _____

    HORIZONTAL ☐   OBLIQUE ☐

    CANT _____

    DISCREPANCY _____ INNER CANTHI _____

MAXILLARY CANINES

    SYMMETRIC ☐   ASYMMETRIC ☐

TONGUE _____

PERIODONTIUM _____

FUNCTIONAL EVALUATION

MANDIBULAR MOVEMENTS (opening) _____

PALPATION OF TMJ _____

AUSCULTATION OF TMJ _____

MUSCLES _____

POSTURAL MEASUREMENTS _____

Bibliography

Bittner C, Pancherz H. Facial morphology and malocclusions. Am J Orthod Dentofacial Orthop 1990;97:308–315.

Burstone CJ. Lip posture and its significance in treatment planning. Am J Orthod 1967;53:262–284.

Cisneros GJ, Kaban LB. Computerized skeletal scintigraphy for assessment of mandibular asymmetry. J Oral Maxillofac Surg 1984;42:513–520.

De Clercq CAS, Abeloos JSV, Mommaerts MY, Neyt LF. Temporomandibular joint symptoms in an orthognathic surgery population. J Craniomaxillofac Surg 1995;23:195–199.

Fellus P. Dynamic and postural changes in the tongue: Influence on facial growth [in Italian]. Mondo Ortod 1989;6:791–798.

Huggins DG, McBride LJ. The influence of incisor position on soft tissue facial profile. Br J Orthod 1975;2:141–146.

Kaban LB, Cisneros GJ, Heyman S, Treves S. Assessment of mandibular growth by skeletal scintigraphy. J Oral Maxillofac Surg 1982;40:18–22.

Kerstens HC, Tuinzing DB, Van der Kwast WAM. Temporomandibular joint symptoms in orthognathic surgery. J Craniomaxillofac Surg 1989;17:215–218.

Laskin BM, Ryan WA, Greene CS. Incidence of temporomandibular symptoms in patients with major skeletal malocclusions: A survey of oral and maxillofacial surgery training programs. Oral Surg Oral Med Oral Pathol 1986;61:537–541.

Moss ML, Salentijn L. The primary role of functional matrices in facial growth. Am J Orthod 1969;55:566–577.

Mutoh Y, Oshashi Y, Uchiyama N, et al. Three-dimensional analysis of condylar hyperplasia with computed tomography. J Craniomaxillofac Surg 1991;19:49–55.

Obwegeser HL, Makek MS. Hemimandibular hyperplasia–hemimandibular elongation. J Maxillofac Surg 1986;14:183–208.

Robiony M, Costa F, Demitri V, Politi M. Iperplasia emimandibolare e allungamento emimandibolare: Ruolo della scintigrafia ossea. Riv Ital Chir Maxillofac 1997;3:17–21.

Rubin R. Mode of respiration and facial growth. Am J Orthod 1980;7:504–510.

Solow B. The dentoalveolar compensatory mechanism: Background and clinical implications. Br J Orthod 1980;7:145–161.

Subtelny JD. A longitudinal study of soft tissue facial structures and their profile characteristics defined in relation to underlying skeletal structures. Am J Orthod 1959;45:481–507.

White CS, Dolwick F. Prevalence and variance of temporomandibular dysfunction in orthognathic surgery patients. Int J Adult Orthodon Orthognath Surg 1992;7:7–14.

Recommended reading

Bell WH, Proffit WR, White RP Jr (eds). Surgical Correction of Dentofacial Deformities. Philadelphia: Saunders, 1980.

Epker BN, Fish LC. Dentofacial Deformities: Integrated Orthodontic and Surgical Correction. St Louis: Mosby, 1986.

Proffit WR, White RP Jr. Surgical-Orthodontic Treatment. St Louis: Mosby, 1991.

2

Cephalometry in Dentofacial Anomalies

with Alberto Guariglia

- Lateral radiography
- Esthetic analysis of the face
- Posteroanterior radiography

Lateral Radiography

An enormous amount of literature has been written on cephalometric analysis for dentofacial anomalies, from Schwarz's analysis of the profile (1954) to the more recent and sophisticated analyses by Arnett and Bergman (1993a and 1993b), with intermediate contributions from Fish and Epker (1980) and Ricketts (1961). Each of these analyses reflects its authors' philosophy and intentions, focusing on skeletal relationships or those of the soft tissues, according to the authors' preference.

Cephalometric analysis on a radiograph taken in lateral projection is without doubt an excellent method to study the relationships between skeletal structures and between these and the soft tissues and teeth. It is useful for orthodontic planning of any extractions and consequent choice of anchorage; it is also a useful tool to verify orthodontic treatment that has been performed for the purpose of profilometric changes. Cephalometry, however, must not be used as the primary component in diagnosis.

> The primary aim of treatment is not to bring cephalometric values within the normal range, but rather to make facial esthetics normal and attractive.

Although these two goals frequently coincide, this is not always the case. In our opinion cephalometric analysis, in the sphere of orthodontic-surgical treatment, must be simple to interpret, both in the diagnostic phase and during treatment planning. It must also be constantly related and integrated with esthetic clinical examination; when there is a discrepancy between the two evaluations, which is always a possibility, the one that is most useful to achieve our specific esthetic or functional goal must be followed, based on the merits of the individual case.

Cephalometric analysis includes angular and linear skeletal measurements, measurement of the relationship between bony bases and the base of the skull, measurement of soft tissues and/or esthetic evaluations, and evaluation of dentoalveolar and dentoskeletal relationships, in all cases respecting the concepts of simplicity and pragmatism described above.

Lateral radiographs must be taken with the teeth in centric relation and the lips in the rest position. Centric relation is used in all cases except those in which there is a marked discrepancy between centric relation and habitual relation. In this case, two radiographs are taken, one in centric relation and the other in the habitual position. The former is used to determine the sagittal relationship between maxilla and mandible, whereas the latter is used to measure the vertical dimensions.

The analysis used by the authors is outlined in Table 2-1. As shown, the values are subdivided into five groups: maxilla, mandible, vertical parameters, dental parameters, and soft tissues. With regard to the bony bases, this analysis takes into consideration three angular measurements to evaluate their position three dimensionally and a linear anthropometric measurement to determine length and development. Evaluation of soft tissues, and that of the vertical dimension, follows the indications given by Fish and Epker (1980), as adapted from Ricketts' analysis (1961). Nevertheless, all strictly cephalometric and geometric considerations must be integrated and compared with clinical and esthetic considerations, and in the case of a discrepancy, the surgeon's or the orthodontist's experience and intuition must, as the case merits, privilege clinical diagnosis or cephalometric analysis. Frequently, the final decision will be based on esthetic considerations.

On the contrary, cephalometric analysis has an irreplaceable, almost dogmatic, value with regard to the position and inclination of the maxillary and mandibu-

TABLE 2-1 Cephalometric angular and linear values considered normal (M = men; W = women)

CEPHALOMETRIC MEASUREMENTS	NORMAL VALUES
Maxilla	
SNA angle	M 82 ± 2 degrees, W 81 ± 2 degrees
Frankfort plane–NA angle	90 ± 3 degrees
Ba-A line	M 94 ± 6 mm, W 88 ± 4 mm
Palatal plane–SN angle	10 ± 3 degrees
Mandible	
SNB angle	M 80 ± 2 degrees, W 78 ± 2 degrees
Frankfort plane–N-Pog angle	89 ± 3 degrees
Ba-Pog line	M 113 ± 5 mm, W 104 ± 4 mm
Gonial angle	130 ± 7 degrees
Vertical parameters	
Go-Me–SN angle	32 ± 4 degrees
S-Go/N-Me ratio	62% ± 3%
Dental parameters	
Maxillary incisor–palatal plane angle	109 ± 5 degrees
Maxillary incisor–SN angle	103 ± 2 degrees
Mandibular incisor–Go-Me angle	90 ± 5 degrees
Soft tissues	
Middle third (G-Sn)/lower third (Sn-Me') ratio	1:1
Length of upper lip (Sn-St)	M 22 ± 2 mm, W 20 ± 2 mm
Interlabial distance (Sts-Sti)	0–3 mm
Distance to line through Sn (perpendicular to Frankfort plane)	
Upper lip (Sts)	–2 to +2 mm
Lower lip (Sti)	–4 to 0 mm
Chin (Pog')	–6 to –2 mm

lar incisors. A normal inclination with regard to their respective bony bases must be rigorously sought and achieved: 109 degrees to the palatal plane for the maxillary incisors and 90 degrees to the mandibular plane (gonion-menton [Go-Me]) for the mandibular incisors.

In the case of significant rotational movements of the maxilla, inclination of the maxillary incisors to the sella-nasion (S-N) plane must also be taken into consideration; this situation comes about especially in cases of open bite, as will be explained in chapter 4.

Compromised solutions over the position of the incisors with respect to their bony bases should only be contemplated where periodontal problems limit the possible orthodontic movement, or in the case of particular esthetic requirements (see chapter 4).

Maxilla

The maxilla is analyzed in relation to the base of the skull in the sagittal and vertical sense by determining

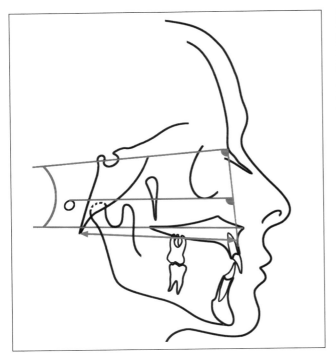

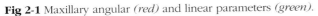

Fig 2-1 Maxillary angular *(red)* and linear parameters *(green)*.

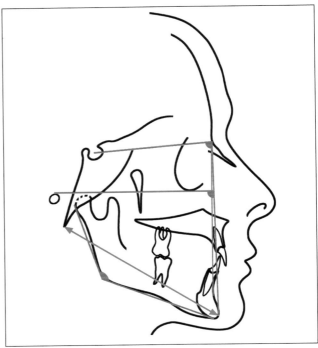

Fig 2-2 Mandibular angular *(red)* and linear parameters *(green)*.

three angles (sella–nasion–point A [SNA], Frankfort plane–NA, and palatal plane–SN) and one linear measurement (the length of the basion [Ba]-A line) (Fig 2-1).

The SNA angle, whose normal value is in the range 82 ± 2 degrees in men and 81 ± 2 degrees in women, can be to some extent conditioned by the inclination of the SN plane; therefore another angular value is also taken into consideration, that at which the Frankfort plane meets the line passing through NA. This value, normally 90 ± 3 degrees, indicates the anteroposterior position of the maxilla and aids interpretation of dentoskeletal anomalies.

The angle between the palatal and SN planes indicates the position of the maxilla with regard to the base of the skull and may reveal any rotation of the maxilla clockwise or counterclockwise; this evaluation is very important in diagnosis and treatment planning for open bite (see chapter 9).

Lastly, the anteroposterior position of the maxilla and its sagittal development are confirmed by measuring the distance between Ba and point A. This value is normally 94 ± 6 mm in men and 88 ± 4 mm in women.

A very important consideration, again with regard to the maxilla, applies to Class II patients. In this anomaly, as confirmed by clinical and esthetic examination and the work of McNamara et al (McNamara 1981; Ellis

et al 1985; Lawrence et al 1985), true skeletal protrusion is only found in exceptional cases; the maxilla is almost always either in a normal or retruded position, whereas the apparent skeletal protrusion is in fact caused by an accentuated vestibularization of the maxillary incisors. These considerations are of particular importance in planning treatment (see also chapter 9).

Mandible

For the mandible the reference values in cephalometric analysis consist of three angular and one linear measurement (Fig 2-2).

The first angle is the SN–point B (SNB) angle; the normal value is 80 ± 2 degrees in men and 78 ± 2 degrees in women. As in the maxilla, this value is confirmed by the angle at which the Frankfort plane meets the N-pogonion (Pog) line. The latter normal value is 89 ± 3 degrees. These values enable determination of the anteroposterior position of the mandible.

The linear distance from the line joining Ba and Pog provides further confirmation concerning size and position of the mandible.

The last measurement taken into consideration is the gonial angle. This value, normally in the range of 130 ± 7 degrees, gives useful indications both for eval-

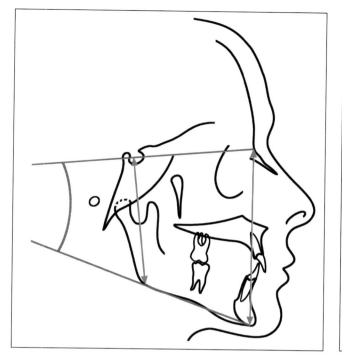

Fig 2-3 Vertical angular *(red)* and linear parameters *(green)*.

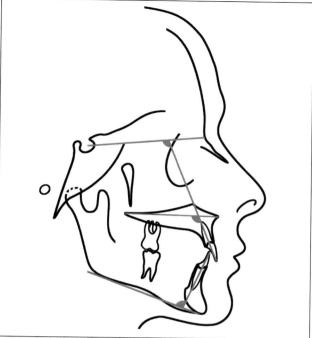

Fig 2-4 Angular parameters *(red)* for the maxillary and mandibular incisors.

uation of the sagittal position of the mandible and, when related to vertical parameters, for studying vertical anomalies and open bite.

Vertical parameters

The vertical dimension, from the skeletal standpoint, is studied by measuring the angle between the mandible and the base of the skull and the relationship between anterior and posterior vertical dimensions (Fig 2-3).

The Go-Me–SN angle is normally equal to 32 ± 4 degrees; wider or narrower values of this angle objectively indicate the presence of open bite or deep bite.

The relationship between anterior and posterior vertical dimension is determined by measuring the segments S-Go and N-Me. This ratio is normally 62% ± 3%. This parameter enables clinicians to establish with some accuracy whether the subject is normal or hyper- or hypodivergent.

Dental parameters

As already stated, the study of dental relationships is undoubtedly the most important component of cephalometric analysis. With rare exceptions, these are the only values that must be brought within the normal range (Fig 2-4). Cephalometric analysis of the relationships between the incisors and their respective bony bases is

the true guide for planning presurgical orthodontic treatment, and the fulcrum of orthodontic decompensation. These values also guide clinicians in the need for any tooth extractions and the choice of anchorage.

As far as the maxillary incisors are concerned, the tooth axis normally forms an angle of 109 ± 5 degrees with the palatal plane, and this value must always be respected. With the few exceptions discussed in chapter 4, the primary task of orthodontic treatment is to bring these values within the normal range. It is known that in cases of dentoskeletal anomaly, the teeth tend to move to compensate for the malocclusion in an attempt to achieve contact. Thus it is common to find an increased value of this angle in Class III subjects, and a lower value in Class II, division 2 subjects.

Another important value is the angle that the axis of the maxillary incisors forms with the anterior cranial base (SN). The normal value is 103 ± 2 degrees, and this serves as a point of reference in cases where surgical rotation of the maxilla is needed to correct open bite. In these cases, obviously the palatal plane also changes, so that a comparison of the two values enables clinicians to modulate the extent of movement of the maxillary incisors (see chapter 4).

Another important value that may be considered in the spatial evaluation of the maxillary incisors is the distance between the perpendicular to the Frankfort plane passing through point A and the most anterior

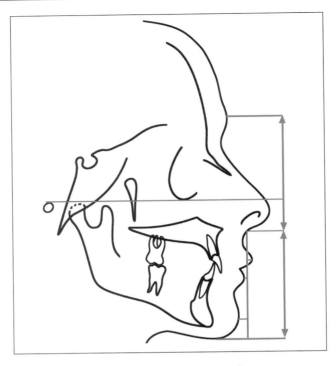

Fig 2-5 Linear parameters *(green)* for the soft tissues.

point of the crown of the maxillary incisor. The normal value for this parameter is 4 mm.

The axis of the mandibular incisor normally forms an angle of 90 ± 5 degrees with the mandibular base (Go-Me). A decrease in this angle is almost always found in Class III subjects as a compensatory factor for malocclusion; in Class II subjects there is usually an increase (see chapter 4).

These are the only cephalometric values that must almost always be normalized, hence the importance of orthodontic planning, because these values will guide clinicians in sagittal movements and in the choice of any necessary extractions to achieve acceptable orthodontic decompensation (see chapter 4).

Soft tissues

The soft tissues are primarily studied clinically, as is discussed in more detail in the next section, but traditional cephalometry can also provide some indications. Different types of profilometric analysis have been proposed for the soft tissues (Burstone 1958 and 1967; Holdaway 1983a and 1983b; Merrifield 1966; Ricketts 1961); Fig 2-5 illustrates the analysis method the authors use, which is extrapolated from analyses by Fish and Epker (1980) and uses the perpendicular to the Frankfort plane.

In the first instance the ratio between the middle third and the lower third of the face is observed, that is, the distances between the glabella-subnasale (G-Sn) and Sn–soft tissue menton (Me'). This ratio is normally 1:1.

The length of the upper lip is then measured, joining Sn to stomion (St). The normal value is 22 ± 2 mm in men and 20 ± 2 mm in women; if these values are lower, the subject is said to have a short upper lip.

Another reference value in studying the soft tissues is the interlabial distance. This is measured as the distance between stomion of the upper lip (Sts) and stomion of the lower lip (Sti), with the lips in the rest position. Normal values vary from 0 to 3 mm, although higher values are now also accepted, up to 5 mm (see the following section). Values greater than 5 mm indicate incompetent lips.

There are also three values that indicate the antero-posterior position of the lips and chin. For these, the distance between Sts, Sti, and soft tissue pogonion (Pog') to a straight line passing through Sn perpendicular to the Frankfort plane is measured. For the upper lip, normal values are between −2 and +2 mm; for the lower lip, normal values are between −4 and 0 mm; and for the chin, normal values are between −6 and −2 mm. Naturally, all these numeric evaluations must be related to the overall esthetics of the face.

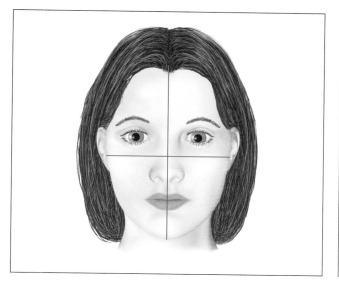

Fig 2-6 Relationship between height and width of the face (1.3:1 for women; 1.35:1 for men).

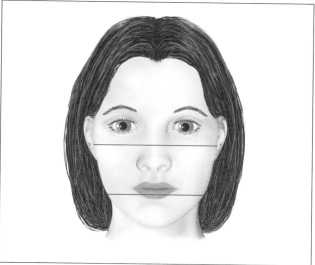

Fig 2-7 The bigonial width should be 30% less than the bizygomatic width.

Esthetic Analysis of the Face

Based on all the above considerations, esthetic analysis is a fundamental and determinant phase with regard to correcting dentofacial anomalies.

As we have seen, there are numerous possible profilometric evaluations of the soft tissues; however, these are almost all incomplete because they are limited to sagittal and vertical measurements and are not three dimensional. The esthetic analysis must be all-encompassing and not simply geometric, but above all it must be clinical. Each face must be evaluated with the proportions between the different structures taken into account: Proportion and harmony are synonymous with beauty, a concept that has been present in art from the earliest times. Furthermore, the relationship between the face and a person's height and build must be considered within a truly complete evaluation. Finally, clinicians must not forget that the concept of beauty is subjective and has undergone significant changes throughout the centuries (see chapter 3).

Clinical examination must be performed with the patient relaxed, in a natural postural position, with the dental arches in centric relation and the lips completely relaxed. Lip relaxation must be stressed from the start, and great care must be taken to ensure the patient relaxes; it is frequently necessary to instruct the patient in detail or to strike the lips repeatedly with the index or middle finger to obtain complete relaxation of the labial muscles.

The examination must be made from the front, profile, and three-quarter profile views, from the hairline to the neck, and must take into consideration all the structures of the face. Chapter 1 examined the salient characteristics that must be determined for each type of dentofacial anomaly. While there is always some subjectivity to the evaluation, and whereas proportion and harmony must dominate over standard reference values, some fundamental indications can be given. In this regard, the esthetic and anthropometric analyses most often followed today are those of Farkas (1981), Farkas and Kolar (1987), and Arnett and Bergman (1993a and 1993b), although in the authors' opinion they are too schematic and mathematical, particularly with regard to some of the reference points.

The maximum width of the face should be evaluated through the bizygomatic width; the ratio between height and width of the face should be 1.3:1 for women and 1.35:1 for men (Fig 2-6); these values may, however, be slightly higher or lower depending on the patient's overall height: in very tall subjects a longer face may be accepted, and vice versa.

Another rather important measurement is the bigonial width: This should be approximately 30% less than the bizygomatic width (Fig 2-7). Nevertheless, today's beauty standards prefer faces in which the bigonial width is wider than the so-called normal range.

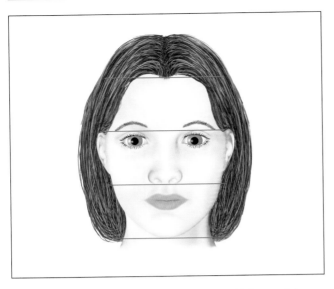

Fig 2-8 Ideal balance between upper, middle, and lower thirds of the face.

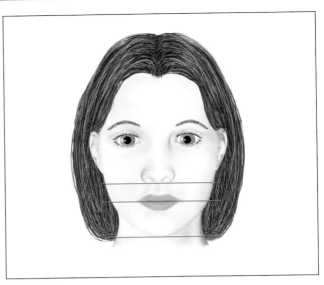

Fig 2-9 The height of the upper lip should be half the total height of the lower lip/chin.

There should be substantial harmony between the upper, middle, and lower thirds of the face (Fig 2-8). The lower third should exhibit a 1:2 ratio between the upper lip and lower lip/chin (Fig 2-9). The length of the lips may be measured, as has already been seen, on a lateral radiograph. In men a slight increase in the lower third may be acceptable, and indeed is sometimes preferable, especially if the increase is created by the lip and chin.

Particular care should be paid to the amount of tooth exposure, both at rest and during smiling. Until a few years ago values were considered normal if they were between 0 and 2 mm; higher values, between 1 and 5 mm, are now proposed (Arnett and Bergman 1993a and 1993b). We believe it is reasonable to accept values between 0 and 4 mm, considering that greater tooth exposure is acceptable in women than in men. During smiling, a 1- to 2-mm exposure of adherent gingiva is usually considered optimal; again, greater exposure is accepted for women than for men.

Similar considerations may be made with regard to labial competence: Until a few years ago this was sought almost as an absolute necessity, but today there is a tendency to favor slight labial incompetence (at rest) in women (according to Arnett and

Bergman, between 1 and 5 mm). The authors are of the opinion that, based on current society and fashion, it is reasonable to propose values between 0 and 3 mm.

The angle of the profile, according to Arnett and Bergman's analysis, should be between 165 and 175 degrees (Fig 2-10); higher values probably indicate a tendency to Class III, lower values indicate Class II malocclusion. However, this value must also be interpreted and integrated with all the other evaluations.

The nasolabial angle must be measured as shown in Fig 2-11; it should be between 85 and 105 degrees, with a tendency to accept higher values in women and lower values in men. Furthermore, there should be substantial balance between the intercanthal distance and the width of the alar base (Fig 2-12), and the width of the mouth should correspond to the distance between the medial margins of the irises (Fig 2-13).

Along with these parameters, which may be measured and quantified as seen in the previous chapter, numerous other clinical evaluations must also be carefully observed: forehead eminences, eyes, orbital rims, zygomas, and thickness of cheeks, as well as soft tissues in general and the nose, paranasal areas, nasogenial fold, muscle tone of lips, and tissues beneath the chin and of the neck specifically.

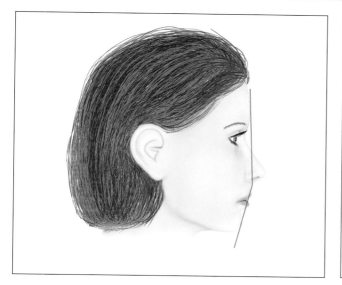

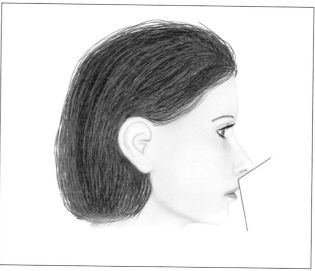

Fig 2-10 Angle of the profile: Ideal value is between 165 and 175 degrees.

Fig 2-11 Nasolabial angle: Ideal value is between 85 and 105 degrees.

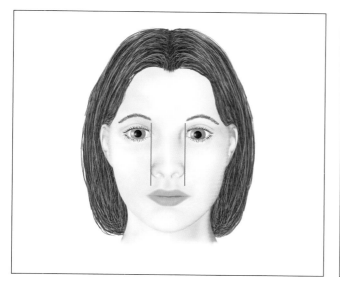

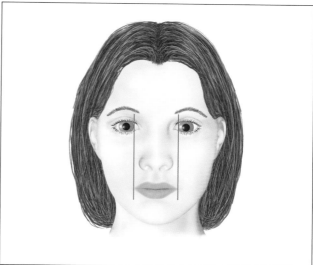

Fig 2-12 The intercanthal width should be the same as the width of the alar base.

Fig 2-13 The width of the mouth should correspond to the distance between the medial margins of the irises.

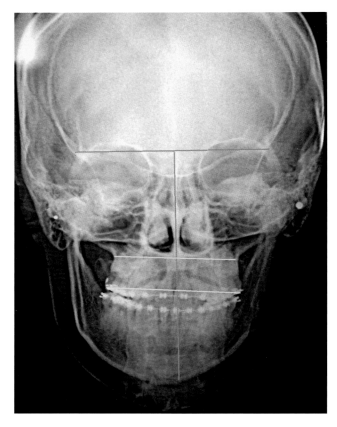

Fig 2-14 Essential planes of reference on the posteroanterior radiograph.

Posteroanterior Radiography

Cephalometric analysis in anteroposterior projection is less widely used than that in lateral projection; it is not part of routine examination but is used only in cases with evident asymmetry. On the radiograph in Fig 2-14 some parallel planes are drawn to extrapolate the asymmetry visually, as it is often partially masked by the soft tissues. Linear or angular measurements are not used; not only do they not provide any important data for diagnosis, but they also might be misleading. The posteroanterior radiograph compared to that in lateral projection is much more sensitive to the inclination of the patient's head.

As reference points the horizontal plane passing through the two frontozygomatic points and the relative axis of symmetry are determined; then planes passing through the common point to right and left are traced to reveal asymmetry and to assign a skeletal or a dental element to that asymmetry (Fig 2-14).

The axis of symmetry is the perpendicular line drawn through the midpoint of the horizontal line joining the two frontozygomatic points and corresponding to the frontozygomatic suture. In rare cases, and particularly with orbital asymmetry, the axis of symmetry is traced perpendicular to a straight line passing through the occipital condyles, at the highest point on the horizontal plane of the upper margin of the occipital foramen magnum.

Bibliography

Arnett GW, Bergman RT. Facial keys to orthodontic diagnosis and treatment planning. Part I. Am J Orthod Dentofacial Orthop 1993a;103:299–312.

Arnett GW, Bergman RT. Facial keys to orthodontic diagnosis and treatment planning. Part II. Am J Orthod Dentofacial Orthop 1993b;103:395–411.

Burstone CJ. The integumental profile. Am J Orthod 1958; 44:1–25.

Burstone CJ. Lip posture and its significance in treatment planning. Am J Orthod 1967;53:262–284.

Butow KW. A lateral photometric analysis for aesthetic-orthognathic treatment. J Maxillofac Surg 1984;12:201–207.

Butow KW, Muller WG, de Muelenaere G. Profilocephalometric analysis: A combination of the cephalophotometric and the architectural-structural craniofacial analysis. Int J Adult Orthodon Orthognath Surg 1989;2:87–104.

Delaire J, Schendel SA, Tulasne JF. An architectural and craniofacial analysis. A new lateral cephalometric analysis. Oral Surg Oral Med Oral Pathol 1981;52:226–238.

Ellis E 3rd, McNamara JA, Lawrence T. Components of adult Class II open-bite malocclusion. J Oral Maxillofac Surg 1985;43:92–105.

Farkas LG. Anthropometry of the Head and Face in Medicine. New York: Elsevier, 1981.

Farkas LG, Kolar JC. Anthropometrics and art in aesthetics of women's faces. Clin Plast Surg 1987;14:599–615.

Fish LC, Epker BN. Surgical-orthodontic cephalometric prediction tracing. J Clin Orthod 1980;14:36–52.

Holdaway RA. A soft-tissue cephalometric analysis and its use in orthodontic treatment planning. Part I. Am J Orthod 1983a;84:1–28.

Holdaway RA. A soft-tissue cephalometric analysis and its use in orthodontic treatment planning. Part II. Am J Orthod 1983b;85:279–293.

Lawrence T, Ellis E 3rd, McNamara JA. The frequency and distribution of skeletal and dental components in Class II orthognathic surgery patients. J Oral Maxillofac Surg 1985; 43:24–34.

McNamara JA Jr. Components of Class II malocclusion in children 8–10 years of age. Angle Orthod 1981;51:177–202.

Merrifield LL. The profile line as an aid in critically evaluating facial esthetics. Am J Orthod 1966;52:804–822.

Ricketts RM. Cephalometric analysis and synthesis. Angle Orthod 1961;31:141–156.

Riedel RA. The relation of maxillary structures to cranium in malocclusion and normal occlusion. Angle Orthod 1952; 22:142–157.

Sassouni V. Diagnosis and treatment planning via roentgenographic cephalometry. Am J Orthod 1958;44:433–463.

Schwarz AM. Ueber eckzahnverlagerung und ihre Behebung. Fortschr Kieferorthop 1954;15:119.

Steiner C. Cephalometrics for you and me. Am J Orthod 1953; 39:729–745.

Steiner C. Cephalometrics in clinical practice. Angle Orthod 1959;29:8–29.

Subtelny JD. A longitudinal study of soft tissue facial structures and their profile characteristics defined in relation to underlying skeletal structures. Am J Orthod 1959;45: 481–507.

Tulloch C, Phillips C, Dann C. Cephalometric measures as indicators of facial attractiveness. Int J Adult Orthodon Orthognath Surg 1993;3:171–179.

Tweed CH. The Frankfort mandibular plane angle (FMIA) in orthodontic diagnosis, treatment planning and prognosis. Angle Orthod 1954;24:121–169.

Wylie GH, Fish LC, Epker BN. Cephalometrics: A comparison of five analyses currently used in the diagnosis of dentofacial deformities. Int J Adult Orthodon Orthognath Surg 1987;2:15–36.

Zucconi M, Ferini-Strambi L, Palazzi S, et al. Craniofacial cephalometric evaluation in habitual snorers with and without obstructive sleep apnea. Otolaryngol Head Neck Surg 1993;109:1007–1013.

Recommended reading

Bell WH, Proffit WR, White RP Jr (eds). Surgical Correction of Dentofacial Deformities. Philadelphia: Saunders, 1980.

Epker BN, Fish LC. Dentofacial Deformities: Integrated Orthodontic and Surgical Correction. St Louis: Mosby, 1986.

Proffit WR, White RP Jr. Surgical-Orthodontic Treatment. St Louis: Mosby, 1991.

3

Treatment
Objectives

- Function
- Esthetics

Function

When treating patients with dentofacial anomalies, an absolute requirement is to obtain normal occlusal, muscular, and joint function; we must thus define what is meant by *normal function*.

From the occlusal standpoint, for the purposes of normal function the goals are correct tooth alignment, Class I occlusion at the canine level, anterior overjet of 1 to 2 mm, anterior overbite of 1 to 2 mm (in general, slight overcorrection with regard to the initial situation is desirable, and thus these values may also be slightly increased), coincidence of the maxillary and mandibular dental midlines and their coincidence with the facial midline axis, and correct transverse relationship.

In cases where the mesiodistal diameter of the incisors differs, and thus the Bolton index calculated in the anterior segments is altered, a compromise of no more than 1.5 mm is permissible at the level of the dental midlines, provided that the canines are in precise Class I occlusion. If the alteration of the Bolton index involves the entire arch, and if the mesiodistal diameters of the maxillary teeth predominate, a position of the maxillary canines that is slightly advanced (1 to 1.5 mm) compared to the classic Class I occlusion may be accepted. On the contrary, if the mesiodistal diameters of the mandibular teeth predominate, mandibular arch stripping will be necessary. The molar relation should be Class I where no extractions are planned or if four premolars are to be extracted; it will inevitably be Class II if the maxillary first or second premolars are to be extracted. In some cases, with extraction of only the mandibular first or second premolars, the molar relation will of necessity be Class III (see chapter 4).

From the muscular standpoint, the muscles most involved in mandibular kinematics must be relaxed in the rest position and must not be contracted or painful. In particular, the following muscles must be examined and palpated: the temporalis muscles, the external and internal pterygoid muscles, the masseter muscles, and the digastric muscles.

In some patients with oral dysfunction, electromyographic examination is undoubtedly a valid diagnostic aid to supplement clinical examination; however, some points must be borne in mind. First and foremost, the type of electromyography commonly applied in the stomatognathic field is surface electromyography, without the use of needles. From the neurophysiologic standpoint its value is limited. Only the temporalis, masseter, and digastric muscles can be investigated with this instrument, whereas the pterygoid muscles escape analysis because only surface electrodes are employed. In addition, electromyography should be performed in specific, shielded locations, and this does not always occur. Despite these limitations, electromyographic examination can be of some use, provided it is interpreted within the overall picture and integrated with the clinical examination. In particular, rather than determine the absolute value for muscular condition expressed in microvolts (mV), it is more important to observe the overall picture and to look for uniform trends in muscle tone, or on the contrary the presence of significant dyskinesia, revealed by marked alterations in the tracings. Figures 3-1 and 3-2 show two tracings, to be considered normal and pathological, respectively, independent of the absolute values in mV. The electromyographic tracing also has unquestionable value in some patients who clearly show dysfunction at the start of treatment. In these cases it is a useful way of checking the treatment that has been begun and a valid instrument for monitoring the patient's musculature during treatment.

In subjectively asymptomatic patients, electromyographic examination may sometimes be a study and

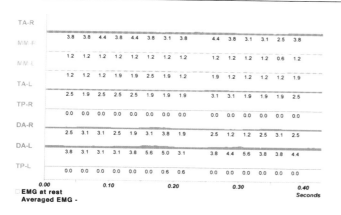

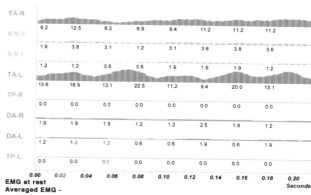

Fig 3-1 Electromyographic tracing that may be considered normal, independent of the absolute values expressed in mV. (TA, anterior temporal muscle; MM, masseter muscle; TP, posterior temporal muscle; DA, digastric muscle; R, right; L, left.)

Fig 3-2 Electromyographic tracing that is clearly pathological, independent of the absolute values expressed in mV. (TA, anterior temporal muscle; MM, masseter muscle; TP, posterior temporal muscle; DA, digastric muscle; R, right; L, left.)

research tool, particularly if applied and interpreted during the pre- and postoperative phases, to evaluate any changes in muscle posture following surgery, but it is certainly not a necessary test in normal clinical practice.

With regard to mandibular kinematics, the functional goal must consider the extent of opening (in millimeters), lateral and protrusive movements, and the presence or absence of marked deviation during opening and closing movements. From this standpoint, kinesiographic examination, usually performed at the same time as electromyography, is a useful and important clinical aid, particularly in patients with dysfunction, both from the strictly diagnostic standpoint and as a way of monitoring the various phases of treatment. It provides information not only on the extent of movement but also on the speed and uniformity of the entire mandibular kinematics. Figures 3-3 and 3-4 show two sets of tracings, the first representing an acceptable situation, the second a clearly pathological state. In this case, too, normality of a tracing must be evaluated overall, and normal function from the kinematic standpoint must be considered only after clinical and instrumental data have been combined.

It is perhaps more difficult to define normal joint function from the static and dynamic standpoints, and the controversy in the field of gnathology surrounding the concepts of centric relation and centric occlusion

is well known. In the sphere of orthodontic-surgical treatment for dentofacial anomalies, *normal* may be defined as a situation in which, from the static and anatomic standpoints, the mandibular condyle is at the center of the glenoid fossa in basal conditions. From the dynamic standpoint there must be no functional limits on opening or during lateral or protrusive movements, and, above all, these movements must occur without pain or even subjectively unpleasant sensations. In the light of these concepts we may therefore examine the goals to be reached in asymptomatic patients and in patients with dysfunction.

In asymptomatic patients, from the subjective and objective standpoints, obviously the situation must remain stable and unchanged over time. For this purpose, it is necessary to monitor the joint situation during the various phases of treatment from the static and dynamic standpoints. From the static standpoint, the condylar position and the condyle-fossa relationship may initially be investigated by simple oblique transcranial radiography, easily performed using any dental radiologic device and a Mongini-Preti–type craniostat (Mongini 1981; Preti and Scotti 1981) integrated with the use of a Gelb diagram (Gelb 1997) (Figs 3-5 and 3-6). This radiologic investigation is undoubtedly very simple, but it is also limited because it does not provide three-dimensional information, as does computerized tomography (CT), nor does it

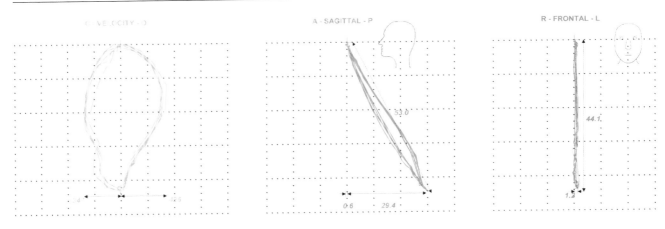

Fig 3-3 Normal kinesiographic tracing. (C, closed; O, open; A, anterior; P, posterior; R, right; L, left.)

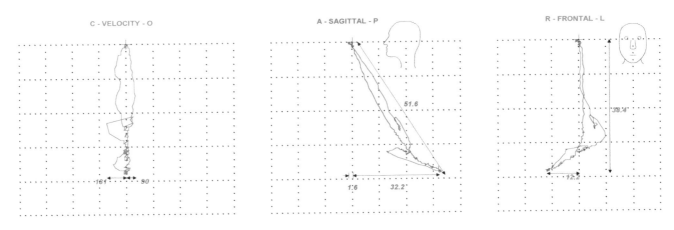

Fig 3-4 Classic example of pathological kinesiographic tracing. (C, closed; O, open; A, anterior; P, posterior; R, right; L, left.)

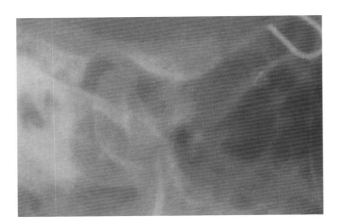

Fig 3-5 Example of oblique transcranial radiograph taken with the Mongini-Preti craniostat.

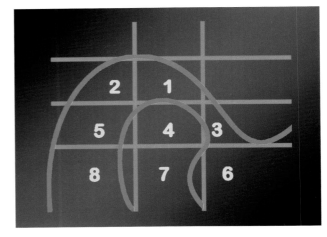

Fig 3-6 Gelb's diagram. The joint cavity is divided into eight compartments. The horizontal lines correspond to the top of the cavity, the articular tubercle, and the point midway between these two references; the vertical lines run through the top of the joint cavity and the intermediate point of the articular eminence. In normal conditions most of the head of the condyle must be within compartment 4.

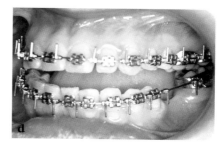

Fig 3-7 *(a)* Evident posterior disloca-tion of the condyle. *(b)* Treatment with anterior repositioning splint.

Fig 3-7 *(c)* Normalized condylar posi-tion. *(d)* Preoperative orthodontic treat-ment eliminates tooth interferences and therefore obviates the need for a main-tenance splint.

provide information on soft tissues or the temporo-mandibular disc, as does magnetic resonance imaging (MRI). Nevertheless, in most cases, if combined with careful clinical examination, oblique transcranial radio-graphy is sufficient for correct management of these patients. Furthermore, if correctly performed after evaluation of the condylar position on an axial radio-graph and subjective determination of the position of the patient's head in the craniostat, it is perfectly re-peatable in the same conditions and thus absolutely comparable over time. The condyle-fossa relationship thus determined must be maintained and checked ra-diographically at the end of orthodontic treatment, im-mediately after surgery (the immediate postoperative checkup is extremely important), at the end of the ac-tive phase of treatment, and during follow-up. From the dynamic standpoint, in normal situations clinical checkups and monitoring are sufficient during treat-ment, and the use of other instrumental examinations is not necessary. The use of electromyography in asymptomatic patients, as mentioned above, may have some value for study and research, especially if focused on controlling the muscle posture in the pre- and postoperative phases.

The case of a patient who is symptomatic and ex-hibits dysfunction at the start of treatment is of course entirely different. First and foremost we must consider that, for example, dysfunction has a much lower inci-

dence among Class III cases than in Class II situations or dentofacial asymmetries. Furthermore, joint and/or muscle symptoms are more frequent in Class III pa-tients with deep bite and in cases where there has been previous extraction of molars with posterior col-lapse and loss of vertical dimension. In any case, when treating a patient who exhibits dysfunction at the start of treatment, it is imperative that clinical symptoms be eliminated through adequate gnathologic treatment with superior or anterior repositioning splints. In a considerable proportion of patients with dysfunction, adequate clinical examination and a simple radiologic evaluation as described above (oblique transcranial ra-diography at rest and at maximum opening) are suffi-cient to plan correct treatment, regaining a normal condyle-fossa relationship, and to maintain adequate monitoring over time (Figs 3-7a and 3-7b).

After the initial use of the superior or the anterior repositioning splint (the duration of this phase is nor-mally between 4 and 6 months), it is usually possible to eliminate the need for the splint since preoperative orthodontic treatment, by eliminating all tooth inter-ferences, itself acts as occlusal and gnathologic treat-ment (Fig 3-7c and 3-7d). Only in the more complex or difficult cases is it necessary to use more sophisti-cated instrumental examinations, such as CT, nuclear magnetic resonance (NMR) imaging, kinesiography, and electromyography (always with the conceptual limitations expressed above). In some cases, a maintenance splint must be worn up to the time of surgery: Some patients, usually those with open bite or dentofacial asymmetry, can only maintain a situation of subjective and objective well-being by wearing the splint. This will entail particular surgical procedures, as will be described in full in chapter 6.

Lastly, it must be stressed that, especially in chronic cases, it is not always possible to completely eliminate all long-term symptoms. This is particularly true of joint noises such as crepitation, which indicate irreversible tissue alteration. The basic concept that must always guide treatment in these patients is to seek a pain-free situation with no functional limitations.

Observation of these concepts, with regard to occlusal, muscular, and joint function, is one of the essential factors, if not the principal one in the absolute sense, to achieve medium- and long-term stability in patients subjected to orthodontic-surgical treatment. In recent years, a possible relationship between malocclusion and posture has frequently been discussed, and naturally dentofacial anomalies have also been related to postural problems. Although, from the theoretical standpoint, direct or indirect connections between the masticatory muscles and the musculature of the neck and spine cannot be excluded, and thus the possibility of descending or ascending associated diseases cannot be ruled out, at present there is no direct scientific evidence to relate dentofacial anomalies and postural disorders. These concepts were clearly expressed at the Consensus Conference of the European Academy of Craniomandibular Disorders, the Italian Society of Orthodontics, and the Italian Society of Physical and Rehabilitative Medicine in 1997; nevertheless, this does not rule out the fact that comparative studies should be done to better interpret the complex equilibrium that regulates muscular posture.

In collaboration with a team of physiotherapists the author undertook a study on a group of patients with dentofacial asymmetry who were thus, at least from the theoretical standpoint, more predisposed than normal subjects to postural problems. No significant muscular or postural problems were found in any of the 10 patients examined, and above all the physiotherapists' evaluation revealed no significant difference between the preoperative and postoperative situations (Ronchi et al, in press).

It may thus be reasonably concluded, in agreement with the aforementioned consensus conference, that at present orthodontic-surgical treatment should not be undertaken with the sole aim of treating and resolving postural problems.

However, this does not preclude the possibility, however theoretical and relatively remote, that postural problems can improve (or in some cases worsen) as a consequence of orthodontic-surgical treatment, and thus this particular aspect must be fully clarified to the patient during the clinical examination.

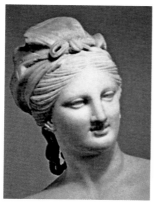

Fig 3-8 Statue of Venus, 100 BC, National Archaeology Museum, Athens.

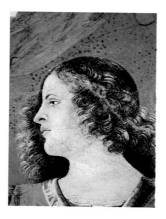

Fig 3-9 Melozzo da Forlì, early 15th-century fresco, Vatican Art Gallery, Rome.

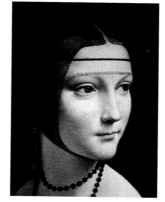

Fig 3-10 Leonardo da Vinci, *Lady with an Ermine*, late 15th century, National Museum, Kraków.

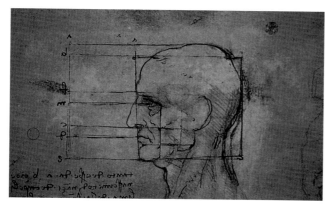

Fig 3-11 Anthropomorphic and cephalometric studies by Leonardo da Vinci, Windsor Castle, Royal Library.

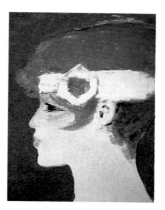

Fig 3-12 Salvatore Fiume, *Gala Cruise* (detail), private collection. (Reprinted with permission.)

Esthetics

The concept of esthetics in dentofacial anomalies is extremely important, and for most patients it is perceived as the chief problem. Nevertheless, the question of esthetics must be tackled from many standpoints. First, how should *esthetics* be defined? The answer is not a simple one, and even if we succeeded in giving a precise and concise definition, are there any rules and parameters that can be quantified and that are universally accepted? Herein lies the problem. We have already seen that numerous types of esthetic, clinical, and cephalometric analyses exist, both for the skeletal base and for the soft tissues, each of which possesses characteristics and reference points that are acceptable. On the other hand, normal cephalometric parameters do not necessarily coincide with pleasing esthetics, and vice versa.

Furthermore, the evolution of esthetics in art, which is the mirror of human taste, shows the continual changes in taste over time. In the history of art there is a continual cyclic alternation of retruded and linear faces and protruded and convex faces, from the Grecian beauty of Venus (Fig 3-8) to the depictions of Melozzo da Forlì in the early 15th century (Fig 3-9) and the portraits by Leonardo da Vinci (Fig 3-10). da Vinci was the first to give wide diffusion to some concepts of anthropometry and cephalometry; nevertheless, his parameters, which would be defined today as biretrusive (Fig 3-11), are very distant from today's trends, which prefer more protruded profiles and more pronounced features. This tendency is also explicit in the scientific literature of recent years; a clear example is found in an article by Auger and Turley (1999). And so, not only in the world of fashion and show business, but also in art, biprotruded and convex profiles prevail (Fig 3-12).

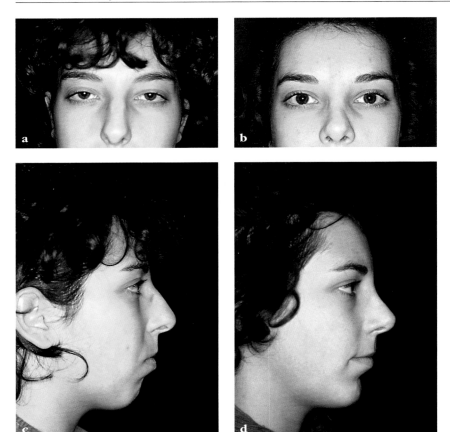

Fig 3-13 *(a and b)* Evident positive change to the expression of the eyes.

Fig 3-13 *(c and d)* Morphologic and profilometric changes obtained in the same patient.

Esthetics is also philosophy and, as Silvio Ceccato has said in his book *La Fabbrica del Bello* [*The Beauty Factory*] (1987), the rules for what is beautiful and for what is pleasing are not always universally true (ie, esthetics for all or for the few). Consequently, two people who exhibit completely different or even diametrically opposed features in a simple cephalometric analysis (for example, a biretruded profile with thin but regular lips and a biprotruded profile with pronounced and fleshy lips) may be equally beautiful or attractive.

So, in the final analysis, what is it that makes a face pleasant and attractive? Certainly not only the profile,

the mouth, or the chin, which of course have their own importance, but many other components as well: the forehead, the nose, the cheekbones, the ears, and in particular the eyes. The eyes are of huge importance in making a face look beautiful and pleasing, not only for their shape or color, but for their lively expression. Often patients with severe dentofacial anomalies have a dull and vacant expression, and in these cases surgery may, within certain limits, help to give the eyes more expression (Fig 3-13). It is, however, true that a dull expression is unlikely to change enough to give the face a lively look, even where significant structural changes to facial esthetics have been made (Fig 3-14).

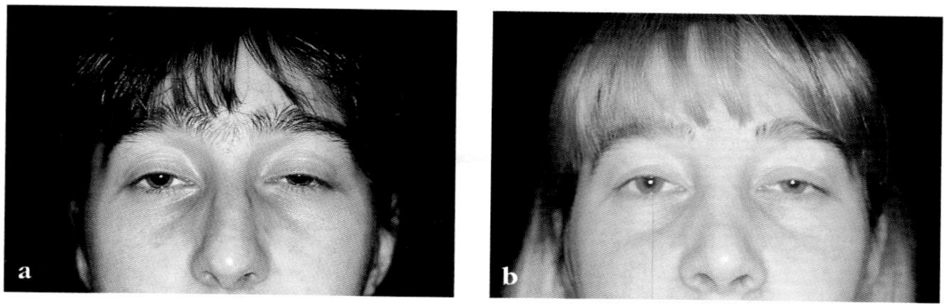

Fig 3-14 *(a and b)* Change to the expression of the eyes is not very significant.

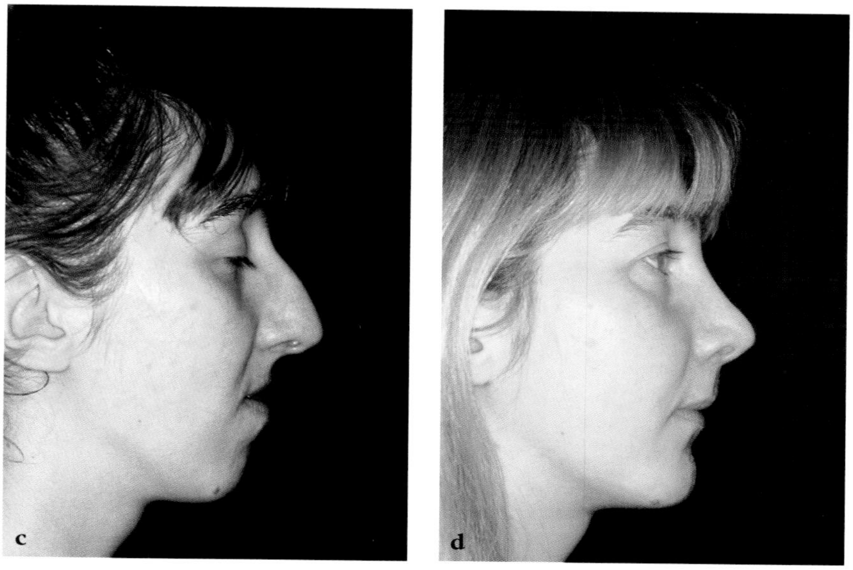

Fig 3-14 *(c and d)* Morphologic and profilometric changes obtained in the same patient.

All these wide-ranging esthetic considerations must naturally be discussed with the patient in an attempt to understand clearly what he or she wants and what his or her expectations are and to explain which goals can be reasonably achieved, without falling into the trap of promising certain and predictable results (see also chapter 10). It must also be considered that some patients want a marked change in their features, while others want the skeletal defect to be corrected without completely transforming their appearance.

The means through which clinicians can have a significant impact on esthetics are the type of osteotomy, rational orthodontic preparation, proper management of the soft tissues, and ancillary surgical procedures (rhinoplasty, genioplasty, and surgery to increase the prominence of cheekbones or paranasal areas). Examination of the soft tissues is of great importance in selecting the type of osteotomy: All surgery to advance the middle third tends to fill out the soft tissues, giving the patient a youthful appearance. On the contrary, excessive mandibular setback will produce an accumulation of soft tissue beneath the chin, giving an appearance of aging. Therefore, the patient's age and the characteristics of his or her soft tissues must be taken into account in selecting surgical procedures (see chapter 9).

Bibliography

Auger TA, Turley PK. The female soft tissue profile as presented in fashion magazines during the 1900s: A photographic analysis. Int J Adult Orthodon Orthognath Surg 1999;14:7–18.

Benech A, Fasciolo A, De Gioanni PP, Madaro E. Evaluation of the posture of patients before and after orthodontic surgery [in Italian]. Minerva Stomatol 1997;46:435–441.

Ceccato S. La Fabbrica del Bello [The Beauty Factory]. Milan: Rizzoli, 1987.

Dunlevy HA, White RP Jr, Turvey TA. Professional and lay judgment of facial esthetic changes following orthognathic surgery. Int J Adult Orthodon Orthognath Surg 1987; 2:151–158.

Ehmer U, Broll P. Mandibular border movements and masticatory patterns before and after orthognathic surgery. Int J Adult Orthodon Orthognath Surg 1992;7:153–159.

European Academy of Craniomandibular Disorders (EACD), Società Italiana di Ortodonzia (SIDO), Società Italiana di Medicina Fisica e Riabilitazione (SIMFER). Consensus Conference on Posture and Occlusion: Evidence or Hypothesis of Correlation. 10 May 1997, Milan.

Farkas LG, Hreczko TA, Kolar JC, Munro IR. Vertical and horizontal proportions of the face in young adult North American Caucasians: Revision of neoclassical canons. Plast Reconstr Surg 1985;75:328–338.

Farkas LG, Kolar JC. Anthropometrics and art in the aesthetics of women's faces. Clin Plast Surg 1987;14:599–616.

Gelb H. Patient evaluation. In: Gelb H (ed). Clinical Management of Head, Neck and TMJ Pain and Dysfunction. Philadelphia: Saunders, 1997.

Jiménez ID. Electromyography of masticatory muscles in three jaw registration positions. Am J Orthod Dentofacial Orthop 1989;95:282–288.

Leonardi R. Potenzialità e limiti dell'elettromiografia nella diagnosi e nel follow-up in ortognatodonzia e gnatologia. Ortognatodonzia Ital 1993;2:817–848.

Leonardi R, Caltabiano M. Valori assoluti ed indici di simmetria elettromiografici dei muscoli masticatori. Analisi della riproducibilità dell'ampiezza intra ed inter-sessione di registrazione. Ortognatodonzia Ital 1996;5:707–716.

Iliffe AH. A study of preference in feminine beauty. Br J Psychol 1960;51:267–273.

Manni A, Brunori P, Lapi A, Raffaelli L, Raffaelli R. Standard electromyographic and kinesiographic parameters in a sample of healthy population [in Italian]. Minerva Stomatol 1995; 44:411–419.

Mongini F. Anatomic and clinical evaluation of the relationship between the temporomandibular joint and occlusion. J Prosthet Dent 1977;38:539–552.

Mongini F. The importance of radiography in the diagnosis of TMJ dysfunctions: A comparative evaluation of transcranial radiographs and serial tomography. J Prosthet Dent 1981;45:186–198.

Moreno A, Bell WH, You ZH. Esthetic contour analysis of the submental cervical region. J Oral Maxillofac Surg 1994; 52:704–713.

Palano D, Molinari G, Salvo C. Electromyographic and computerized magnetic gnathokinesiographic studies of normal subjects [in Italian]. Minerva Stomatol 1990a;39: 967–975.

Palano D, Molinari G, Salvo C. Electromyography and computerized magnetic gnathokinesiography in the diagnosis and therapy of craniomandibular disorders [in Italian]. Minerva Stomatol 1990b;39:977–987.

Preti G, Scotti R. Importance of the correct incidence in temporomandibular joint radiography with an oblique transcranial projection [in Italian]. Minerva Stomatol 1981;30: 437–442.

Ricketts RM. Divine proportions in facial esthetics. Clin Plast Surg 1982;9:401–422.

Rigsbee OH 3rd, Sperry TP, BeGole EA. The influence of facial animation on smile characteristics. Int J Adult Orthodon Orthognath Surg 1988;3:233–239.

Ronchi P, Colombo L, Cassi M, Balzaretti E, Meroni M. Anomalie dento-facciali e postura: Evidenze o ipotesi di correlazione? Valutazioni kinesiologiche e posturali in pazienti affetti da asimmetrie maxillo-mandibolari sottoposti a trattamento ortodontico-chirurgico. Ortodonzia Clinica (in press).

Stempel GH 3rd. Visibility of blacks in news and news-picture magazines. J Quart 1971;48:337–339.

Van der Dussen FN, Egyedi P. Premature aging of the face after orthognathic surgery. J Craniomaxillofac Surg 1990;18: 335–338.

Recommended reading

Proffit WR, White RP Jr. Surgical-Orthodontic Treatment. St Louis: Mosby, 1991.

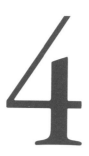

Preoperative Orthodontic Treatment

with Luigi Colombo and
Alberto Guariglia

- General guidelines
- Class III malocclusion
- Class II malocclusion
- Dentofacial asymmetry
- Open bite

General Guidelines

The previous chapter addressed the idea that correct muscle and joint function is one of the dominant factors for a stable result. Another concept affecting long-term stability that must guide the clinician throughout treatment is that of putting everything in the correct place. This principle, which is both dogmatic and philosophical, requires surgery to reposition the bony bases correctly in all three dimensions, whereas the task of orthodontics is to replace the teeth in their ideal position with respect to the supporting alveolar base, creating synergism among all components and respecting muscles and joints. Thus, preoperative orthodontic treatment must aim to obtain two ideal arches capable of being coordinated with each tooth in the correct position, always treating the two arches separately and bearing in mind the goals of the subsequent surgical repositioning.

To correctly approach preoperative orthodontic treatment, careful study of the casts is fundamental. Initially they must be analyzed separately: the shape of the arch (parabolic, triangular, square), the extent of crowding, tooth rotation, and the curve of Spee must be evaluated (Fig 4-1). Only after this preliminary examination should the relationship between the two arches be examined. It is sufficient initially to position the casts manually with the molars in Class I occlusion, so as to evaluate discrepancies between the two arches that impede their coordination and to identify the first general indications concerning the requirements and goals of preoperative orthodontic treatment (Fig 4-2). These are the guidelines underlying the whole of preoperative orthodontic treatment, and they will be discussed in more detail with all the necessary variables in the different sections in this chapter. After this brief and general indication, the first thing to be examined is the position of the maxillary and mandibular incisors, as well as any crowding. The entire orthodontic treatment plan will be developed from these evaluations (which differ depending on the pathological situation), as will be explained in this chapter.

With regard to the type of equipment and techniques to be used, the authors believe that standard equipment and the simplest and most widely used orthodontic techniques are preferable. Brackets cemented directly onto the teeth are perfectly acceptable even for orthodontic-surgical treatment. This is limited, however, to the premolars and to the anterior segment. Brackets must not be too small and should always consist of twin attachments that are large enough to enable optimal control of tooth rotation and bodily movement of the tooth. Ceramic brackets may be used in the maxilla from canine to canine, whereas metallic attachments are preferable in the mandibular arch.

The first and second molars must always be banded. In the mandibular arch this must be done from the start of treatment with a single band on the second molars and a wide twin attachment on the first molars. In the maxillary arch it is sufficient initially to fit a double band to the first molars for extraoral traction if required, whereas in the final phases of preoperative treatment the second molars should be fitted with a single band and the first molars with wide twin attachments. In addition, lingual buttons or wings should always be applied to the molars to correct any crossbite using crossed elastics in the pre- or postoperative period.

With regard to preplanned inclination on the attachments, in the mesiodistal sense or with regard to torque, this obviously depends on the type of orthodontic technique used. It is clear that if the straight-wire technique is used, inclination should be planned on the attachments from the start. If the classic edgewise technique (still the most suitable for orthodontic-surgical treatment) is used, the attachments must all be standard passive attachments. For other techniques,

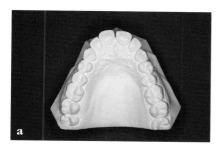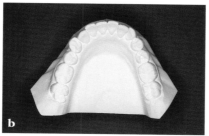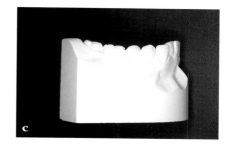

Fig 4-1 *(a to c)* Preliminary separate examination of casts.

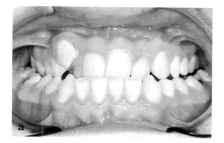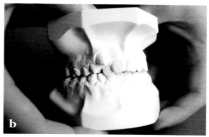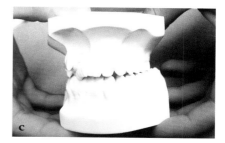

Fig 4-2 *(a to c)* Initial simple, manual maneuver to evaluate lack of coordination between the arches.

preinclination on attachments should, in any case, be reduced to a minimum, and tooth movement should be managed through archwires as much as possible. With regard to the height at which to cement the brackets, on the mandibular arch they must be placed 0.5 to 1.0 mm more apically than normal to allow for intraoperative and immediate postoperative requirements.

Hooks integrated into the brackets are not recommended for the surgical phases, and thus their use must be dictated by orthodontic considerations alone. For the surgical arches required during the operation (intraoperative maxillomandibular fixation, immediate postoperative phase), preformed hooks fixed onto the arches, or alternatively those prepared and welded onto the orthodontic wire, are indicated (see chapter 10).

In recent years, the lingual technique has become widespread, especially to meet the esthetic and social requirements of adult patients. However, it is not generally recommended for presurgical treatment because of the difficulty of achieving ideal three-dimensional control over tooth movements. Furthermore, the presence of attachments on the lingual side often interferes with the study of surgical feasibility on the plaster casts, and requires laborious laboratory work on them. In any case, the buccal appliance must be positioned immediately prior to surgery and maintained during the postoperative phases (see chapter 11). However,

in cases with particular requirements there is no absolute contraindication to the lingual technique, at least for the first phases of treatment, and the use of buccal attachments can be delayed to the later phases.

The third molars also deserve comment. Extraction of third molars is normally recommended in cases where therapeutic extraction of the premolars is not required; in cases requiring extraction of the premolars, maintenance of the third molars must be evaluated case by case depending on type of occlusion, position, type of osteotomy planned, and their shape and relationship with the opposing arch. In the case of dysodontiasis or impaction, third molars should always be extracted. The mandibular third molars must be extracted at least 6 months before surgery if osteotomy of the mandibular angle is planned, because if the two procedures are done simultaneously complications may arise, such as undesired fracture and/or failure of the osteotomy to consolidate. The maxillary third molars may be extracted during a Le Fort I osteotomy; however, if posterior ostectomy is planned for vertical repositioning (see chapter 7), it is recommended that they be extracted at least 6 months prior to the procedure.

The goals and basic concepts of orthodontic preparation may be subdivided as: *position of incisors, transverse coordination, dental midlines, symmetry of canines,* and *curve of Spee.* Each aspect will be analyzed separately for each type of anomaly.

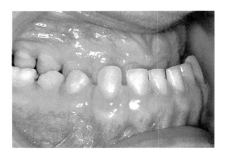

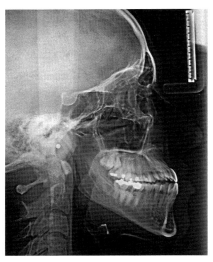

Fig 4-3 Evident lingualization of the mandibular incisors, which can be evaluated clinically.

Fig 4-4 In another patient, the lateral radiograph clearly demonstrates the marked vestibularization of the maxillary incisors.

Class III Malocclusion

Position of incisors

As already stated, there is a natural mechanism in most Class III cases that compensates for the sagittal skeletal discrepancy, so that during growth a lingualization of the mandibular incisors develops together with a vestibularization of the maxillary incisors in an attempt to achieve anterior tooth contact. Inclination can be extremely marked, as shown in Figs 4-3 and 4-4, and may have significant periodontal implications. Furthermore, frequently what does not occur naturally may occur as the consequence of previous orthodontic treatment, carried out in the vain attempt to resolve orthodontically an underlying skeletal discrepancy that in reality could only be corrected surgically.

Restoration of the correct inclination of the incisors in respect to their bony bases thus becomes absolutely essential in preoperative orthodontic treatment. Reference parameters for correct evaluation are exclusively of the cephalometric type. Since the goal of orthognathic surgery is to reposition the skeletal bases in their ideal position three dimensionally, the most suitable and reliable cephalometric values are

the inclination of the maxillary incisors on the palatal plane and that of the mandibular incisors on the mandibular plane (generally gonion-menton). It is obvious that if the bony bases are in the correct position at the end of treatment, and likewise the incisors are correctly inclined with regard to the bases, then the incisors themselves will automatically be in the correct position with regard to all the other structures (cranial base, Frankfort plane, etc). This is why the position of the incisors becomes an essential, dogmatic issue, the only true and absolutely necessary cephalometric reference point of the entire treatment (see chapter 2).

Restoration of the correct position of the incisors, also defined as *decompensation*, together with correction of crowding, of necessity dictates whether tooth extractions will be required. Normally, mild to moderate crowding of the mandibular arch can be resolved through vestibularization of the incisors without requiring extraction. In general, crowding of 2 to 3 mm per hemiarch can be resolved in this way; in most cases, correction of the inclination of the incisors is achieved simply by using increasingly heavy square or rectangular archwires (Fig 4-5). Obviously, in calculating spaces to correct crowding, the starting position

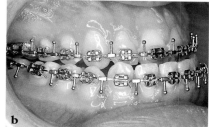
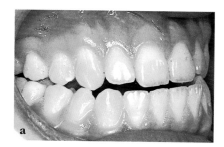

Fig 4-5 *(a and b)* Decompensation of the mandibular incisors.

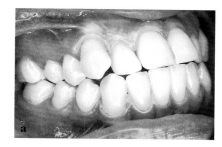
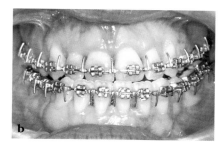

Fig 4-6 *(a and b)* Marked mandibular crowding that requires extraction of the premolars.

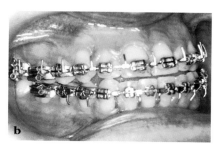

Fig 4-7 *(a and b)* Vestibularization of the maxillary incisors that will require extraction of the premolars to achieve full decompensation.

and the planned final position of the mandibular incisors must be taken into consideration. In more severe crowding, more than 4 mm per hemiarch, the first or second premolars are extracted, depending on whether the crowding is more marked in the anterior or posterior arch segments (Fig 4-6). In some situations, the dental condition (extensive caries, endodontic therapy) may dictate extractions.

Similar considerations apply to the maxillary incisors. Because they are markedly vestibularized in a high percentage of cases, decompensation requires an amount of space that can often be gained only by extracting the first premolars (Fig 4-7). Whether or not therapeutic extraction of premolars is planned obviously affects the final molar relationship. If extractions are limited to the

maxillary arch, the final molar relationship will be Class II; if no teeth are extracted, or if they are extracted from both arches, the final molar relationship will be Class I. Therapeutic extraction of the mandibular first premolars in Class III cases of necessity also involves extracting the maxillary first or second premolars.

In some selected cases it is possible to recover 1 to 2 mm on each side through extraoral traction on first or second molars; in other cases, the existence of interincisal diastemas or spaces due to prior extractions enables the maxillary incisors to be lingualized sufficiently to achieve the ideal inclination (Fig 4-8). If the maxillary anterior teeth are to be retruded, this almost always requires maximum posterior anchorage and/or use of Class II elastics (Fig 4-9). In any

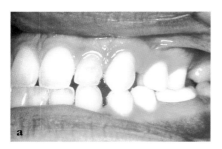 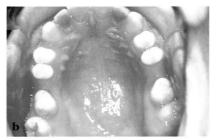 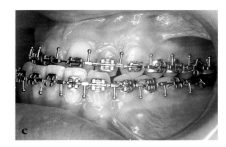

Fig 4-8 *(a to c)* Spaces in the maxillary arch due to prior extractions facilitate lingualization of the anterior teeth.

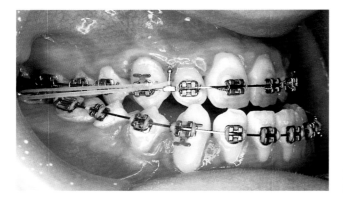

Fig 4-9 Use of Class II elastics to lingualize the mandibular incisors.

case, perfect control of torque on the incisors with appropriate rectangular archwires is essential.

Where the maxillary arch is well aligned, with no transverse problems and with teeth in good condition, a slight vestibularization of the maxillary incisors may be acceptable (not more than 115 degrees on the palatal plane) to avoid extraction of the premolars and the inevitable extension of the time required for orthodontic treatment. In these cases the mandibular incisors should be overcorrected, by a similar angular value, so that the case may be completed with slight dental bimaxillary protrusion, the same amount on both arches.

The orthodontic procedures required to prepare these patients for surgery (ie, extraction of maxillary teeth, but frequently not of mandibular teeth, and Class II elastics) are the exact opposite of corrective orthodontic treatment, and thus produce a temporary worsening of the situation. It is therefore essential to explain this temporary worsening of the functional and esthetic situation to the patient.

It therefore becomes essential to immediately outline the correct plan for combined orthodontic-surgical treatment, and never to begin exclusive orthodontic treatment without being absolutely certain that the case can be resolved without surgery (in these cases

the choice of timing for orthodontic treatment is also essential). Otherwise, the consequences can be very serious for the patient.

In some cases, decompensation of the maxillary and mandibular incisors may even go beyond ideal values (109 degrees for maxillary incisors, 90 degrees for mandibular incisors) if bone and periodontal conditions permit it. This produces a negative overjet that is even more accentuated, and thus the bony bases must and can be repositioned surgically to a greater extent, with greater esthetic impact (Fig 4-10). The concept is that of the surgical operation that can be modified as a function of the position of the incisors and the desired esthetic goals.

Although the position of the incisors was previously described as dogmatic, in some cases it may, and indeed must, be necessary to accept compromised solutions where periodontal problems and limitations are evident. This occurs more frequently with the mandibular incisors than with the maxillary incisors: There may be little adherent gingiva in the anterior segment of the mandibular arch, and furthermore the shape and thickness of alveolar bone and of the mental symphysis may prevent extensive vestibularization of the incisors. In these cases a smaller degree of decompensation must be accepted (Fig 4-11).

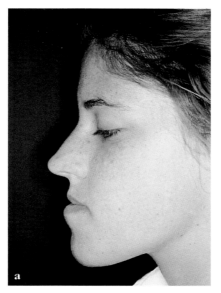

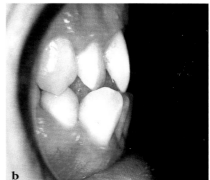

Fig 4-10 *(a and b)* Class III malocclusion with dental compensation.

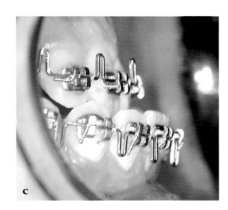

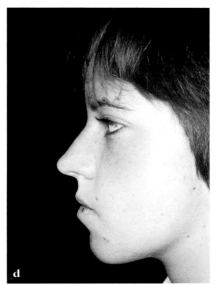

Fig 4-10 *(c and d)* In this patient, accentuated mandibular and maxillary decompensation has enabled the mandible to be set back considerably, with greater esthetic impact.

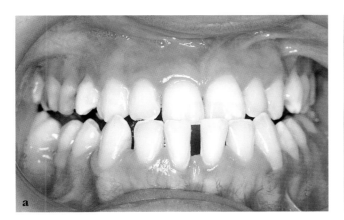

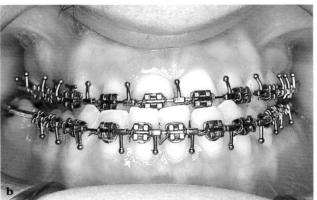

Fig 4-11 *(a and b)* The precarious periodontal condition does not, in this case, enable full decompensation, so a compromise must be accepted.

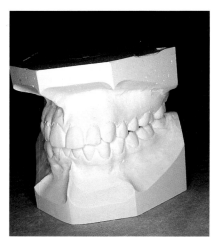

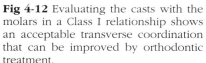

Fig 4-12 Evaluating the casts with the molars in a Class I relationship shows an acceptable transverse coordination that can be improved by orthodontic treatment.

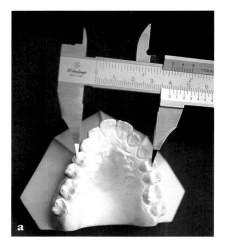

Fig 4-13 (a and b) Preestablished methods used to evaluate transverse coordination of the two arches.

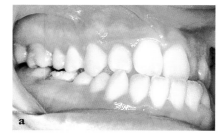

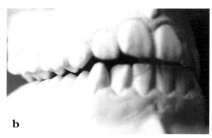

Fig 4-14 Initial Class III malocclusion (a) and evaluation on the casts (b), where the need to contract the maxillary arch is apparent.

Transverse coordination

With regard to transverse coordination, two fundamental concepts must be taken into account: how to evaluate for a lack of it and how to correct it.

As mentioned in chapter 1, right from the start of treatment clinicians must become accustomed to looking at each arch independently; therefore the transverse relationship must be evaluated on each plaster cast singly and never during the intraoral clinical examination. Furthermore, this step must only be done after having decided whether any premolars are to be extracted, and thus after having established what the molar relationship will be at the end of treatment (molar Class I or Class II, as discussed above). At this point, simply by taking hold of the plaster casts and placing the molars in the planned final relationship, we have a clear view of the transverse relationship and of any need to correct it (Fig 4-12). Various tables also exist that relate intermolar and interpremolar widths to determine correct transverse coordination (Fig 4-13), but it is the authors' opinion that simple handling is quicker, more immediate, and more reliable.

In a Class III malocclusion an apparent contraction of the maxilla frequently resolves spontaneously simply through sagittal displacement of the bony bases. Furthermore, in a certain number of cases, only the maxillary first premolars are extracted and thus a Class II molar relationship is obtained; in these patients an apparent lack of transverse coordination, even if severe, may resolve spontaneously. In these situations it is often necessary, in the preoperative phase, to slightly contract the width of the maxilla through buccopalatal torque applied to the posterior segments, if necessary together with linguobuccal torque applied to the mandibular molars (Fig 4-14).

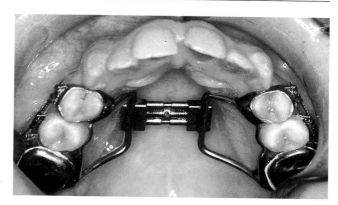

Fig 4-15 Purely orthopedic expansion of the maxillary arch with the expansion device.

Fig 4-16 The various phases of surgically assisted expansion: *(a)* lateral osteotomies; *(b)* tracing of the median osteotomy; *(c)* pterygomaxillary disjunction; *(d)* median osteotomy with an osteotome; *(e)* activation of the expansion device.

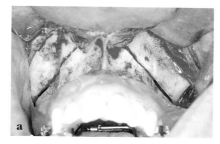
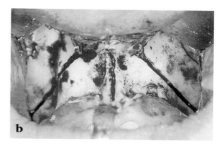
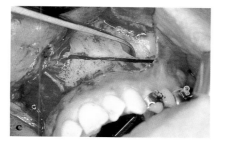
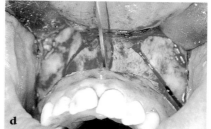
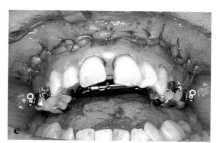

In cases in which there is true contraction of the maxilla, the extent of the required expansion must be established, and a decision made about how it can best be achieved. A basic concept is to apply approximately 20% overcorrection of the transverse defect; if the transverse deficiency, as measured on the plaster casts, is 3 mm, then orthodontic expansion should be 4 mm. Even in a patient who has completed growth, expansion of up to 4 mm can generally be obtained orthodontically (through expansion arches, palatobuccal torque in posterior segments, and quad-helix). However, for values greater than 4 mm, orthopedic ap-

proaches, such as disjunction of the palatine suture, are necessary. This procedure may easily be performed in patients up to 16 years of age with the classic palatal-torque expansion device cemented onto premolars and molars (Fig 4-15). Surgically assisted expansion (Fig 4-16), which employs osteotomy lines similar to those of the Le Fort I osteotomy, is always necessary for patients older than 20 years (see chapter 7). In patients between the ages of 16 and 20 years, the choice of orthopedic or surgically assisted expansion must take the following factors into consideration: the patient's skeletal structure (whether the patient has

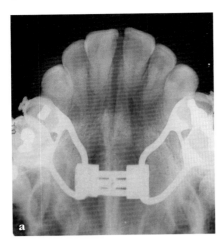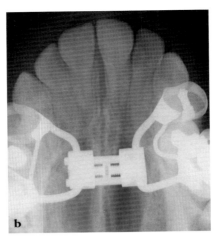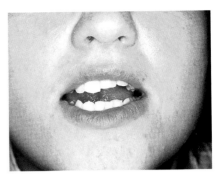

Fig 4-17 *(a)* Insufficient orthopedic expansion, despite the interincisal diastema: The suture has not fully opened. *(b)* Complete and efficacious orthopedic expansion: The suture has opened completely.

Fig 4-18 Evident deviation of the maxillary dental midline with regard to the midline axis of the upper lip and face.

large bones and shows clinical or radiographic signs that growth is complete); in some cases, evaluation of the carpal index; the radiographic appearance of the suture on occlusal radiographs (a suture that is not serrated opens more easily; a suture that is significantly interdigitated may indicate that surgical disjunction is required); whether the expansion will be greater than 8 mm; and whether orthopedic expansion alone previously failed. However, an extremely important consideration must be borne in mind in these cases: Opening of the palatine suture must always be verified by occlusal radiography and never only by the clinical appearance of the interincisal diastema, which in some cases may be misleading (Fig 4-17).

Once expansion has been achieved, the expansion device must be kept in place for approximately 4 months. Fixed appliance therapy must follow immediately. The two steps must always take place in a single appointment to avoid the risk of early relapse.

In general, if rapid palatal expansion is required, it should be the first procedure of preoperative treatment.

Dental midlines

The concept that must guide the orthodontist and surgeon through all planning and operative phases is that, once treatment is completed, the two dental

midlines must not only coincide with one another but also fall in line with the facial midline axis. The *facial midline axis* is the axis drawn perpendicular to the bipupillary line at its midpoint in clinical evaluation, or the axis drawn perpendicular to the line that joins the frontozygomatic suture at its midpoint in posteroanterior cephalometric evaluation. Furthermore, the point that characterizes the mental symphysis must also coincide with the facial midline axis. A discrepancy of 1 mm between the two dental midlines and the facial midline axis may be tolerated.

Thus the ideal and the theoretical goal of all preoperative orthodontic treatment is that the maxillary dental midline should coincide with the facial midline axis; this condition becomes imperative when mandibular osteotomy alone is planned. Should insuperable orthodontic limits make this impossible, it will be necessary to perform maxillary osteotomy to achieve this goal even though this procedure is not strictly necessary from esthetic or cephalometric standpoints. In general, initial deviation of the dental midline above 3 mm requires surgical repositioning, and in these cases it is useless to attempt to reposition the dental midline orthodontically, as this challenges some insuperable biologic limits that apply to orthodontic movements (Fig 4-18).

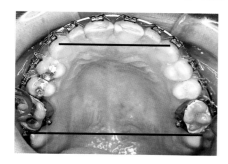

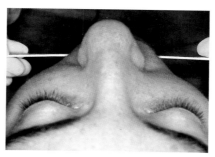

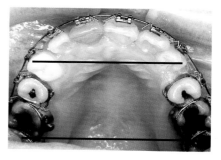

Fig 4-19 Clinical evaluation of canine symmetry, from below.

Fig 4-20 Clinical evaluation of canine symmetry, from above, using a wooden tongue depressor.

Fig 4-21 The absence of the maxillary right canine, due to prior extraction, means that symmetry must be evaluated with the right premolar: The left canine must be distalized by an additional 2 mm.

Similar considerations hold for the mandibular dental midline: It must coincide with the line of the mental symphysis on completion of preoperative orthodontic treatment. The surgical operation to reposition the mandible will obviously make these two lines coincide with the facial midline axis. In cases where orthodontic limitations make it impossible to align the dental midline with the mental symphysis, this goal can and must be pursued through genioplasty for lateral repositioning (see chapter 5). Also with regard to the mandibular dental midline, initial deviation of more than 3 mm is indicative of corrective genioplasty.

Finally, in cases where maxillary osteotomy alone is planned, it is imperative that orthodontic preparation of the mandibular arch perfectly center the mandibular dental midline with regard to the facial midline axis of the face; should this involve deviation from the line of the symphysis, genioplasty for lateral repositioning also will be required.

Symmetry of canines

The position of the canines constitutes another key point in preoperative orthodontic treatment. It is imperative that these teeth occupy a symmetric position in the two arches. Indeed, an asymmetric position of the canines would inevitably cause lateral deviation or some form of dentofacial asymmetry.

The position of the maxillary canines may be evaluated by examining the patient from below (Fig 4-19) or from above with the help of a tongue depressor linking the two canines (Fig 4-20). This symmetry is also required because any surgical rotation of the maxilla on the horizontal plane to bring the canines into symmetry would inevitably lead to an even less balanced position of the molars, which could not be reconciled with an acceptable occlusion. Thus symmetry of the canines must be obtained through suitable mesiodistal or distomesial orthodontic tooth movement. In cases of accentuated asymmetry, strategic unilateral extraction of the premolars may be necessary to achieve this goal correctly.

This concept is further complicated in cases of agenesis of one or both maxillary lateral incisors, where it is decided to close the space orthodontically with relative transformation of the canine to a lateral incisor and the first premolar to a canine. The evaluation and search for symmetry in such cases must clearly be based on the first premolars; similar considerations must be made in cases where a canine is missing (Fig 4-21).

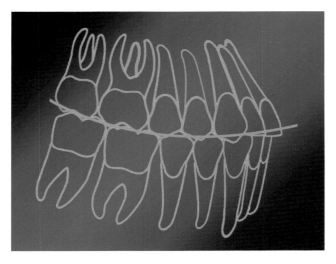

Fig 4-22 Preparation of the curve of Spee in Class III cases.

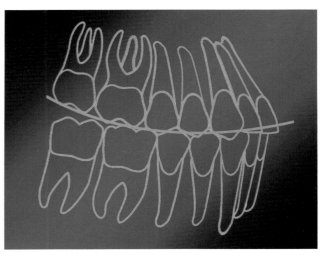

Fig 4-23 Preparation of the curve of Spee in Class III cases with reduced vertical dimension.

Curve of Spee

Analysis and management of the curve of Spee in preoperative orthodontic treatment is of particular strategic importance. First of all, it must be remembered that in Class III cases with mandibular dental compensation and tendency to deep bite, there is often an accentuated curve of Spee. The decompensation of the mandibular incisors and leveling of the corresponding tooth arch automatically bring about a flattening of this curve; nevertheless the flattening must not be complete, and some curvature, which could be defined as physiologic, must be maintained in order to simplify management of the occlusion immediately after surgery. Maintenance of some curvature of the mandibular arch enables the postsurgical occlusion to be obtained with a slight overbite (2 to 3 mm) that facilitates immediate postsurgical physiotherapy (see chapter 11) and helps to control any tendency to relapse in subsequent weeks and months (Fig 4-22).

This concept of a "physiologic" curve of Spee associated with an anterior overbite necessarily implies that the position of the brackets on the mandibular teeth must be 0.5 to 1.0 mm more apical than usual, at the least from the first premolars forward.

In cases with particularly deep bite and posterior vertical deficit, the maxillary arch should be prepared with an accentuation of the curve in the posterior segments, thus leaving some posterior lateral open bite in the postoperative occlusion (Fig 4-23); this will be closed during postoperative orthodontic treatment using vertical elastics, which will help to maintain the vertical height achieved and impede relapse of the deep bite.

In patients with anterior open bite, the physiologic curve of Spee must be further accentuated to obtain an overbite of 3 mm. The position of the mandibular brackets must also be adequate for this purpose. Furthermore, the curvature of the maxillary arch must be maintained and perfectly adapted to the mandibular arch, carefully avoiding creation of any posterior lateral open bite, which would bring a high risk of postoperative relapse. Frequently, in patients with anterior open bite, the curve of Spee is initially flat or even inverse, and preoperative orthodontic treatment must of necessity recreate a physiologic curve of Spee. These concepts will be explored in greater depth in treating open bite.

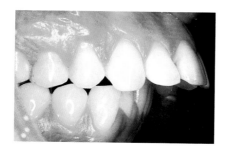

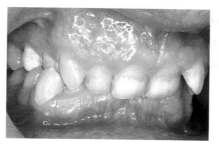

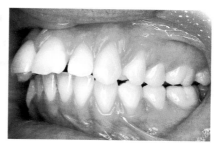

Fig 4-24 Vestibularized maxillary incisors in a Class II, division 1 case.

Fig 4-25 Highly lingualized maxillary incisors in a Class II, division 2 case.

Fig 4-26 Vestibularized mandibular incisors in a Class II, division 1 case.

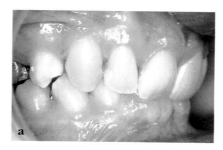

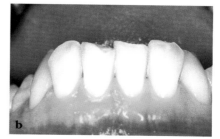

Fig 4-27 *(a and b)* Lingualized mandibular incisors in a Class II, division 2 case.

Class II Malocclusion

Position of incisors

The position of the incisors and their inclination with regard to the bony bases also constitutes a fundamental point in presurgical preparation of Class II cases. The principle of decompensation, which also holds for Class II cases, here too frequently involves a temporary worsening of occlusal relationships, which presupposes the application of orthodontic criteria that are practically the opposite of those normally used in classic orthodontic treatment for Class II cases.

Naturally, within Class II, division 1 and division 2 malocclusions must be distinguished. Division 2 cases are essentially hypodivergent, with deep bite, whereas division 1 cases may present varying characteristics (normal, deep, or vertical open bite). Furthermore, Class II, division 2 cases must not be confused with Class I cases with severe deep bite. The latter are a

well-defined clinical situation resulting from skeletal deep bite and are discussed in chapter 12.

The maxillary incisors are generally vestibularized in Class II, division 1 cases (Fig 4-24), whereas they are characteristically inclined toward the palate in Class II, division 2 cases (Fig 4-25). The mandibular incisors are usually vestibularized in division 1 cases (Fig 4-26), whereas they are lingualized to varying extents in division 2 cases with deep bite (Fig 4-27).

Preoperative orthodontic treatment, if necessary with extraction of premolars, is thus rather different in the two situations. In Class II, division 1 cases, as also seen in chapter 2, the maxillary incisors and especially the mandibular incisors are vestibularized to varying extents. Correction of the maxillary incisors usually requires palatal movement of these teeth by a few degrees, and in most cases this can be achieved without extracting the premolars, or at most with the help of extraoral traction on maxillary first or second molars. However, when there is also tooth crowding, even if

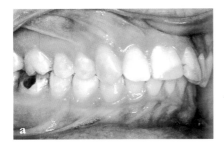 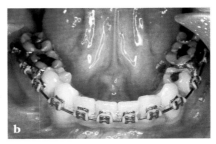 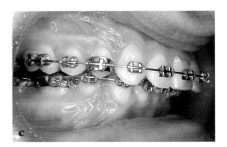

Fig 4-28 *(a to c)* Extraction of mandibular first premolars in a Class II, division 1 case to correct the axis of the incisors and to level the curve of Spee.

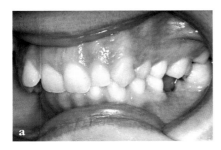 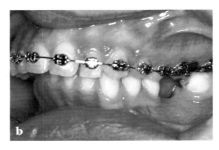

Fig 4-29 Orthodontic transformation of a Class II, division 2 malocclusion *(a)* into a Class II, division 1 malocclusion *(b)*.

only slight (2 to 3 mm per hemiarch), extraction, usually of the first premolars, becomes necessary. Correction of vestibularized mandibular incisors frequently requires extraction of the first premolars: This procedure is also necessary to reduce crowding, as frequently occurs, and to correct an excessive curve of Spee (Fig 4-28) (see sections below). Nevertheless, the periodontal condition of the incisors themselves is of great importance in evaluating what movement of the mandibular incisors will be required, as well as the thickness and characteristics of the mental symphysis; in some situations periodontal treatment may be indicated before orthodontic treatment.

In a small number of cases some compromise must be accepted with regard to inclination of the incisors. However, in most cases lingualization of the mandibular incisors is accompanied by an improvement of the periodontal condition of these teeth. Furthermore, in some cases, the extent of skeletal movement required may be modified by altering the inclination of the mandibular and/or maxillary incisors, accepting a slight vestibularization of the maxillary incisors and an angle somewhat less than 90 degrees for the mandibular incisors. This can be useful in clinical situations characterized by severe mandibular hypodevelopment, in which considerable surgical advancement is desirable. Obviously, extractions condition the final molar relationship; in cases in which extraction only

involves the mandibular arch, a final Class III molar relationship is inevitable; in other cases (with no extractions or extractions in both tooth arches), the final molar relationship will be Class I. In any case, the canine relationship must be rigorously Class I.

In Class II, division 2 cases, presurgical orthodontic treatment must transform the malocclusion to division 1. This entails vestibularizing the maxillary incisors, sometimes to a considerable extent. This is usually the initial orthodontic procedure, before attachments can be applied to the mandibular arch. In most cases correction of the axis of the incisors, up to 109 degrees on the palatal plane, may be obtained by using increasingly heavy arches, gradually replacing round archwires with rectangular archwires. In parallel with the vestibularization of the incisors, leveling and alignment of the entire arch is also automatically achieved. Treatment of the mandibular arch begins as soon as the bite has been opened to some extent: Normally the mandibular incisors must be slightly intruded and vestibularized to reach a 90-degree inclination of their axis on the gonion-menton plane (Fig 4-29). In some cases it may be useful to begin with the lingual technique at the mandibular arch, then proceed to the vestibular technique in later phases. In order to flatten the curve of Spee it is necessary to extrude the premolars and sometimes also the first molars; the extent of crowding in these cases will dictate the need for

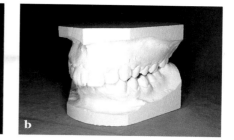

Fig 4-30 *(a and b)* Evident lack of transverse coordination, revealed by testing the casts manually, in a Class II, division 1 case.

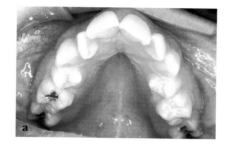

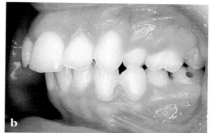

Fig 4-31 Typical triangular shape of a contracted palate *(a)*, in a Class II, division 1 case *(b)*.

premolar extractions. For crowding of 3 to 4 mm per hemiarch the usual approach is extraction of the first and second premolars, partly in consideration of the need to level the curve of Spee, which is notoriously an orthodontic procedure requiring a certain amount of space. In these (infrequent) cases, too, the final molar relationship will be Class III. Frequently the curve of Spee cannot be completely corrected preoperatively, and thus will be postponed to postsurgical treatment (see also sections below).

Transverse coordination

With regard to transverse coordination, the concepts described for Class III cases also hold for Class II cases. However, in Class II cases, unlike in Class III cases, transverse coordination of the arches may, misleadingly, appear adequate at intraoral clinical examination alone. In these cases, a correct evaluation of the arches on the plaster casts may reveal varying extents of maxillary transverse deficit. Naturally, the plaster casts are studied by placing them manually into the planned final molar relationship (Class I or, more rarely, Class III), which of necessity will be dictated by the decision whether to extract the premolars. Thus the decision to expand the maxillary arch is made after planning the position of the incisors, arch alignment, and correction of crowding (Fig 4-30).

A transverse discrepancy can also be detected through a simple clinical maneuver: When the patient protrudes the mandible until the canines are brought into Class I occlusion, a contraction of the maxilla be-

comes visible. In general it may be said that the need for expansion of the maxillary arch is more frequent in Class II than in Class III cases.

Clinical parameters indicating orthodontic, orthopedic, or orthodontic-surgical expansion are exactly the same as those considered for Class III cases. Thus for transverse discrepancies less than 4 mm it is possible to achieve correction through orthodontics alone, expanding the maxillary arch, and if necessary contracting the mandibular arch (this is possible primarily where extractions are planned) and acting suitably on the torque applied to lateroposterior segments. For values greater than 4 mm it will be necessary to apply orthopedic or orthodontic-surgical expansion, depending on the patient's age and with consideration of the factors described above with regard to patients between 16 and 20 years of age. For patients older than 20 years it is always better to consider surgical-orthodontic expansion.

An important consideration concerning Class II cases is that a careful evaluation must be made of which segment or segments most require transverse expansion (canine, premolar, molar, or throughout). In practice, this evaluation may influence the choice of surgical technique to be adopted and/or the design of the device to be used for expansion. Thus pterygomaxillary disjunction may or may not be performed, depending on whether the contraction is anterior or posterior, or alternatively orthodontic devices that include the canine may be selected. In many Class II cases the greatest contraction is at the level of the canines (Fig 4-31).

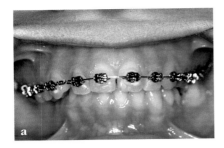

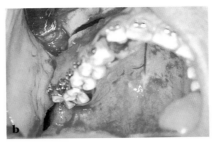

Fig 4-32 Evident unilateral Brodie syndrome *(a)*, corrected by lateroposterior segmental osteotomy of the maxilla *(b)*.

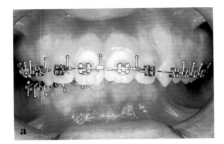

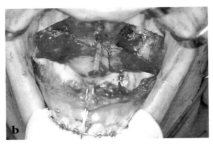

Fig 4-33 Evident unilateral Brodie syndrome *(a)*, corrected with total osteotomy of the maxilla in two pieces *(b)*.

A particular situation that may occur, though rarely, in Class II cases consists of the Brodie syndrome, also known as *scissors-bite* or *buccal occlusion*; this is a rare condition characterized by excessive transverse development of the maxilla (DeFreece 1984). This maxillary excess may be unilateral or bilateral. In the less severe cases presurgical correction of this anomaly may be achieved through orthodontics, acting with suitable rectangular archwires and/or modulating the torque in the lateroposterior segments. In more severe cases, which are prevalently unilateral, surgery will be necessary, such as the lateroposterior segmental osteotomy-ostectomy developed by Perko (1972) and modified by Bell et al (1980) (see chapter 7). This osteotomy can be performed alone, in association with osteotomy to advance the mandible (Fig 4-32), or during a Le Fort I maxillary osteotomy, when planned, with segmentation of the maxilla (Fig 4-33; see also chapter 7).

Dental midline and symmetry of canines

In presurgical orthodontic treatment for Class II cases, exactly the same principles described for Class III cases are valid and should be consulted. In brief, it is fundamental that, on completion of presurgical orthodontic treatment, the maxillary dental midline coincides with the facial midline axis, and that the mandibular dental midline coincides with the point characterizing the mental symphysis. In cases in which there is an initial deviation greater than 3 mm—and this holds for both

the maxillary and mandibular arches—it will be necessary to plan an osteotomy to reposition the maxilla laterally, or, alternatively, genioplasty with lateral repositioning. Symmetry of the canines is also a requirement, as was seen in Class III cases.

Curve of Spee

Full control over the curve of Spee is also fundamental in presurgical orthodontic preparation for Class II cases. Management of spaces in the arch, postsurgical occlusal stability (and thus any tendency to relapse), and vertical dimension of the lower third of the face may all depend on this factor. In general it may be said that in Class II cases, except for hyperdivergent cases with open bite, presurgical preparation must tend to level the curve of Spee (Fig 4-34).

Leveling the maxillary curvature does not normally create any particular difficulty in Class II, division 1 cases; in Class II, division 2 cases, in which the initial maxillary curvature is inverted, more time and more careful modulation of the orthodontic arches may be required, especially with regard to the transition from round wires to rectangular wires.

With regard to the mandibular arch, normally in skeletal Class II normal-divergent, normal vertical bite and, even more, in hypodivergent, deep overbite cases, the curve of Spee is relatively accentuated. Thus, in general, presurgical orthodontic preparation will require this curve to be leveled, completely if possible. Since this operation requires some space, it

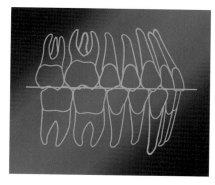

Fig 4-34 Preparation of the curve of Spee in Class II cases.

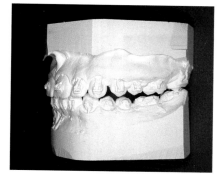

Fig 4-35 Good surgical feasibility with lateral open bite in a Class II, division 2 case: The open bite will be closed during the postoperative orthodontic treatment.

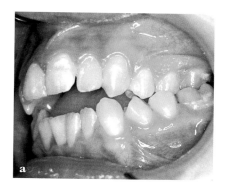

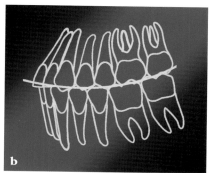

Fig 4-36 Class II, division 1 case with open bite *(a)* and preparation of the curve of Spee *(b)*.

is often necessary to extract the first or second premolars, especially where there is some degree of crowding (3 to 4 mm) or when the mandibular incisors are to be lingualized. Furthermore, leveling of the curve of Spee may quite often be very difficult in cases of deep bite, partly due to the characteristics of these patients' muscles, which oppose the planned tooth movements. In these cases it is nevertheless possible to achieve a stable occlusal relationship during surgery, with contacts at the incisor, canine, and molar levels, obviously after flattening the maxillary curvature if necessary (Fig 4-35). The lateral open bite thus formed can easily be closed during postoperative orthodontics, with vertical elastic bands (see chapter 11). It should be remembered that this way of proceeding produces a vertical increase in the lower third of the face, which is generally desirable in these patients.

Lastly, in cases that are particularly complex from the orthodontic standpoint, complete correction of the curve of Spee may require segmental surgical repositioning of the anterior group, from canine to canine (see chapter 5). In these situations, orthodontic treatment must be segmental, and its goals must be to re-

create sufficient tooth alignment in the three segments, the two lateral and the anterior, and to create a minimum interdental diastema between canines and first premolars to facilitate interdental osteotomy. Naturally, the roots and apexes must also be diverged, and this cannot be achieved initially by applying a simple compressed spring to the arch, but rather requires careful management of the bodily movement of the teeth with suitable control of second-order bends and mesiodistal uprighting of the roots.

The approach must be different in hyperdivergent Class II cases with anterior open bite. First and foremost it is important to remember that, in these patients, the maxillary curvature is generally relatively accentuated, whereas the curve of Spee may be flattened or even inverted (Fig 4-36a). In these cases it is recommended to prepare the two arches with some degree of physiologic curve of Spee in order to achieve greater occlusal stability in the immediate postsurgical period and to be able to cope with the possible tendency to relapse (Fig 4-36b). These concepts are covered in greater detail in the section dedicated to open bite.

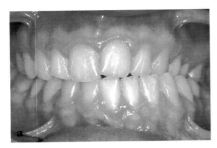 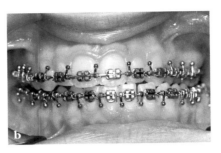 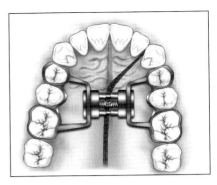

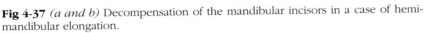

Fig 4-37 *(a and b)* Decompensation of the mandibular incisors in a case of hemimandibular elongation.

Fig 4-38 Asymmetric, surgically assisted expansion of the maxilla.

Dentofacial Asymmetry

Position of incisors

In patients with dentofacial asymmetry, too, the common goal is that of eliminating dental compensation and normalizing the axis of the incisors with respect to their bony bases. The maxillary and mandibular incisors may be vestibularized or lingualized to varying extents, and there may also be mesiodistal inclination depending on the skeletal situation. This is especially frequent for the mandibular incisors. However, decompensation is relatively simple in these cases (Fig 4-37).

Management of spaces, with regard to the two arches, must of necessity take two fundamental factors into account: the extent of crowding and the periodontal condition, in particular that of the incisors. Thus the decision when planning therapeutic extractions for arch alignment must depend on the need for vestibularization or lingualization of the incisors, on crowding, and on periodontal conditions. Extractions may be needed in both arches or in a single arch. This will obviously dictate the final molar relationship, which may therefore be Class I, Class II, or, more rarely, Class III (see above).

Transverse coordination

For dentofacial asymmetry, as for all other types of anomalies, transverse diameters must be evaluated by placing the casts in the planned final molar relationship, after having drawn up the plan with regard to the incisors and any therapeutic extractions. Normally, in dentofacial asymmetry, whether in the form of hemimandibular hyperplasia or hemimandibular elongation, there are no particular problems in obtaining adequate coordination of transverse diameters. The general principles concerning the need for expansion of the maxillary arch follow the guidelines given above.

In a small percentage of cases the asymmetry may also influence the shape of the maxillary arch. In these cases orthodontic-surgical expansion of the asymmetric type may be useful and should be achieved through lateroposterior osteotomy according to Schuchardt (1942 and 1959) (see chapter 7) combined with the application of an orthopedic expansion device (Fig 4-38). In this way, symmetry of the maxillary arch may be achieved.

In all other cases, when maxillary expansion greater than 4 mm is required, and when it must occur symmetrically, the classical orthodontic-surgical expansion described above is used.

Dental midlines

Clearly, problems relating to symmetry are of special importance in this group of dentoskeletal anomalies. In cases of simple hemimandibular elongation, in which mandibular osteotomy alone is planned, it is imperative that at completion of preoperative orthodontic treatment the maxillary dental midline coincide perfectly with the facial midline axis (Fig 4-39a). To achieve this, asymmetric and unilateral extraction of premolars will be necessary. With regard to the mandibular arch, from the purely theoretical standpoint it would be appropriate for the dental midline to coincide with the point characterizing the mental symphysis. Nevertheless, due to the considerable tooth compensation that occurs during growth, this is not always possible orthodontically. In these cases, compensatory genioplasty will be necessary with lateral repositioning equal to the extent of discrepancy present between the mandibular dental midline and the mental symphysis. It must also be considered that, when early orthodontic-orthopedic treatment is indicated in cases of positional mandibular laterodeviation, in most cases resulting from premature tooth contacts and transverse contraction of the maxilla, the mandibular dental midline may be modified

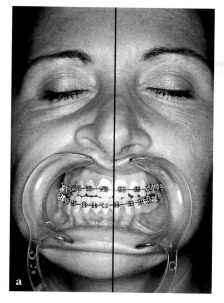
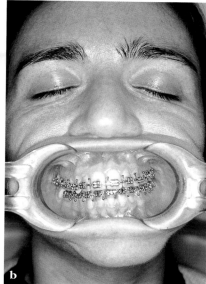

Fig 4-39 Surgery to the mandible alone is sufficient in hemimandibular elongation cases *(a)*; a two-jaw operation is needed in cases of hemimandibular hyperplasia with canting of the occlusal plane *(b)*.

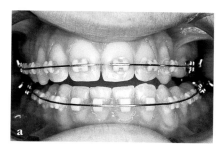
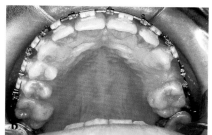

Fig 4-40 *(a and b)* Evaluation of the symmetry of the canines in a case of dentofacial asymmetry with absence of left maxillary premolars.

because of the orthodontic and orthopedic treatment that is applied.

In cases of hemimandibular hyperplasia with canting of the occlusal plane where osteotomy is planned, of necessity involving both jaws, it is clear that coincidence between the maxillary dental midline and the facial midline axis will only be achieved in the surgical phase, and thus control of the maxillary midline during presurgical orthodontic treatment is of only relative importance (Fig 4-39b). In these cases, symmetry must, on the contrary, be carefully achieved with regard to position of the canines (see next section).

In these cases, too, the above considerations hold true with regard to the mandibular arch.

Symmetry of canines

As already mentioned, with dentofacial asymmetries it is crucial to control the canines; this constitutes the key focus of preoperative orthodontic treatment in these patients (Fig 4-40). It is imperative to achieve a symmetric position of the canines on the two arches, even if this must involve asymmetric extraction of premolars and, thus, a different final molar relation-

ship on the two sides. This is a necessary compromise in order to achieve a symmetric position of the bony bases during surgery, and thus a morphologically and esthetically satisfactory end result. Symmetry of the canines may be evaluated clinically, as described in full in the section on Class III cases.

Curve of Spee

Correction of the curve of Spee must be aimed at achieving normal values for both the maxilla and the mandible. With regard to the maxillary arch, this can generally be obtained in the preoperative phase with no particular problem. With regard to the mandibular arch, in some cases compensatory mechanisms exist with dentoalveolar intrusion or extrusion that may make it impossible to achieve this goal through preoperative orthodontics alone. In these situations it may be convenient to plan an intraoperative occlusion characterized by a unilateral open bite, of such a size as to permit adequate postsurgical eruption, with the help of vertical elastics, thus achieving normalization of the curve of Spee in the final phases of treatment.

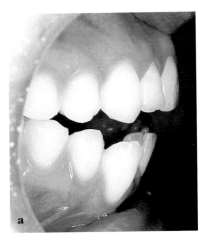
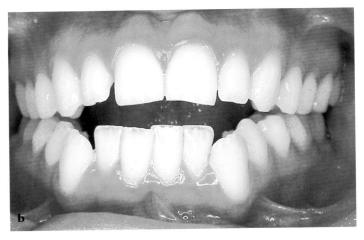

Fig 4-41 *(a and b)* Maxillary and mandibular incisors are vestibularized in open bite.

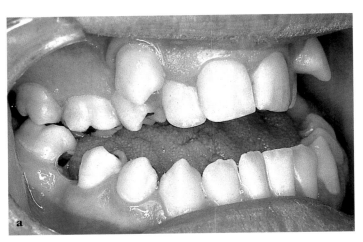
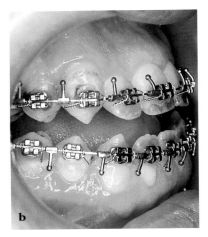

Fig 4-42 *(a and b)* Orthodontic preparation of the two arches with open bite, with normalization of the axes of the incisors.

Open Bite

Position of incisors

In open bite, the maxillary and mandibular incisors are, in general, vestibularized to some extent (Fig 4-41). The presence of some degree of maxillary transverse deficit is also not uncommon, with associated problems of space. The underlying concept is in any case always the same: The incisal axes must be in the correct position in relation to the bony bases. This may or may not involve therapeutic extraction of premolars, depending on the space available and on the planned orthodontic lingualization, but periodontal conditions also must al-

ways be considered, especially those of the maxillary incisors (Fig 4-42).

However, a clarification is necessary: In cases of total open bite (which are the majority) the maxillary posterior vertical excess requires surgical correction through posterior osteotomy–cuneiform ostectomy of the entire maxilla, which makes it possible to reposition the posterior part of the maxilla (Fig 4-43). This necessarily entails a clockwise rotation of the palatal plane, and thus also of the maxillary incisal axis. Therefore, in these cases the position of the maxillary incisors must be evaluated not on the palatal plane but on the anterior cranial base (sella-nasion) or with regard to the perpendicular from nasion to the Frank-

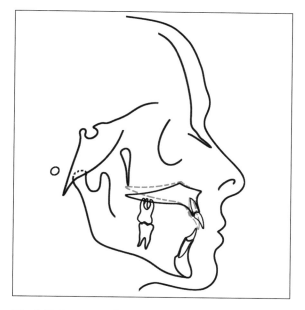

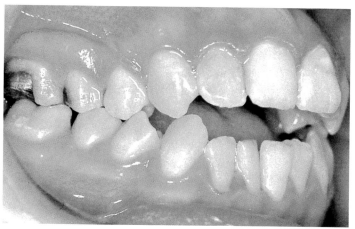

Fig 4-43 Diagram of the clockwise surgical rotation of the maxilla. The change that will occur to the axis of the maxillary incisors is clear.

Fig 4-44 Accentuation of the maxillary curve of Spee and vestibularization of the incisors.

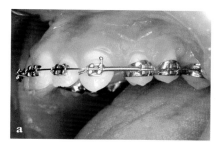

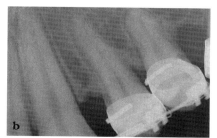

Fig 4-45 (a and b) Creation of an adequate diastema between canine and premolar for the interdental osteotomy.

fort plane. In practice it becomes necessary to leave some degree of vestibularization of the maxillary incisors, of an extent proportional to the planned maxillary rotation.

In cases characterized by anterior open bite with an excessively accentuated maxillary curvature and marked vestibularization of the incisors (Fig 4-44) multiple-piece osteotomy of the maxilla may be indicated (see chapter 7). In these cases, preoperative orthodontic treatment must be segmental and thus correction of the axis of the maxillary incisors will only be completed during surgery. In these patients, preoperative orthodontics must be limited to leveling and aligning, separately, the segments planned for

the multiple-piece osteotomy. In these cases it is indicated to create a slight diastema between canines and first premolars to facilitate the interdental osteotomy. Naturally, a simple compressed spring on the orthodontic arch will not suffice: The bodily movement of the teeth and the mesiodistal uprighting of the roots must be carefully controlled to achieve correct deviation that continues to the apexes (Fig 4-45).

Lastly, in some patients, again characterized by anterior open bite, vestibularization of the mandibular incisors and abnormally inverted curve of Spee (Fig 4-46), an anterior subapical osteotomy according to Kole (1959) may be necessary, in association with

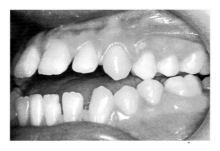

Fig 4-46 Inverted curve of Spee and vestibularization of the incisors.

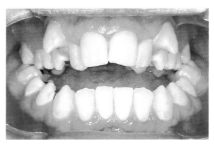

Fig 4-47 Evident transverse contraction of the maxilla with open bite.

maxillary and mandibular osteotomies (see chapter 5) to normalize surgically a curve of Spee that otherwise could not be corrected. In these cases, the inclination of the mandibular incisors can also be corrected with this type of osteotomy. Preoperative orthodontic treatment will be segmental, with the minimum aim to achieve correct leveling and tooth alignment in the two lateral and the anterior segments. In these patients, diastemata normally already exist in the mandibular arch, and thus segmental orthodontic treatment to achieve good tooth alignment in each of the three segments is in a certain sense facilitated. Nevertheless, bodily tooth movement and mesiodistal uprighting of the roots must always be carefully controlled so as to deviate not only the crowns of the canine and first premolar but also the roots.

Transverse coordination

In patients with open bite there is almost always a fairly conspicuous maxillary contraction, often with a narrow triangular palate (Fig 4-47). In all these patients, correction of the maxillary transverse deficit plays an essential role throughout treatment. First and foremost, maxillary expansion greatly improves breathing in these subjects, eliminating oral respiration and with it one of the chief causes of the anomaly. Furthermore, it must be considered that, from the dynamic standpoint, relapse of this expansion produces lateroposterior premature contacts that inevitably also produce a vertical relapse and thus a return to open bite. Hence the need to perform this expansion with approximately 20% overcorrection. Clearly this means that surgical-orthodontic expansion, performed at the start of treatment, rather than purely orthodontic or orthopedic expansion, may be preferable. In this regard

some clarification may be necessary. We have seen that in some cases it may be necessary. to use a multiple-piece maxillary osteotomy to correct the position of the incisors and/or the curve of Spee if they are abnormally altered. It might be thought that surgical expansion could be performed at the same time as the osteotomy. However, a cornerstone article by Proffit et al in 1996 clearly showed that, in an ideal hierarchy of stability, purely surgical expansion of the maxilla has the highest rate of relapse among orthognathic surgical operations. This is due on one hand to the nonelasticity of the palatine fibromucosa, which is to a great extent responsible for the relapse, and on the other hand to the geometric type of expansion. In brief, surgical-orthodontic expansion is the more reliable method to achieve valid and stable expansion of the maxilla, even if it involves a second operation to the maxilla itself. Obviously, it is up to the surgeon to trace the osteotomy lines for the preliminary surgical-orthodontic expansion at the same points that will be planned and required for the subsequent and definitive total osteotomy of the maxilla.

Lastly, this way of proceeding, ie, with initial and preliminary expansion of the maxilla, brings a marked improvement in the patient's respiration, eliminating oral respiration and also regaining some muscle tone in the perioral muscles. This undoubtedly predisposes the patient to optimal conditions with regard to postoperative rehabilitation, and thus also rapid functional adaptation to the new skeletal configuration, with unquestionable advantages in terms of long-term stability and control of relapse.

Dental midlines and symmetry of canines

Normally, in cases of open bite in the classic sense, dentoskeletal anomalies are chiefly or exclusively in

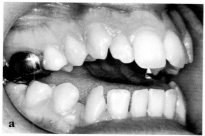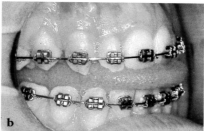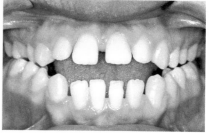

Fig 4-48 *(a and b)* Preparation of the curve of Spee in maxillary and mandibular arches with open bite; note also the lingual interposition.

Fig 4-49 Marked accentuation of the maxillary curve and inversion of the curve of Spee. In these cases a three-piece osteotomy of the maxilla is necessary, along with an anterior subapical osteotomy of the mandible.

the vertical direction. Thus, problems of symmetry are generally slight or nonexistent. However, this does not make it less important to rigorously apply both the concept of coincidence of dental midlines with the respective skeletal midlines and that of symmetry of the canines. From the standpoint of preoperative orthodontic treatment, exactly the same concepts considered for skeletal Class III and Class II anomalies hold here as well and should be consulted.

Curve of Spee

The proper management of the curve of Spee in open bite is of particular importance with regard to the risk of relapse. The final and necessary goal is that of achieving a physiologic curve of Spee or one that is only slightly accentuated, with congruency between the two arches, or with slight anterior overbite (2 to 3 mm) as seen in the cases of preparatory orthodontics for Class III or Class II cases with open bite tendency (see Figs 4-22 and 4-36b). From the orthodontic standpoint this requires first and foremost that the attachments on the mandibular incisors be positioned slightly more gingivally than normal.

Furthermore, as previously mentioned, the maxillary curvature in these patients is accentuated to varying degrees, whereas the curve of Spee is frequently flat or even inverted. Orthodontic correction of these problems involves extrusion of the incisors and/or intrusion of the premolars in the simpler cases, in which the initial defects are not quantitatively marked, which is chiefly the case of patients with total open bite (Fig 4-48). In other cases, with more accentuated initial defects of the maxillary curvature and the curve of Spee, as is frequently present in patients with anterior open bite, segmental orthodontic treatment should be planned, opting for surgical correction of the maxillary

curvature and the curve of Spee with multiple-piece osteotomy of the maxilla (see chapter 7) and subapical osteotomy according to Kole (1959) for the anterior mandibular group (see chapter 5) (Fig 4-49). In these situations, the goals of orthodontic treatment are to recreate sufficient tooth alignment in the three segments, the two lateral and the anterior, and to create a minimum interdental diastema between canines and first premolars to facilitate interdental osteotomy.

As explained above, it is most important that the roots and apexes be deviated, which cannot be achieved with a simple compressed spring on the arch; rather, the bodily movement of the teeth must be carefully managed, with suitable control over the second-order bends and mesiodistal uprighting of the roots. These considerations especially apply for the maxillary arch. In these patients, diastemata in the mandibular arch normally already exist, especially in the anterior segment, so that to some extent segmental orthodontic treatment is facilitated. However, this does not mean that the bodily movement of the teeth must not be equally rigorous.

Bibliography

Bays RA, Greco JM. Surgically assisted rapid palatal expansion: An outpatient technique with long-term stability. J Oral Maxillofac Surg 1992;50:110–113.

Bell WH, Proffit WR. Maxillary excess. In: Bell WH, Proffit WR, White RP Jr (eds). Surgical Correction of Dentofacial Deformities. Philadelphia: Saunders, 1980:341–343.

Bolton WA. Disharmony in tooth size and its relation to the analysis and treatment of malocclusion. Angle Orthod 1981;28:113–130.

Capelozza L, Martins A, Mazzotini R, Da Silva OG. Effects of dental decompensation on the surgical treatment of mandibular prognathism. Int J Adult Orthodon Orthognath Surg 1996;11:165–180.

DeFreece GA. Treatment of Class II, division I malocclusion with full buccal occlusion of the maxillary teeth (Brodie syndrome): A case report. J Charles H. Tweed Int Found 1984;12:112–129.

Garino GB, Capurso U. Biomeccanica applicata alla preparazione ortodontica prechirurgica delle III Classi scheletriche. Ortognatodonzia Ital 1993;2:401–414.

Hoppenreijs TJM, Van der Linden FPGM, Freihofer HPM, et al. Stability of transverse maxillary dental arch dimensions following orthodontic-surgical correction of anterior open bites. Int J Adult Orthodon Orthognath Surg 1998; 13:7–22.

Jacobs J, Sinclair P. Principles of orthodontic mechanics in orthognathic surgery cases. Am J Orthod 1983;84:399–407.

Jager A, Luhr HG. A longitudinal study of combined orthodontic and surgical treatment of Class II malocclusion with deep overbite. Int J Adult Orthodon Orthognath Surg 1991;6:29–38.

Kole H. Formen des offenen Bisses und ihre chirurgische Behandlung. Dtsch Stomatol 1959;9:753–766.

Kraut RA. Surgically assisted rapid maxillary expansion by opening the midpalatal suture. J Oral Maxillofac Surg 1984;42:651–655.

Lew K. Orthodontic considerations in the treatment of bimaxillary protrusion with anterior subapical osteotomy. Int J Adult Orthodon Orthognath Surg 1991;6:113–122.

Perko M. Maxillary sinus and surgical movement of maxilla. Int J Oral Surg 1972;1:177–184.

Phillips C, Medland WH, Fields HW, Proffit WR, White RP. Stability of surgical maxillary expansion. Int J Adult Orthodon Orthognath Surg 1992;7:139–146.

Pogrel MA, Kaban LB, Vargervik K, Baumrind S. Surgically assisted rapid maxillary expansion in adults. Int J Adult Orthodon Orthognath Surg 1992;7:37–41.

Proffit WR, Turvey TA, Phillips C. Orthognathic surgery: A hierarchy of stability. Int J Adult Orthodon Orthognath Surg 1996;11:191–204.

Schuchardt K. Ein beitrag zur chirurgischen kieferorthopädie unter berücksichtingung ihrer bedeutung für die behandlung angeborener und erworbener kieferdeformitäten bei soldaten. Dtsch Zahn Mund Kieferheilkd 1942;9:73.

Schuchardt K. Experience with the surgical treatment of deformities of the jaws: Prognathia, micrognathia and open bite. In: Wallace AG (ed). Second Congress of the International Society of Plastic Surgeons. London: Livingstone, 1959:73.

Shetty V, Caridad JM, Caputo AA, Chaconas SJ. Biomechanical rationale for surgical-orthodontic expansion of the adult maxilla. J Oral Maxillofac Surg 1994;52:742–749.

Silvestri A, Iaquaniello M, Fadda M. Changes and long-term evaluation of incisal angle in surgical-orthodontic treatment of skeletal Class III [in Italian]. Mondo Ortod 1991; 14:51–56.

Sperry TP. The role of tooth extrusion in treatment planning for orthognathic surgery. Int J Adult Orthodon Orthognath Surg 1988;4:197–211.

Stromberg C, Holm J. Surgically assisted, rapid maxillary expansion in adults. A retrospective long-term follow-up study. J Craniomaxillofac Surg 1995;23:222–227.

Tompach PC, Wheeler JJ, Fridrich KL. Orthodontic considerations in orthognathic surgery. Int J Adult Orthodon Orthognath Surg 1995;10:97–107.

Zachrisson S, Zachrisson BV. Gingival condition associated with orthodontic treatment. Angle Orthod 1972;42: 26–34.

5

Mandibular Surgery

with Andrea Di Francesco

This chapter illustrates the methods in the field of mandibular surgery that are most commonly used to correct dentofacial anomalies. Some methods that are now obsolete have been deliberately excluded, such as osteotomy-ostectomy of the body of the mandible. Others that are no longer indicated because of the advent of the new distraction osteogenesis methods, such as inverted L osteotomy of the ramus, have also been left out. Methods that are very rarely used, at least in Italy, because they are excessively laborious and involve a high risk of damaging the vascular-nervous bundle or tooth roots, have also been omitted. In particular, these include subapical total osteotomy and subapical posterior osteotomies, which can be easily replaced by less risky methods that may also give a better therapeutic result (eg, bilateral split or median osteotomy, genioplasty, anterior subapical osteotomy). The reader can obtain detailed information about these methods from the books and articles listed in the bibliography.

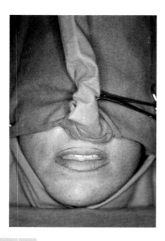

Fig 5-1 Preparation of the operative field for surgery on the mandible alone (mandibular laterodeviation).

Positioning the Patient

The patient is intubated nasotracheally and a nasogastric tube is inserted; this will remain in place for several hours after awakening to reduce the risk of postoperative vomiting. The head is placed in normal extension, then fixed to the head of the operating table with hypoallergenic plaster extending to 1 cm above the eyebrows. The eyes are protected with ophthalmic ointment and covered with a hypoallergenic plaster. Intraoral disinfection is performed with chlorhexidine and the skin is disinfected with povidone-iodine, after which the sterile sheets are put in place, leaving the chin, the angles of the mandible, and the zygomatic region exposed. If surgery is confined to the mandible, since in this case the maxilla comprises the fixed reference point, the eyes may remain covered with sheets (Fig 5-1).

Obwegeser–Dal Pont Bilateral Split Osteotomy

This is the most commonly used technique, both for mandibular advancement and for setback. Lateral movements and those in the three directions in space are also possible. It was first described in 1957 by Trauner and Obwegeser, and was then modified by Dal Pont in 1958. (For further details on the surgical technique, see the enclosed DVD.)

The tissue is infiltrated with anesthetic and vasoconstrictor diluted in physiologic solution (adrenaline 1:200,000 to 1:400,000). Infiltration follows the oblique external line of the mandible, subsequently also involving both the vestibular side up to the second molar and the lingual side in correspondence with the mandibular spine. After waiting about 5 minutes, a

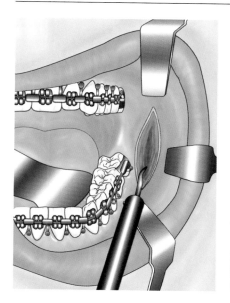

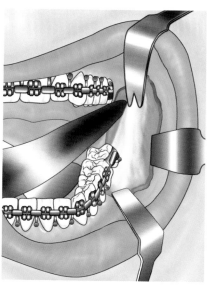

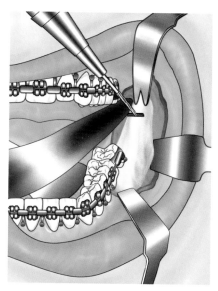

Fig 5-2 The incision to expose the fibers of the buccinator muscle.

Fig 5-3 Exposure of the mandibular ramus while protecting the vascular-nervous bundle.

Fig 5-4 Osteotomy groove on the internal cortex of the ramus.

mucosal incision is made along the infiltrated zone to expose the fibers of the buccinator muscle (Fig 5-2). The incision must be made with an electrosurgical knife or with a no. 15 blade. The muscle fibers are subjected to bipolar coagulation and then sectioned. The external cortex of the body of the mandible is exposed with the help of a periosteal elevator, from the molar region to 1 cm below the sigmoid notch; this can be located precisely with a curved elevator. Particular attention must be paid when exposing the inferior border of the body of the mandible, and likewise the posterior border of the mandibular ramus, taking care to keep the periosteum intact.

Dissection continues in the cranial direction to expose the inferior part of the coronoid process and the insertion of the temporal muscle tendons. After these tendon fibers have been exposed and detached, a special swallowtail retractor can be inserted to maintain adequate retraction of the soft tissue. The next step is a careful and delicate detachment of the periosteum from the medial face of the mandibular ramus downward to expose the mandibular spine, below which runs the vascular-nervous bundle. With the help of a periosteal elevator, the bones are completely exposed medially to

the posterior border of the mandible, and a protector is inserted straddling the mandibular border. This provides good visualization of the medial face of the ramus above the mandibular spine and, at the same time, protects the vascular-nervous bundle (Fig 5-3). Nevertheless, care must be taken not to incline the protector excessively so as not to risk compressing the bundle.

With a long Lindemann bur, a groove is made on the internal cortex of the mandibular ramus, approximately halfway between the sigmoid notch and the mandibular spine (Fig 5-4). Obviously, this location may vary slightly depending on the shape and anatomy of the mandibular ramus. The groove must extend from the base of the coronoid process almost to the posterior border of the mandible. If a sagittal osteotomy is planned, the groove must also involve the posterior border of the mandible; if an oblique osteotomy is preferred (see below), then the osteotomy groove must stop 4 to 5 mm before reaching the posterior border of the mandible. Since the mandibular ramus is not of uniform thickness, the groove must be of proportional depth. The bur is used to make it deeper in the more anterior part of the ramus at the base of the coronoid process, where the bone is thicker; it becomes much

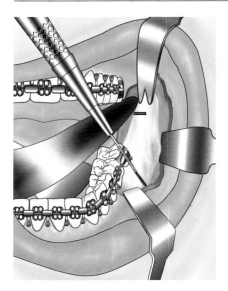

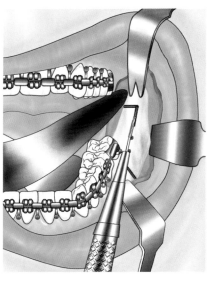

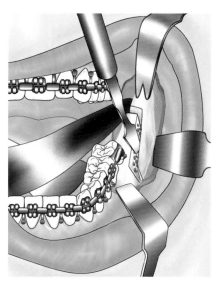

Fig 5-5 Osteotomy groove on the external cortex of the body of the mandible.

Fig 5-6 Completion of the osteotomy groove.

Fig 5-7 Performance of the osteotomy using scalpels.

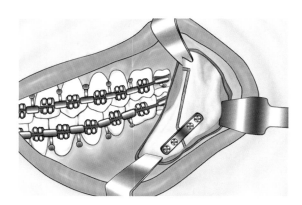

Fig 5-8 Osteosynthesis with miniplates and monocortical screws.

more superficial as it moves downward toward the posterior border of the ramus.

Once this first phase is completed, the protector is removed and positioned anteriorly at the level of the second molar, straddling the inferior margin. With the same long Lindemann bur, the osteotomy groove is continued on the external cortex of the body of the mandible to reach the inferior mandibular border, which must be sectioned very carefully (Fig 5-5). Next, with a very fine Lindemann bur and starting from the groove made on the lingual side, the osteotomy groove is completed, descending down the anterior border of the mandibular ramus to join the groove made on the vestibular cortex (Fig 5-6).

After completing this step, the osteotomy itself is performed. Initially very fine osteotomes are used, followed by thicker ones, with small enlargement movements, whereby the vascular-nervous bundle becomes visible, and if necessary can be protected with a peri-

osteal elevator. By progressively enlarging the opening with a wedge-shaped osteotome and a thin osteotome, the osteotomy is completed (Fig 5-7). In difficult cases, should the nerve remain adherent to the external osteotomy segment, it must be detached very gently so that it remains free toward the distal segment. In case of lesions occurring to the vascular-nervous bundle, suturing with very fine nylon can be attempted, although it is very laborious and does not have a high success rate. It is often preferable to gently replace the nerve and give it some continuity with fibrin glue (eg, Tissucol [Baxter]).

The osteotomy is sagittal when the section exactly follows the posterior border of the ramus. The osteotomy is oblique when the fracture does not follow the posterior border of the ramus and mandibular angle, but runs approximately 5 mm below the mandibular spine, which in practice almost corresponds with the mylohyoid line. A sagittal osteotomy

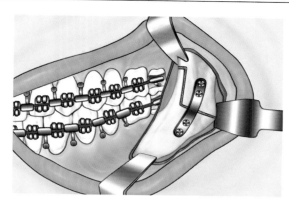

Fig 5-9 Gotte osteotomy tracing.

is generally preferred to correct Class III cases, freeing and detaching the internal pterygoid muscle along the posterior border of the body of the mandible. Conversely, an oblique osteotomy is generally preferred to correct Class II cases, in this case leaving the insertions of the internal pterygoid muscle on the posterior border of the body of the mandible. In reality, in some cases the osteotomy line may be dictated by the particular anatomic shape of the ramus, which may indicate or even require one of the two variants.

Once the two segments are fully mobilized and independent, and after the same surgical procedures are completed on the other side of the mandible, the mandible is fixed to the maxilla at the planned occlusion. At this point, the engagement of the two segments is checked. In Class III cases the proximal segment will have to be suitably reshaped. In Class II cases the osteotomy gap will be visible and thus also the extent of advancement. In severe Class II cases with mandibular advancement greater than 8 mm, myotomy of the suprahyoid muscles may be indicated and should be performed intraorally at the level of the mental symphysis after a mucosal incision similar to that used for genioplasty has been made (see below).

The next step is wire osteosynthesis between the cortical bone of the proximal and distal segments, taking care to correctly position the condyle in the glenoid fossa. The proximal segment must be pushed slightly back and upward to correct Class III cases; to correct Class II cases with deep bite and/or pronounced condyles, more force may be needed. In cases with a disposition to condylar resorption (see chapter 13) it is essential not to apply any compression to the condyles. The next step is definitive rigid fixation, which may be through bicortical screws or miniplates with monocortical screws (Fig 5-8; further considerations on this point may be found in chapter 6).

The maxillomandibular fixation is now removed, and occlusion, mandibular movements, and condylar mobility are checked. Two maxillomandibular elastic bands should now be positioned as a canine-to-canine guide. Surgery is completed by suturing the mucosal plane and, if necessary, inserting bilateral intraoral rubber drainage which may be removed after 48 hours.

Gotte Bilateral Split Osteotomy of the Mandibular Angle

This variant was described by Gotte in 1966. In practice it differs from the method described above with regard to the osteotomy line, which is traced on the vestibular side. The osteotomy line in this modified method follows the line bisecting the mandibular angle (Fig 5-9). In this case, the osteotomy is rigorously sagittal. In the original method, this osteotomy required no fixation, other than being completed with maxillomandibular fixation and exploiting the line itself, which bisected the angle, together with the sandwich effect of the masseter and internal pterygoid muscles, which held the two segments of the mandible in place. As surgical instruments have been miniaturized, and with the introduction of miniplates with monocortical screws, this technique can also easily be used with rigid fixation. With this type of osteotomy, curved miniplates are suitable because they adapt very well to the osteotomy line (see Fig 5-9).

The advantage of using this method rather than the Obwegeser–Dal Pont technique lies in the greater simplicity and lower risk of lesions to the mandibular nerve due to the reduced space of the osteotomy. Nevertheless, since the engaging surfaces are smaller, it is indicated more for mandibular setback and in cases of laterodeviation. In these cases, at least from the theoretical standpoint, it should also reduce the risk of condylar dislocation (see chapter 6).

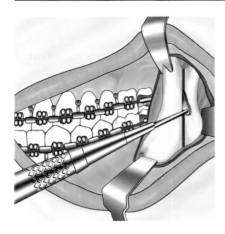

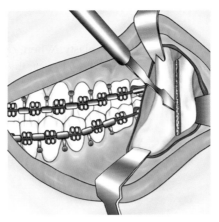

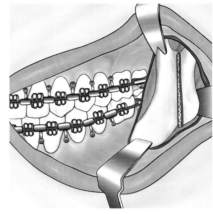

Fig 5-10 Osteotomy tracing for vertical osteotomy of the ramus.

Fig 5-11 Completion of the osteotomy with a thin scalpel.

Fig 5-12 Lateralization of the proximal segments.

Vertical Osteotomy of the Mandibular Ramus by the Intraoral Approach

Vertical osteotomy of the mandibular ramus was described by Hebert et al in 1970. Previously performed through the extraoral approach, it may now be performed intraorally, thanks to the existence of appropriate instrumentation.

After the usual infiltration, as described above, a vestibular incision is made starting from the molar region and extending to the anterior border of the mandibular ramus, so that the tissues can be dissected subperiosteally to expose the entire lateral surface of the ramus of the mandible, from the neck of the condyle to the angle of the mandible, including the molar region of the body of the mandible. The special protector for vertical osteotomy is positioned to straddle the posterior border of the ramus of the mandible, and an angled oscillating saw is used to perform a vertical osteotomy of the mandibular ramus, starting from the sigmoid notch and ending slightly in front of the mandibular angle (Fig 5-10). In performing this osteotomy, care must be taken to guide the osteotomy behind the external mandibular tubercle, which identifies the position of the mandibular foramen on the lingual side and thus the entrance of the inferior alveolar nerve. Furthermore, to avoid vascular complications,

careful attention must also be paid to the depth of the osteotomy, since it is not possible to protect the medial soft tissues. Thus it is advisable to use a thin osteotome to complete the osteotomy (Fig 5-11). Once the osteotomy section is complete, the small segment is lateralized using an elevator. The insertions of the internal pterygoid muscle are now visible, and an elevator is used to detach them. After the osteotomy on the other side is completed, the distal segment is checked to ensure that it is fully mobile with regard to the two proximal segments. The mandibular arch is then placed according to the planned surgical occlusion, and maxillomandibular fixation is applied. During this maneuver, the two proximal segments are held in a lateralized position, with care taken not to cause significant condylar dislocation (Fig 5-12).

Suturing concludes the surgery. The maxillomandibular fixation is kept in place for 4 weeks. This technique has the undoubted advantage of a lower risk of lesions to the mandibular nerve, while its disadvantage is the need for maxillomandibular fixation and thus the impossibility of early mobilization (see chapter 6). It is also only applicable to skeletal Class III cases where significant retraction of the mandible is not required. Lastly, it may be used unilaterally in cases of severe mandibular asymmetry on the side of the mandibular retrusion in conjunction with an Obwegeser–Dal Pont or Gotte bilateral split osteotomy on the opposite side (see chapter 9).

Median Mandibular Osteotomy

This type of osteotomy may be used to correct transverse discrepancies that cannot be corrected orthodontically and is always used in association with bilateral split osteotomy.

The first step is bilateral osteotomy of the mandibular ramus with one of the above techniques, after which the anterior vestibular fornix is infiltrated with anesthetic and vasoconstrictor diluted with physiologic solution (adrenaline 1:200,000 to 1:400,000). The vestibular mucosa is then incised horizontally from canine to canine (Fig 5-13). The incision is made about 3 mm in front of the base of the vestibular fornix and proceeds superficially in the more lateral zones, whereas in the mental symphysis zone the incision is deep, sectioning the insertions of the mentalis muscles and the periosteum. At this point, subperiosteal dissection is performed to completely expose the mental symphysis to the inferior border of the mental protuberance. Subsequently, a flexible spatula or a special retractor is positioned so as to provide ample vision of the entire mental symphysis region. The right and left mental foramina are then identified and the mental nerves adequately protected. Only after the position of the nerves has been determined is it possible to continue dissection of the previously incised soft tissues to expose not only the mental symphysis but also the vestibular cortex of the mandibular body bilaterally (Fig 5-14). The vertical osteotomy line is traced (Fig 5-15), or alternatively an inverted *T* is traced (Fig 5-16). In the case of an inverted T osteotomy, the vertical branch stops about 1.5 cm from the inferior border, where it meets the horizontal osteotomy line, which runs through the inferior portion of the mental symphysis (see Fig 5-16). This configuration enables changes to be made to the mental protuberance that are similar to those achieved with genioplasty. When, on the contrary, no changes are required in that area, the simple vertical tracing may be used.

After the necessary tracing has been determined, the osteotomy begins. An oscillating saw is used, beginning with the horizontal line, in the case of the inverted T osteotomy. The vertical osteotomy is then made, taking care to stop a few millimeters below the upper margin. The more cranial part of the vertical osteotomy is made with a thin scalpel after the vestibular cortex has been prepared with a very thin Lindemann bur. At this point a small portion of external or internal cortex is removed, depending on whether it is intended to increase or reduce the posterior transverse diameter. In both cases, this procedure will avoid formation of an interincisal diastema.

Once the mandibular tooth arch has been dissected at the median line, the two mandibular hemiarches, now mobile, are placed in the planned occlusion with the maxillary arch. It is important at this stage to have the occlusal splint available. Rigid fixation is then applied with miniplates in the mental symphysis region (Fig 5-17).

At this point the two proximal segments resulting from the sagittal osteotomy are positioned and their synthesis achieved by rigid fixation with miniplates or wiring plus maxillomandibular fixation (see chapter 6).

With this type of osteotomy the bigonial width can also be altered, either increasing or reducing the intermolar diameter. Naturally this requires correct orthodontic preparation of the two arches, in particular with regard to transverse diameters. However, the changes to be obtained cannot be particularly accentuated if condylar problems are to be avoided (see chapter 6), and thus there can only be a slight change in intergonial width in the esthetic sense.

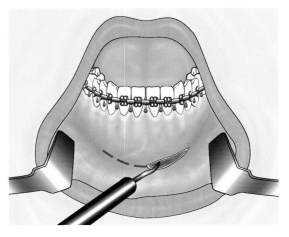

Fig 5-13 Incision for access to the mental symphysis region.

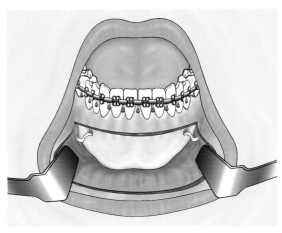

Fig 5-14 Dissection and exposure of the entire region of the mental symphysis.

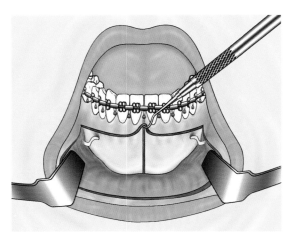

Fig 5-15 Tracing of the vertical median osteotomy.

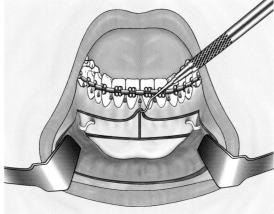

Fig 5-16 Tracing of the inverted T vertical median osteotomy.

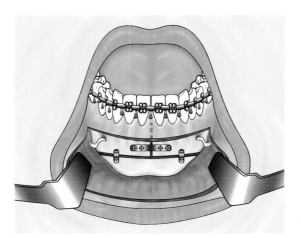

Fig 5-17 Fixation with miniplates and monocortical screws.

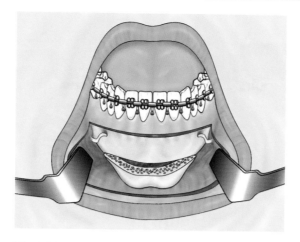

Fig 5-18 Basic osteotomy tracing for genioplasty.

Genioplasty

From the standpoint of the morphology of the mental symphysis, there is great variability in all three planes: sagittal, vertical, and transverse. Each skeletal type (for example, deep bite or open bite in Class II malocclusion) tends to have a typical morphology. On the other hand, there are also persons who, while presenting the same type of dentofacial deformity, may be characterized by widely differing morphology of the mental symphysis. The chin must therefore be considered independently in planning overall surgery to achieve optimal esthetic and functional results.

Genioplasty enables the osteotomy segment to be repositioned in the three dimensions of space, correcting vertical and sagittal defects and asymmetry of the symphysis. In general, the operation is associated with other osteotomies. In particular clinical situations, genioplasty may be postponed by approximately 6 months (see chapter 9).

The basic technique follows that described by Trauner and Obwegeser (1957). The vestibular mucosa is incised horizontally from canine to canine. The incision runs about 2 to 3 mm in front of the bottom of the vestibular fornix, as described above for median osteotomy. The incision continues superficially toward the more lateral parts; in the central zone a deep incision is made that directly sections the insertions of the mentalis muscles and the periosteum to reach the underlying bone. The bone is completely exposed in the entire region of the mental symphysis, including the inferior mandibular margin. A flexible spatula, or alternatively a hook-shaped retractor, is then inserted. Subperiosteal dissection continues laterally toward the mental foramina. Once the emergence points of the two nerves have been identified, detachment continues above and below them. The incision may now be extended laterally, taking care to protect the two nerves, and the periosteum may be cut around the bundle to facilitate distension and minimize the tensions created during retraction. At this point, two thin flexible spatulas are inserted beneath the two nerves so that they straddle the inferior mandibular border bilaterally, providing ample visibility to trace the osteotomy (see Fig 5-14).

It is useful to make a small vertical notch in correspondence with the mental symphysis as a reference point to maintain centrality of the osteotomized segment or to correct any asymmetry as needed. The horizontal osteotomy line must run 4 to 5 mm below the apices of the canines and 3 mm below the mentalis nerves (Fig 5-18). The osteotomy is performed with an oscillating saw, checking the lingual side with a finger, and, if possible, completed with the saw (a longer and narrower blade can be used if necessary) below the mental foramen. Use of osteotomes to complete the osteotomy section should be minimized to avoid unpredictable fracture lines at the inferior mandibular border, posterior to the mandibular foramina, that might make it difficult to reposition and fix the osteotomized segment. Once the osteotomy is complete and the segment is fully mobilized (see Fig 5-18), he-

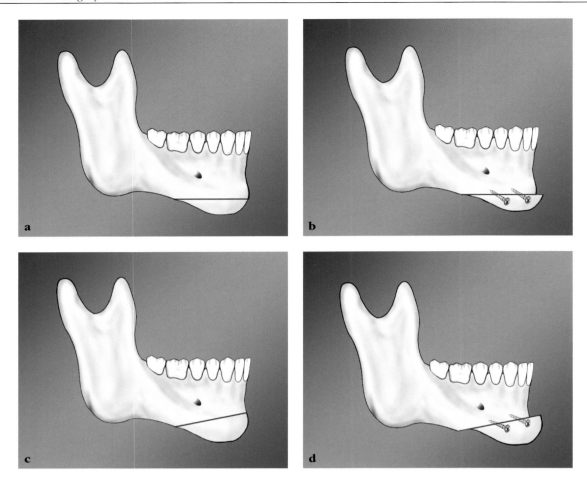

Fig 5-19 In advancement genioplasty, the height of the lower third of the face may remain unchanged *(a and b)* or be reduced *(c and d)* by varying the angle of the osteotomy.

mostasis must be carefully controlled on the lingual side with bipolar coagulation.

In case of sagittal movements, usually in the posteroanterior direction, the angle given to the osteotomy section can alter the anterior facial height to some extent. The angle of the cut must be planned from the cephalometric prediction tracing. The height of the inferior third of the face may be altered by varying the angle of cut (Fig 5-19). In cases of severe hypoplasia of the mental symphysis region, to achieve the maximum possible advancement the osteotomy segment may be advanced to overlap the underlying part. Naturally this procedure produces some reduction in the vertical dimension, which must be taken into account when planning surgery (Fig 5-20). Lastly, in extreme cases a two-piece osteotomy may be used, and the two segments can be positioned with one above the other (Fig 5-21).

In some cases a vertical increase may also be necessary. After the osteotomy has been made and the bone segment mobilized, the segment is rotated

clockwise and an autologous bone graft, or alternatively alloplastic material such as hydroxyapatite, is interposed (Fig 5-22).

With regard to genioplasty for reduction in the anteroposterior sense, it must be borne in mind that this type of operation carries the risk of leaving excessive soft tissue beneath the chin, with very unsatisfactory esthetic results. Thus this type of osteotomy must only be used in particular cases, with extreme care, and for moderate reduction. An alternative may be that of contouring the mental symphysis region. This does not require any osteotomy section, but simply a reduction of the profile, using a fissure bur or a pear-shaped bur; however, care should always be taken to make reference points or notches so as to achieve symmetric reduction on both sides (Fig 5-23). Naturally, this procedure may be used only for reduction of a few millimeters.

Where a vertical reduction is planned, two parallel osteotomy lines must be made, depending on the planned vertical reduction (Fig 5-24). This type of

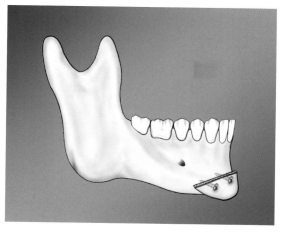

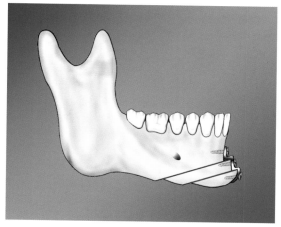

Fig 5-20 Extreme advancement of the entire osteotomy fragment.

Fig 5-21 Two-piece advancement genioplasty.

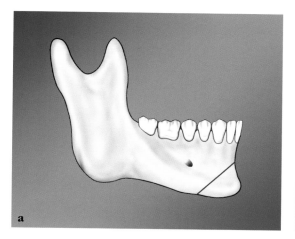

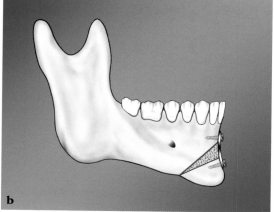

a

b

Fig 5-22 *(a and b)* Genioplasty for vertical increase, with interposition of autologous bone or alloplastic material.

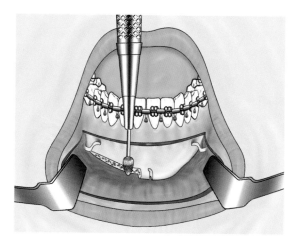

Fig 5-23 Sagittal reduction genioplasty by bone contouring.

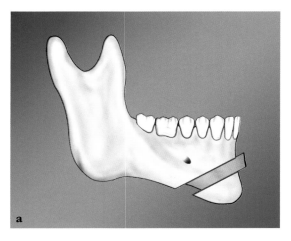
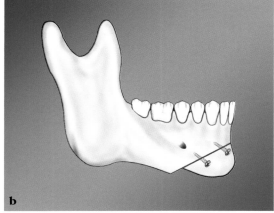

Fig 5-24 *(a and b)* Vertical reduction genioplasty.

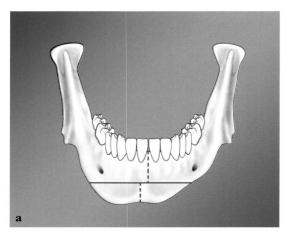
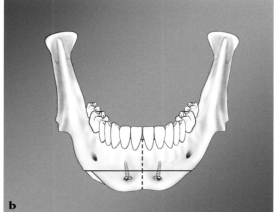

Fig 5-25 *(a and b)* Genioplasty to correct asymmetry.

procedure naturally may be associated with any type of sagittal movement, in the posteroanterior direction or, much more rarely, in the opposite direction.

In cases of dentofacial asymmetry where there is also asymmetry in the mental symphysis region, or in cases in which the dental midline does not exactly correspond to the line of the symphysis, genioplasty with lateral translation will be needed. This operation involves meticulous surgical planning and rigorously precise osteotomy lines. Again, it is also necessary to mark reference lines, both for the dental midline and for the symphysis line of the osteotomized segment, which must perfectly coincide at the end of the operation (Fig 5-25). In some cases, in the more severe forms of dentofacial asymmetry, a cuneiform ostectomy is also needed to achieve good final symmetry (Fig 5-26). Lastly, in particular and selected cases, it is possible to perform a hemigenioplasty, as proposed by Raffaini et al (1994) (Fig 5-27).

Independent of the type of osteotomy used and the type of movement achieved, the inferior segment can be stabilized by applying microplates with screws of 1.5-mm diameter, or bicortical screws of 2-mm diameter, which provide better stability. This is particularly important during the first phases of early mandibular mobilization.

The incision is then closed with two layers of absorbable sutures. The first suture of each layer is placed at the facial midline axis and the mentalis muscle, so as to correctly reposition the soft tissues.

In the case of marked advancement, it is useful to make a release incision on the periosteum at the labial side to achieve some relaxation, which will bring the lip and chin tissues upward. If this is not done, the lower lip may appear retracted with subsequent fibrosis and retraction downward during healing, producing excessive exposure of the mandibular teeth and difficulty in closing the lips. A pressure dressing is applied to the chin to contain and support the soft tissues and lip, eliminating empty spaces to reduce swelling and achieve better definition of the labiomental fold (Fig 5-28).

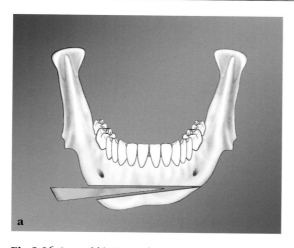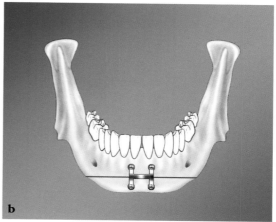

Fig 5-26 *(a and b)* Genioplasty with cuneiform ostectomy in asymmetry cases.

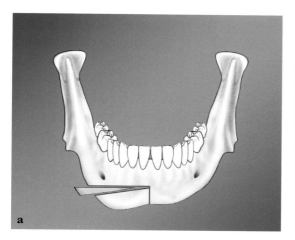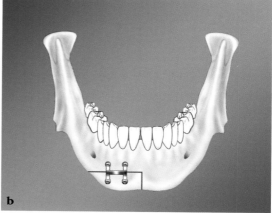

Fig 5-27 *(a and b)* Diagram of hemigenioplasty according to Raffaini et al (1994).

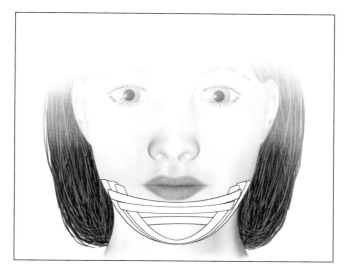

Fig 5-28 Pressure dressing with plaster after surgery at the mental symphysis.

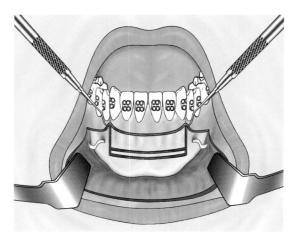

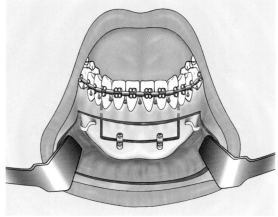

Fig 5-29 Tracing of the Kole anterior subapical osteotomy.

Fig 5-30 Repositioning of the osteotomy fragment and fixing with miniplates or microplates.

Kole Anterior Subapical Osteotomy

This technique, described by Kole in 1959, enables the anterior group from canine to canine to be repositioned and is chiefly used to correct a curve of Spee that cannot be modified orthodontically (for example, in open bite or severe Class II, division 2 cases), and then primarily with vertical movement. Alternatively it is used to normalize the axis of the mandibular incisors when this cannot be done by preoperative orthodontics alone; in such cases it entails a rotary movement in the vestibular or lingual direction. In all these cases the anterior subapical osteotomy is associated with other osteotomy operations. More rarely it may be used alone to correct a dentoalveolar Class III situation, in which case the mobilized segment is moved bodily in the sagittal sense, in the anteroposterior direction.

In cases in which a fairly large posterior movement is planned, the first premolars must be extracted. In all other situations (for example, in chiefly vertical movements) a very small diastema between canine and first premolar is sufficient and can be achieved through adequate preoperative orthodontic treatment (see chapter 4).

Incision and dissection are as described for genioplasty and median osteotomy (see above and Fig 5-14). Once the operative field is adequately exposed with suitable retractors, the osteotomy lines are traced (Fig 5-29).

The subapical horizontal osteotomy line is 5 mm beneath the tooth apexes. While the horizontal section is being cut, a finger is held on the lingual side to detect when the osteotomy reaches the lingual cortex. The mucoperiosteum and adherent gingiva are then gently detached by tunneling distally to the canines, and the vertical osteotomy is made with a thin, narrow oscillating saw and completed with a small interdental osteotome. If the first premolars have been extracted, the osteotomy can easily be made with a fissure bur in correspondence with the postextraction alveolus. In any case, during this maneuver a finger must always be held on the lingual side to check progress.

Once the osteotomized segment is fully mobile, and after all areas of interference have been removed, the dentoalveolar segment is passively positioned in the occlusal splint. This is fixed with wire to an orthodontic arch, prepared previously on plaster models during the surgical simulation phase and put in place in the operating room at this stage of surgery. Rigid fixation with mini- or microplates follows (Fig 5-30). If the planned movement entails creating an osteotomy gap, as occurs in superior repositioning, a bone graft is inserted in the gap. For this purpose, bone taken from the iliac crest, or from the proximal mandibular segments after bilateral split osteotomy, may be used. If bilateral split osteotomy is also planned, the operation is completed by fixing the two segments as described above.

The incision is sutured on two planes, muscle and mucosa. Suturing begins with detached stitches at the median line and the muscle layers, taking care to ensure lip symmetry. A pressure dressing is applied as for genioplasty (see Fig 5-28) for 5 to 7 days to hold the tissues of the chin and lower lip in a raised position and to avoid healing taking place with the lower lip in a lowered position.

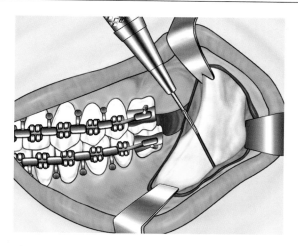

Fig 5-31 Tracing of the corticotomy for mandibular distraction.

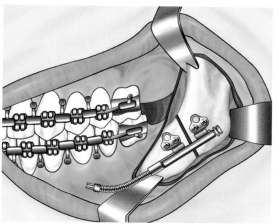

Fig 5-32 Temporary adaptation and fixation of the distractor.

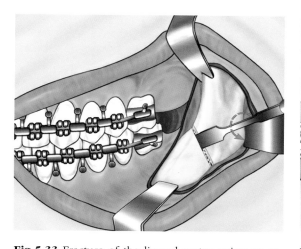

Fig 5-33 Fracture of the lingual cortex using an osteotome.

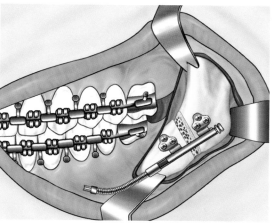

Fig 5-34 Definitive fixation of the distractor and checking of the distraction vector.

Mandibular Distraction Osteogenesis

The concepts of distraction osteogenesis, which were conceived by Codivilla (1905) and then developed by Ilizarov et al (1980) have only recently been applied to the oral maxillofacial area. The principle is that of achieving a gradual lengthening of the mandible and, consequently, also of the soft tissues. Intraoral distractors are now available that have been sufficiently tested and are fairly reliable.

The surgical technique entails making an intraoral incision similar to that for bilateral split osteotomy; subperiosteal dissection is limited to the external side of the body and ramus of the mandible. With a long Lindemann bur, an incision is then made right through the external cortex in the retromolar area, slightly in front of the angle. This incision must extend to include the entire inferior mandibular border and the superior part of the cortex (Fig 5-31). At this point the distractor is adapted and fixed temporarily in place with screws (Fig 5-32); it is then removed and, using an osteotome and taking advantage of its rotary movements, the lingual cortex is fractured (Fig 5-33). The two segments must be fully mobilized; the procedure is repeated on the contralateral side, and the distractors are fixed definitively. Correct functioning and precision of the distraction vector are checked (Fig 5-34). The distractors are then set to zero and a first distraction of 1 mm is applied. After a latent period of 5 to 7 days, active distraction begins at a rate of 1 mm per day (in practice, two turns of the distractor screw). During this phase surgeon and orthodontist should check the patient jointly.

As with all methods, especially those that have been recently introduced, there are both advantages and disadvantages. The main disadvantage, and it is a significant one, consists of the difficulty of properly checking the distraction vector, both at the moment of application and during distraction. Patient compliance may also be less than optimal in terms of tolerability of the device. Partly to counterbalance these drawbacks, some authors, chief among them Hoffmeister and Wangerin (1997), suggest early removal of the distractor, 2 weeks after the end of active distraction, with consequent manipulation of the bone callus before it is completely calcified, by appropriate maxillo-mandibular elastics to bring the mandibular arch into correct occlusion. In practice this is an application of the so-called floating bone concept to the distraction technique. Nevertheless, if the callus is already partially calcified, this procedure may produce significant stress and can potentially be dangerous for the temporomandibular joint, causing condylar dislocation with the possibility of resorption and/or short-term relapse. The advantage of distraction osteogenesis (associated with the floating bone technique if necessary) consists of a gradual lengthening of both the mandible and the soft tissues; thus the technique may be indicated when considerable lengthening is needed, certainly more than 10 mm. However, at present no reliable studies exist concerning the long-term stability of the result as compared with traditional osteotomy.

It is therefore the opinion of the authors that this method, at present, is indicated in cases of hemifacial microsomy or in situations of severe mandibular hypoplasia that require advancement of more than 10 mm and in which a traditional osteotomy cannot be used or would also require bone grafts (for example, inverted L osteotomy). In all other cases in which good results can be achieved with traditional osteotomies the authors believe those procedures are still preferable.

Bibliography

Alexander CD, Bloomquist DS, Wallen TR. Stability of mandibular constriction with a symphyseal osteotomy. Am J Orthod Dentofacial Orthop 1993;103:15–23.

Bell WH, Brammer JA, McBride KL, Finn RA. Reduction genioplasty: Surgical techniques and soft-tissue changes. Oral Surg Oral Med Oral Pathol 1981;51:471–477.

Codivilla A. On the means of lengthening in the lower limbs, muscles and tissues which are shortened through deformity. Am J Orthop Surg 1905;2:353–369.

Dal Pont G. L'osteotomia retromolare per la correzione della progenia. Minerva Chir 1958;14:1138–1145.

Diner PA, Kollar E, Martinez H, Vazquez MP. Intraoral distraction for mandibular lengthening: A technical innovation. J Craniomaxillofac Surg 1996;24:92–95.

Diner PA, Kollar E, Martinez H, Vazquez MP. Submerged intraoral device for mandibular lengthening. J Craniomaxillofac Surg 1997;25:116–123.

Fridrich L, Casko S. Genioplasty strategies for anterior facial vertical dysplasias. Int J Adult Orthodon Orthognath Surg 1997;12:35–41.

Gotte P. On the surgical therapy of prognathism. Experiences and results of a modification of Obwegeser's intraoral method [in Italian]. Minerva Stomatol 1966;15:12–27.

Hebert JM, Kent JN, Hinds EC. Correction of prognathism by intraoral vertical subcondylar osteotomy. J Oral Surg 1970; 28:651–663.

Hinds EC, Kent JN. Genioplasty: The versatility of horizontal osteotomy. J Oral Surg 1969;27:690–701.

Hoffmeister B, Wangerin K. Callus distraction technique by an intraoral approach: The floating bone concept. Int J Oral Maxillofac Surg 1997;26(suppl 1):76.

Hurmerinta K, Hukki J. Vector control in lower jaw distraction osteogenesis using an extra-oral multidirectional device. J Craniomaxillofac Surg 2001;29:263–270.

Ilizarov GA, Devyatov AA, Karnerim VK. Plastic reconstruction of longitudinal bone defects by means of compression and subsequent distraction. Acta Chir Plast 1980;22:32–41.

Kawamoto HK Jr. Discussion of reduction mentoplasty. Plast Reconstr Surg 1982;70:151–167.

Kole H. Formen des offenen Bisses und ihre chirurgische Behandlung. Dtsch Stomatol 1959;9:753–766.

McTavish J, Marucci D, Bonar SF, Walsh WR, Poole MD. Does the sheep mandible relapse following lengthening by distraction osteogenesis? J Craniomaxillofac Surg 2000;28: 251–257.

Merlini C, Piasente M, Roghi M, Amelotti C, Antonioli M. Il ruolo della osteotomia verticale del ramo mandibolare nella correzione chirurgica della III Classe. Ortognatodonzia Ital 1996;5:361–391.

Obwegeser HL. Surgery of the maxilla for the correction of prognathism [in German]. SSO Schweiz Monatsschr Zahnheilkd 1965;75:365–374.

Obwegeser HL, Makek MS. Hemimandibular hyperplasia—Hemimandibular elongation. J Maxillofac Surg 1986;14: 183–208.

Rachmiel A, Levy M, Laufer D. Lengthening of the mandible by distraction osteogenesis: Report of cases. J Oral Maxillofac Surg 1995;53:838–846.

Raffaini M, Monteverdi R, Sesenna E. L'emimentoplastica: Una tecnica per correggere le asimmetrie del mento. Riv Ital Chir Maxillofac 1994;5:9–11.

Rubio-Bueno P, Villa E, Carreno A, et al. Intraoral mandibular distraction osteogenesis: Special attention to treatment planning. J Craniomaxillofac Surg 2001;29:254–262.

Samchukov ML, Cope JB. The effect of sagittal orientation of the distractor on the biomechanics of mandibular lengthening. J Oral Maxillofac Surg 1999;57:1214–1222.

Trauner R, Obwegeser H. Surgical correction of mandibular prognathism and retrognathism with consideration of genioplasty. Oral Surg Oral Med Oral Pathol 1957;10: 677–697.

Recommended reading

Bell WH, Proffit WR, White RP Jr (eds). Surgical Correction of Dentofacial Deformities. Philadelphia: Saunders, 1980.

Brusati R, Sesenna E. Chirurgia delle deformità mascellari. Milan: Masson, 1988.

Epker BN, Wolford LM. Dentofacial Deformities: Surgical-Orthodontic Correction. St Louis: Mosby, 1980.

Proffit WR, White RP Jr. Surgical-Orthodontic Treatment. St Louis: Mosby, 1991.

6

Mandibular Osteotomies: Type of Fixation and Condylar Position

There are still two schools of thought concerning the type of fixation that should be used after mandibular osteotomy (bilateral split osteotomy or at the mandibular angle): *(1)* rigid internal fixation (RIF) with three bicortical screws or with plates and monocortical screws, without maxillomandibular fixation (see chapter 5), or alternatively *(2)* wiring with maxillomandibular fixation for a period varying between 4 and 6 weeks. Further questions include: If RIF is utilized, which type should be preferred? And, are the devices to maintain condylar position, which have recently been applied clinically, indispensable or not?

The use of RIF undoubtedly offers a series of advantages for the surgeon, the orthodontist, and the patient. First and foremost it offers greater safety at the moment when the patient regains consciousness and during the immediate postoperative period: It enables the airways to be checked, and likewise guarantees access in the (rare) event of hemorrhage or vomiting. There are also undeniable advantages for the patient during convalescence in terms of greater comfort and convenience, most obviously in eating, drinking, speaking, and oral hygiene. RIF enables the surgeon to achieve immediate control over occlusion on the operating table, which is extremely important. During surgery a limited amount of selective grinding can be performed, or, if necessary, bone segments that have inadvertently been positioned improperly can be corrected. The freedom of movement of the mandibular condyles may also be evaluated, though within the limits given by the patient's position and muscular relaxation. There is no doubt that, with RIF, counterclockwise rotation of the proximal segment can be avoided, which is always a possible occurrence if fixation is by wiring.

From the biologic standpoint, RIF appears to accelerate bone healing. The healing process with wire

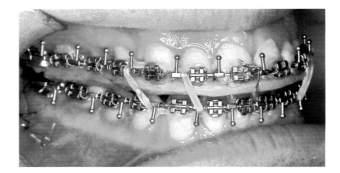

Fig 6-1 Immediate postoperative rehabilitation guided by an occlusal splint.

osteosynthesis comes about through the formation of endosteal callus and secondary bone: only later does new osteoblast activity occur. With RIF the bone appears to heal to a greater extent by first intention, with less endosteal and periosteal callus formation and immediate osteoblast activity.

But the greatest advantage of RIF is from the standpoint of postoperative rehabilitation and orthodontic treatment: It enables immediate active and passive treatment and a gradual but rapid progression toward normal mandibular mobility. This improves the return to all stomatognathic system activities (these aspects will be dealt with in more detail in chapter 11). Lastly, regaining function at an early stage appears to facilitate the natural biologic remodeling of the temporomandibular joint (TMJ), through which optimal neuromuscular and condylar adaptation may be achieved in the phases following surgery.

With regard to skeletal stability, although RIF undoubtedly provides better stability in the immediate postsurgical period, this does not appear to be true in the long term. From this standpoint other factors pre-

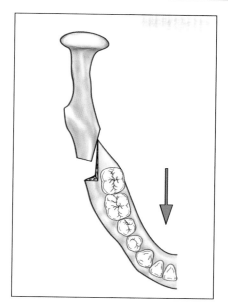

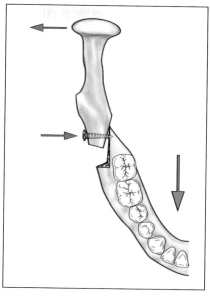

Fig 6-2 Diagram of a mandibular advancement: Note the dihedral angle formed between the two segments.

Fig 6-3 Rigid fixation with bicortical screws may cause rotation of the proximal segments and thus of the condyle.

dominate, such as muscle equilibrium, stability of occlusion, and condylar position, as we have already mentioned in some of the previous chapters.

Nevertheless, to counterbalance the numerous positive aspects, RIF may also have some disadvantages. First and foremost, a perfect orthodontic preparation is necessary and the surgical occlusion attained must be as stable as possible. Splints may only be used to optimize this stability and to provide the patient with a guide for the immediate postsurgical period (Fig 6-1). The splint cannot and must not be a tool to resolve severe occlusal defects. It follows that RIF may not be indicated in cases with severe and extensive edentulism, especially if this affects posterior segments, and/or in cases with a significant lack of occlusal stability.

Another disadvantage that is far from negligible in modern times is the economic factor: The cost of plates and screws is still quite high. Furthermore, their removal also represents both an economic and a biologic cost. Absorbable plates for mandibular surgery do not at present appear to be adequately reliable. Lastly, although removal of a plate with monocortical screws is a simple matter even under local anesthesia, the same may not be said for bicortical screws, which require a transbuccal approach.

But undoubtedly the most serious contraindication, in the opinion of supporters of wiring, is the risk that RIF may cause condylar malpositioning that may lead to TMJ disorders or cause relapse.

If we look at the dynamics of mandibular advancement with Obwegeser–Dal Pont osteotomy, it is clear that a dihedral angle is formed between the two segments (Fig 6-2). For this reason, with rigid fixation there may be a risk of excessive compaction of the two segments. This would inevitably lead to a rotation of the condyle with increased intercondylar width, which in its turn would predispose the patient to TMJ disorders. The risk of causing this type of condylar distortion is obviously higher with the use of bicortical screws than with miniplates and monocortical screws (Fig 6-3). The danger is also increased in cases of asymmetric movements of the mandible (as in laterodeviation and dentofacial asymmetry) and is directly proportional to the degree of asymmetry. With plates and monocortical screws the risk is reduced provided that the plates are passively contoured to a perfect fit and that the screws are strictly monocortical (5 to 6 mm). In this way, damage due to compression of the vascular nervous bundle or tooth roots will also be avoided. Miniaturization and angulation of surgical instruments makes it relatively simple to put this type of fixation in place with an intraoral approach (Fig 6-4). Use of bicortical screws, on the contrary, frequently also requires an extraoral transbuccal approach, with minimal but inevitable permanent esthetic damage (Fig 6-5). With some experience and good manual dexterity, the proximal and distal segments can be stabilized without altering the position of the condyles. Data reported in the literature show that

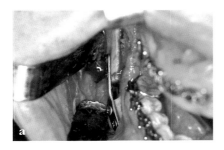
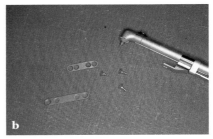

Fig 6-4 Rigid internal fixation with miniplates and monocortical screws *(a)*. The angled screwdriver makes this procedure possible in all cases with a rigorously intraoral approach *(b)*.

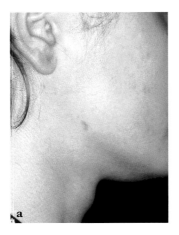
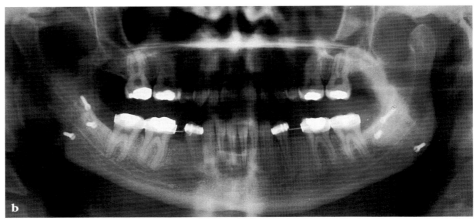

Fig 6-5 Esthetic outcome *(a)* with the use of bicortical screws *(b)*.

it is fundamental to maintain the proximal segment and the condyles as close as possible to their preoperative position to achieve the best results from the standpoints of short- and long-term stability.

Coming now to the geometric model relating to mandibular setback according to Obwegeser–Dal Pont or Gotte osteotomies, we see that distortion of the proximal segment will chiefly depend on the posterior movement of the distal segment. This tends to favor outward rotation of the anterior part of the proximal segment and inward rotation of the condyle, decreasing the intercondylar width and compressing the medial structures of the TMJ (Fig 6-6). To prevent this from happening, the posterior part of the distal segment must be suitably reshaped, freeing it of all interferences. This is increasingly important as the extent of mandibular setback increases (Fig 6-7). In general, the risk is much smaller with Gotte osteotomies, and the distal segment much less frequently needs significant contouring. In any case, also in regard to mandibular setback, fixation with passive miniplates and monocortical screws appears to be more reliable than with bi-

cortical screws, in terms of maintaining the preoperative condylar position. In cases requiring considerable asymmetric movement of the mandible (for example, in severe dentofacial asymmetries), the risk of causing some degree of condylar displacement is probably higher, even in experienced hands.

Lastly, if we use a median mandibular osteotomy with significant variation of the transverse diameter at the molar and premolar levels, there will inevitably be repercussions on the condylar position (Fig 6-8). In these circumstances it is indispensable to make an in-depth evaluation of these changes to select the most suitable type of fixation and not to risk long-term TMJ disorders. With the intention of resolving these problems, Luhr et al (1986) and Luhr (1989) developed a special device (Fig 6-9) that maintains the condyle in the preoperative position with three-dimensional control of the condyle. The device consists of a sufficiently rigid T-shaped plate. It is passively adapted, and one end of it is fixed before completion of the mandibular osteotomy, to the external surface of the mandibular ramus, while the other end is attached to a fixed struc-

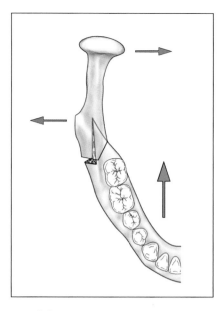

Fig 6-6 Diagram of mandibular setback: Repositioning of the distal segment posteriorly may cause rotation of the proximal segment and thus of the condyle.

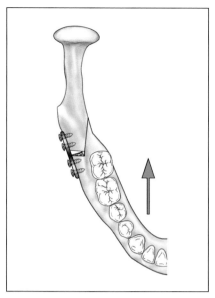

Fig 6-7 Suitably reshaping the distal segment in its posterior part and using miniplates with monocortical screws greatly reduces the risk of condylar dislocation.

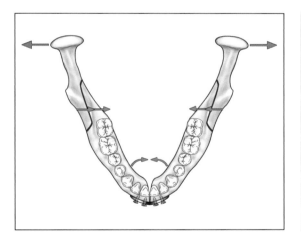

Fig 6-8 Diagram of a median osteotomy with contraction of the transverse diameter; the risk of rotating and dislocating the condyles is clear.

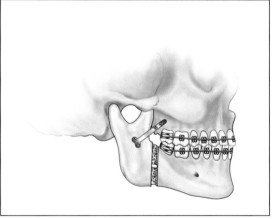

Fig 6-9 Diagram of the device described by Luhr.

ture not involved in the osteotomy (the maxillary tooth arch in the case of mandibular osteotomy alone, or the zygomaticomaxillary ridge in the case of double-jaw osteotomy). Obviously, during this maneuver the two arches must be provisionally fixed in the preoperative centric occlusion (according to a previously prepared wax bite) without dislocating the condyle heads. The plate is then removed, the osteotomy of the mandible is completed bilaterally, and maxillomandibular fixation is put in place at the planned occlusion. The proximal segment is then repositioned with the help of the above device, fixing it in the same holes used previously. In this way, the condyle-fossa relationship should be perfectly maintained (Fig 6-10). The last step is definitive rigid fixation, preferably with miniplates, after which the device is removed.

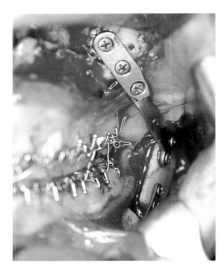

Fig 6-10 The device in situ with application of rigid fixation.

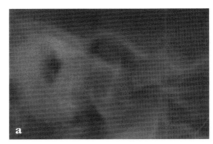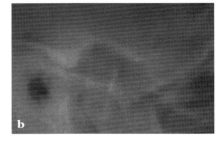

Fig 6-11 Preoperative radiograph *(a)* and postoperative checkup *(b)* by oblique transcranial radiography using a craniostat. Note the exact maintenance of the condylar position.

Other devices have since been proposed, and a number of studies have dealt with this problem. Nevertheless, one question arises: Are such devices really necessary?

In milestone research on this subject, Ellis (1994) suggested that, before answering this question, a whole series of other questions must be clarified and resolved. How much may the condyles actually move after mandibular osteotomy? Is the extent of this displacement proportional to the onset of TMJ disorders and any medium- or long-term instability? To what extent do anesthesia and muscle relaxation influence condylar position? Is there only one condylar position compatible with normal function? (This is undoubtedly the most important question.) And if this single condylar position does exist, can it really be reproduced, and if so, how? Are the devices described truly able to maintain condylar position exactly in three dimensions? And lastly, to what extent can contouring and morphostructural adaptation of the condyles after surgery compensate for any positional changes?

These questions are still awaiting replies. It would therefore seem reasonable to conclude that at present devices of this sort are not strictly indispensable, or at least not in most cases. Their application is relatively complex (especially in double-jaw osteotomies, where their perfect rigidity is also debatable) and their use extends the length of the operation. Nevertheless, they undoubtedly help to minimize errors in main-

taining condylar position. Thus their use in particular clinical situations may be supported: in patients with dysfunction who are using superior or anterior repositioning splints, including during the preoperative orthodontic phase, and who achieve or maintain a physiologically acceptable and subjectively asymptomatic situation only with such devices and in patients with severe dentofacial asymmetry or mandibular laterodeviation, with transverse displacement of the mandible of 5 mm or more, in which, as already seen, there is a greater risk that the condyles will be severely displaced after surgery.

In any case, using RIF, it is good practice to check the pre- and postoperative condylar position (on day 1 or 2) with an oblique transcranial radiograph of the TMJ. Although this type of examination has its limitations, as discussed in chapter 3, it is a simple, rapid, and inexpensive way to evaluate and monitor condylar position that in most cases is sufficient and indispensable (Fig 6-11). It would be most useful to be able to use intraoperative radiography; however, the impossibility of using the same craniostat on the operating table and the characteristics of radiologic devices for intraoperative use (brilliance amplifiers) make this type of control both difficult and somewhat risky. The neuronavigator might provide useful elements to solve this problem, but at present the method's cost and complexity make it of little practical use. Clearly this does not mean that in the future,

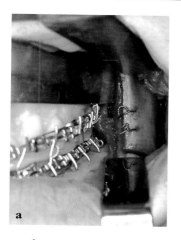
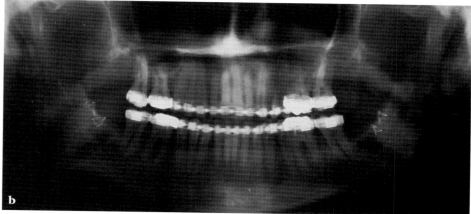

Fig 6-12 Fixation by wiring *(a)* and radiographic checkup *(b)*.

simple, rapid, safe, and economic methods (perhaps using ultrasonography) may not become available for intraoperative monitoring of the condylar position.

With regard to wiring, supporters of this method maintain that it greatly decreases the risks of TMJ disorders following orthognathic surgery. From the purely theoretical standpoint, the mandibular condyles do possess some freedom to reposition themselves under the influence of muscles and the central nervous system during the period of maxillomandibular fixation, which would undoubtedly be an advantage. Nevertheless, convincing and significant studies have not yet been published that compare the two methods from this standpoint in comparable clinical situations. Furthermore, the condition of the musculature in the days and weeks immediately following surgery is clearly not the same as it was beforehand, nor is it optimal or definitive. Surgical procedures such as detachment and subsequent reinsertion of muscles, postoperative edema, maxillomandibular fixation, and fibrosis if it occurs, all contribute to making the muscle status very different than in preoperative conditions, and also different from the conditions that must be reinstated at complete healing, both for skeletal and for soft tissue structures.

With wiring (Fig 6-12), even when it is correctly performed (if necessary also with double wiring and/or circumferential ligature), there is never complete certainty of preventing the proximal segment from rotating in a counterclockwise direction. This ro-

tation, under the action of particularly strong temporalis muscles, may become so marked as to create significant changes in condylar position, with repercussions including compression of the joint structures.

Lastly, it has been shown that even a short period of maxillomandibular fixation (limited to 4 weeks) causes a decrease, including in the long term, in mandibular range of movements. It also decreases the condyles' ability to undergo remodeling and adaptation, aspects that are essential to proper recovery and return to functioning after orthognathic surgery.

All these arguments and considerations do not therefore appear sufficient to prefer wiring over RIF, even taking into account the hypothetical risk of positional modifications to the condyles, especially in light of the significant advantages offered by RIF with regard to postoperative management, patient comfort, and rapid recovery of function. Undoubtedly RIF must be applied with utmost care and judgment, as described above.

Wiring might, however, be useful in particular clinical situations, as already mentioned: in patients with some posterior edentulism and occlusal instability and in those with marked dentofacial asymmetry in which extensive asymmetric movement is produced in both jaws. Lastly, a good surgeon must in any case possess exquisite mastery of both methods, from both the theoretical and the dexterity standpoints, so as to be able to exploit and use them for the best in all the different clinical situations.

Bibliography

Anucul B, Waite PD, Lemons JE. In vitro strength analysis of sagittal split osteotomy fixation: Noncompression monocortical plates versus bicortical position screws. J Oral Maxillofac Surg 1992;50:1295–1299.

Burye MT, Stella JP. An innovative method for accurate positioning of the proximal segment in sagittal split osteotomies. Int J Adult Orthodon Orthognath Surg 2000; 15:59–63.

Ellis E 3rd, Reynolds S, Carlson DS. Stability of the mandible following advancement: A comparison of three postsurgical fixation techniques. Am J Orthod Dentofacial Orthop 1988;94:38–49.

Ellis E 3rd, Hinton RJ. Histologic examination of the temporomandibular joint after mandibular advancement with and without rigid fixation: An experimental investigation in adult *Macaca mulatta*. J Oral Maxillofac Surg 1991;49: 1316–1327.

Ellis E 3rd, Carlson DS, Billups J. Osseous healing of the sagittal ramus osteotomy: A histologic comparison of rigid and nonrigid fixation in *Macaca mulatta*. J Oral Maxillofac Surg 1992;50:718–723.

Ellis E 3rd. Condylar positioning devices for orthognathic surgery. Are they necessary? J Oral Maxillofac Surg 1994; 52:536–552.

Foley WL, Beckman TW. In vitro comparison of screw versus plate fixation in the sagittal split osteotomy. Int J Adult Orthodon Orthognath Surg 1992;7:147–151.

Harris MD, Van Sickels JE, Alder M. Factor influencing condylar position after the bilateral sagittal split osteotomy fixed with bicortical screws. J Oral Maxillofac Surg 1999;57: 650–654.

Helm G, Stepke MT. Maintenance of the preoperative condyle position in orthognathic surgery. J Craniomaxillofac Surg 1997;25:34–38.

Luhr HG, Schauer HW, Jäger A, Kubein-Meesenburg D. Changes in the shape of the mandible by orthodontic surgical techniques with stable fixation of the segments [in German]. Fortschr Kieferorthop 1986;47:39–47.

Luhr HG. The significance of condylar position using rigid fixation in orthognathic surgery. Clin Plast Surg 1989;16: 147–156.

Magalhães AEO, Stella JP, Tahasuri TH. Changes in condylar position following bilateral sagittal split ramus osteotomy with setback. Int J Adult Orthodon Orthognath Surg 1995; 10:137–145.

Merten HA, Halling F. A new condylar positioning technique in orthognathic surgery. J Craniomaxillofac Surg 1992; 20:310–312.

Rotskoff KS, Herbosa EG, Villa P. Maintenance of condyle-proximal segment position in orthognathic surgery. J Oral Maxillofac Surg 1991;49:2–7.

Schwestka-Polly R, Engelke D, Kubein-Meesenburg D. Application of the condylar positioning appliance in mandibular sagittal split osteotomies with rigid skeletal fixation. Int J Adult Orthodon Orthognath Surg 1992;7:15–21.

Stroster TG, Pangrazio-Kulbersh V. Assessment of condylar position following bilateral sagittal split ramus osteotomy with wire fixation or rigid fixation. Int J Adult Orthodon Orthognath Surg 1994;9:55–63.

Van Sickels JE, Tiner BD, Keeling SD, Clark GM, Bays R, Rugh J. Condylar position with rigid fixation versus wire osteosynthesis of sagittal split advancement. J Oral Maxillofac Surg 1999;57:31–34.

Recommended reading

Tucker MR, Terry BC, White RP Jr, Van Sickels JE (eds). Rigid Fixation for Maxillofacial Surgery. Philadelphia: Lippincott, 1991.

7

Maxillary Surgery

with Giorgio Novelli

- Positioning the patient
- Classic Le Fort I maxillary osteotomy
- Multiple-piece Le Fort I osteotomy
- Bell high osteotomy
- Maxillomalar osteotomy
- Schuchardt lateroposterior segmental osteotomy
- Maxillary distraction osteogenesis

Positioning the Patient

As was described in chapter 5, the patient is intubated nasotracheally, and a nasogastric tube is also put in place, particularly in cases of double-jaw osteotomy. The tube will be kept in place for several hours after the patient regains consciousness to reduce the risk of postoperative vomiting. The head is positioned in normal extension and fixed to the head of the operating table with hypoallergenic plaster extending to 1 cm above the eyebrows. The eyes are protected with ophthalmic ointment and allowed to close spontaneously. After the oral cavity and face have been disinfected, the operating field is carefully prepared, with the tubes fixed in place and the eyes left uncovered so that the three-dimensional position of the maxilla can be evaluated, using glabella, inner canthi, and palpebral fissure as reference points (Fig 7-1). In cases in which displacement of the maxilla will be limited to the sagittal plane, or in which vertical displacement will be minimal and strictly symmetric (for example, see the case presented in the DVD), the eyes may also be covered.

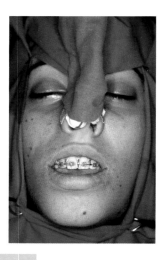

Fig 7-1 Preparation of the operative field for a double-jaw operation, which will include three-dimensional repositioning of the maxilla.

Classic Le Fort I Maxillary Osteotomy

This type of osteotomy was described and used for the first time for orthognathic purposes by Wassmund in 1927 and later reviewed and codified by Obwegeser in 1969. The Le Fort I maxillary osteotomy in its classic version enables most skeletal deformities of the maxilla to be effectively corrected.

In this type of operation, close collaboration with the anesthetist is necessary in order to maintain optimal hypotension (generally systolic pressure should be 90 mm Hg or less) to reduce intraoperative bleeding to a minimum. Where extensive bleeding is expected or if some anemia is present, the patient may be invited to bank some blood a few days before surgery. For further clarification of the technique, see the enclosed DVD.

After the patient is positioned and the operative field prepared as described (the exact position of the head is of great importance in these operations), anesthetic and vasoconstrictor diluted with physiologic solution (adrenaline 1:200,000 to 1:400,000) is infiltrated locally.

The incision is now made, using a scalpel or an electrosurgical knife, at the level of the maxillary vestibular fornix above the mucogingival junction. This incision extends from the zygomatic process, at the level of the first molar on one side, to the corresponding contralateral point, taking great care not to damage the parotid ducts (Fig 7-2).

Once the mucosa, muscle, and periosteum are dissected, the soft tissues and periosteum are carefully retracted to expose the anterior and lateral parts of the maxilla, the zygomatic process, the emergence of the infraorbital nerve, and, posteriorly, the area toward the tuberosity and the pterygoid processes of the sphenoid. During this phase, great care must be taken not to expose the buccal fat pad, and to remain beneath

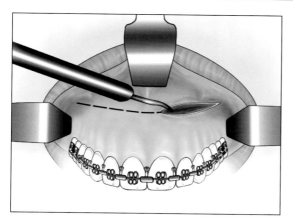

Fig 7-2 Incision for access to the maxilla and the middle third of the face.

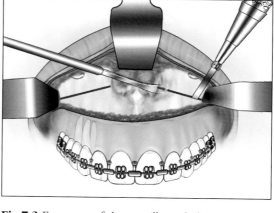

Fig 7-3 Exposure of the maxilla and classic Le Fort I osteotomy line.

the periosteum particularly in the tuberopterygoid region because of the presence of the upper part of the internal maxillary artery. The next phase of preparation for osteotomy entails exposing the piriform rim and, again subperiosteally, dissecting at least 2 cm of the nasal floor including the lateral wall and the anterior nasal spine. During this phase, care must be taken not to lacerate the nasal mucosa to minimize bleeding and cicatricial healing in this area. It may be useful to insert a small hemostatic gauze (Surgicel [Johnson & Johnson] or similar).

Once dissection of the soft tissues is completed, the reference points needed for the osteotomy must be placed. First and foremost, reference points are marked with a small lance-shaped bur at the piriform rim and at the zygomatic ridge. If the maxilla is to be repositioned superiorly, or if a cuneiform posterior osteotomy is planned, reference points must be established for how much bone will need to be removed to achieve the planned result. The osteotomy is now begun with oscillating saws or surgical burs. The classic osteotomy line starts from the anterior nasal opening, the nasal mucosa protected by insertion of an elevator along the lateral wall of the nose. The osteotomy line continues through the canine fossa and, posteriorly, along the lateral wall of the maxilla, passing at the base of the maxillary zygomatic process and extending posteriorly to the pterygomaxillary junction (Fig 7-3).

During this phase, the incision should be kept 4 to 5 mm above the tooth apexes to prevent damage to them. Classic reference distances from the occlusal plane are 34 mm from the cusp of the canine and about 24 mm from the second molar. It is clear that this numeric information must be adapted to the specific surgical case and the anatomic characteristics of different maxillas. In this phase it is also possible to place marker points (usually small holes) that will be used to quantify the movements made.

Once the osteotomies have been completed, the lateral walls of the nose are sectioned using an osteotome with protection on the nasal side (Fig 7-4). Since the lateral walls of the nose are very thin, it is necessary to proceed with care and to stop when the sound of the cutting becomes more blunted. The risk is that of damaging the palatine blood vessels with consequent hemorrhage, which would be difficult to check until the maxilla is fully mobilized.

The next phase is to determine the anterior insertion point of the nasal septum on the maxilla. Once this has been located, a special osteotome is used to dissect the septum from the maxilla for its entire length, taking care not to lacerate the nasal mucosa (Fig 7-5). The maxilla is now separated from the pterygoid processes. The index finger is placed palatally as a reference point, and a sharp, curved osteotome is inserted at the level of the pterygomaxillary junction and advanced with light and continual hammer taps until the index finger feels the tip of the osteotome palatally. At this point disjunction is complete (Fig 7-6).

The maxilla is now fully mobilized, and downfracture can be completed simply by applying progressive finger pressure downward on the anterior zone (Fig 7-7). By positioning a wire at the level of the anterior nasal spine and applying suitable traction, complete mobilization may be achieved using a specific blunt instrument, interposed at the level of the pterygomaxillary junction; this pushes the maxilla forward. In cases in which considerable advancement is required, Rowe forceps may be used to increase mobilization (see the footage on the DVD).

With mobilization completed, the next step is to smooth the bone surfaces, which is very important in cases where the maxilla will be impacted or advanced; any interference that might hinder the planned movement must be eliminated. Then, with bone nippers or rosette burs, the lateral walls of the nasal cavities are

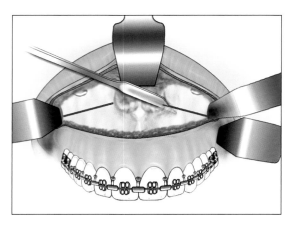

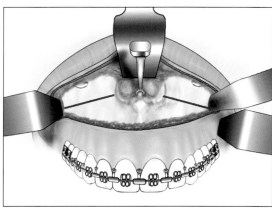

Fig 7-4 Osteotomy of the medial walls of the maxillary sinus using an osteotome with protection at the nasal side.

Fig 7-5 Osteotomy of the nasal septum, at the base, using an osteotome with double protection.

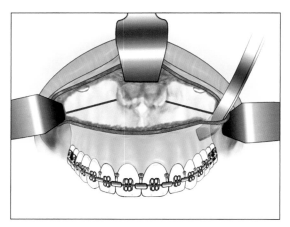

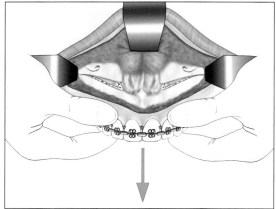

Fig 7-6 Retrotuberal osteotomy with a curved osteotome.

Fig 7-7 Manual downward mobilization of the maxilla (downfracture).

smoothed (taking great care not to damage the palatine blood vessels), as is the septal bone and, in the case of superior repositioning, the posterior and medial areas of the maxilla (Fig 7-8). Great attention must be paid during this phase to the cartilage of the nasal septum, which must be carefully shaped and/or corrected (if deviated) to aid repositioning of the maxilla. Any bony spurs must also be removed. In cases where superior repositioning will be significant (8 to 10 mm), it may be useful to reduce the turbinates surgically. To obtain access to these, a bilateral incision of the nasal mucosa will suffice and will enable the two turbinates to be exposed. These are now suitably reduced with scissors and/or an electrosurgical knife, as required. The nasal planes and any lacerations are now sutured. The piriform rim and the anterior nasal spine are shaped using a rosette bur (Fig 7-9), and the maxilla is placed in the planned position.

Repositioning may be achieved using the definitive occlusal splint if mandibular osteotomy is not planned;

once maxillomandibular fixation has been put in place, the two jaws as a unit must be positioned passively, held by the mandibular angles, so that the condyles are correctly positioned in their respective fossae (Fig 7-10). Once the vertical position of the maxilla has been checked, definitive fixation may be done using four titanium microplates (Fig 7-11) or two anterior microplates and, posteriorly, wiring with zygomatic suspension (Fig 7-12).

If mandibular osteotomy is also planned, repositioning may be done using an intermediate splint, and on this guide, temporary maxillomandibular fixation is put in place. Alternatively, the position may simply be based on clinical and esthetic evaluation of the operative field (see chapter 10 for indications, advantages, and disadvantages of these two methods). In either case, temporary fixation with four wires (two anterior and two posterior) is always recommended, and the position and orientation of the maxilla should be carefully checked on the sagittal and vertical planes before

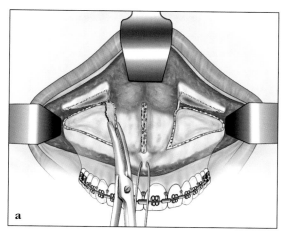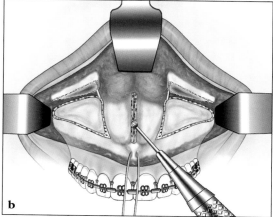

Fig 7-8 A bone nipper is used to smooth the medial walls of the maxillary sinus *(a)*, and a rosette bur is used to smooth the septal crest *(b)*.

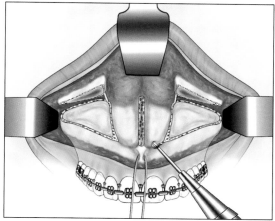

Fig 7-9 The piriform apertures are contoured with a bur.

proceeding to definitive fixation. The reference points may be the inner canthi or the palpebral fissures. The distance between these points and the occlusal plane or, even better, the orthodontic arch, is now measured (see chapter 10, Fig 10-13). In some cases it may be advantageous to check the exact horizontal position of the maxilla, using a particular instrument derived from the Fox plane and used in prosthodontics (see chapter 10, Fig 10-14). Once the desired position has been achieved, definitive internal rigid fixation follows, as described above.

In cases in which significant advancement or lowering of the maxilla is required, autologous bone grafts may be used to fill the bone gaps. Such grafts encourage the bone healing process at the osteotomy site and therefore increase the stability of the result. Donor sites are the iliac crest, the calvaria, or, in cases of mandibular setback, the mandible (inferior-medial border or ex-

ternal cortex of the ramus). In these cases, fixation must be done with four microplates.

Suturing of the surgical access completes the operation and requires particular care. Since the alar base is always enlarged after maxillary osteotomy (see chapter 8), it must be sutured. Using surgical tweezers, one side of the alar base is grasped and pulled downward and medially (Fig 7-13). Several attempts are often required to find the right point. A nonabsorbable suture material is then inserted. The same maneuver is next performed on the other side, and the two ends of the thread are tied together tightly, while verifying that the alar base has effectively been cinched (Fig 7-14). The mucosal layer may be closed with a V-Y flap, the width of which may be varied, influencing the extent of advancement of the soft tissues and offering the possibility of achieving a fuller and better-shaped upper lip (Fig 7-15) (see chapter 8).

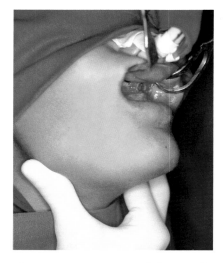

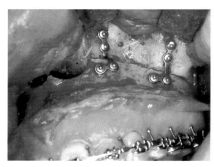

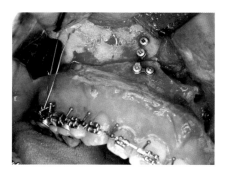

Fig 7-10 In osteotomy of the maxilla alone, the maxillomandibular complex is manually repositioned by applying pressure at the mandibular angles. In this way a correct physiologic position of the condyle in the glenoid fossa is favored.

Fig 7-11 Fixation with two miniplates of 0.5-mm thickness on each side.

Fig 7-12 Fixation with a miniplate at the level of the anterior pillar of the maxilla and wiring with suspension at the zygomatic ridge posteriorly.

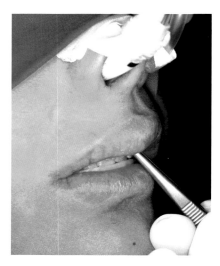

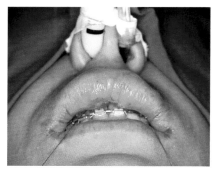

Fig 7-13 Traction applied to the alar base with surgical forceps to pass the nonabsorbable suture.

Fig 7-14 After performing the same maneuver on the contralateral side, check that the alar base has been cinched before tying the suture.

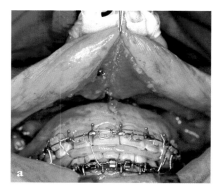

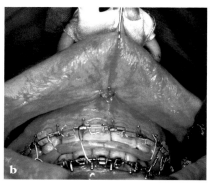

Fig 7-15 Closing the mucosal access (*a*) with a V-Y suture (*b*).

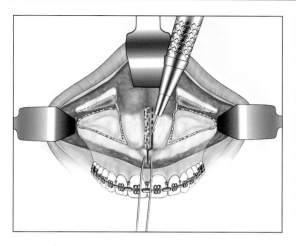

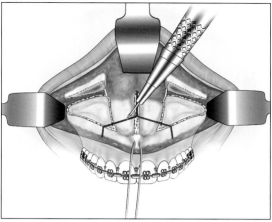

Fig 7-16 Paramedian osteotomy for subdivision into two segments.

Fig 7-17 Osteotomy lines for segmentation into three pieces.

Multiple-Piece Le Fort I Osteotomy

As was already said in chapter 4, in some cases, especially cases of open bite, a maxillary osteotomy in two or three pieces may be useful. With this surgery, the maxilla is first fully mobilized and then split into segments, guided by model surgery (an absolute necessity in these cases) and fixation devices (resin plates, occlusal splints) prepared on the casts (see chapter 10).

If the maxilla is split into two segments, when an expansion is necessary (which, however, cannot be more than 3 to 4 mm because of resistance from the palatine fibromucosa), it is sufficient to make a median osteotomy using a very thin Lindemann bur, at a point immediately lateral to the line of the median palatine suture, where the bone is thinner (Fig 7-16). Naturally, great care must be taken not to damage or perforate the palatine fibromucosa. The osteotomy begins in the premaxillary area, using the bur to pass precisely between the two central incisors, and is then completed with a thin interdental osteotome; mobilization of the two pieces is completed manually, and the previously prepared resin plate is applied. This must always be removed after definitive

rigid fixation is applied to avoid compression on the palatine fibromucosa and possible postoperative vascular complications (see chapter 13).

A split into more than two pieces normally involves an anterior segment, comprising the canines and the incisors, and two posterior segments, comprising the premolars and molars, although in particular cases asymmetric or "personalized" segments may be planned to meet the specific requirements of the case. For preference, the classic subdivision follows orthodontic preparation that slightly deviates the roots of the canines and premolars (see chapter 4) to facilitate interdental osteotomy. After the maxilla has been completely mobilized, the interdental osteotomies are performed with a thin Lindemann bur, and are completed using thin interdental osteotomes (Fig 7-17). Once the pieces are fully mobilized, the temporary resin plate is inserted before definitive rigid fixation. Above all, in cases of multiple segments, the plate must always be removed at the end of surgery.

A particular type of osteotomy, in two pieces, which is indicated in Class II cases with concomitant unilateral Brodie syndrome, involves mobilizing the posterior segment involved in the anomaly, including premolars and molars, with medial dislocation of this segment, made possible by a suitable ostectomy of the palate (see chapter 4, Fig 4-33).

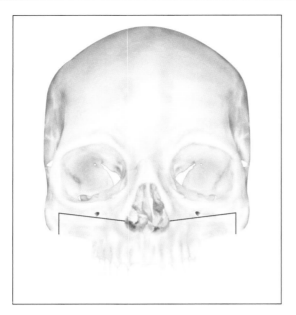

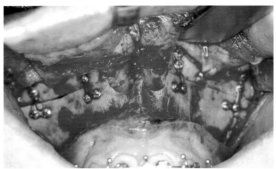

Fig 7-18 Osteotomy tracing for a Bell high osteotomy.

Fig 7-19 In high osteotomy, fixation should preferably be with four microplates of 0.5-mm thickness, two anterior and two posterior.

Bell High Osteotomy

This type of osteotomy, described by Bell et al (1988), is shown in Fig 7-18. Its purpose is to achieve better engagement of the bone segments than is possible in the classic Le Fort I osteotomy, where engagement is often poor, particularly in the lateroposterior region. An even more important advantage of this type of osteotomy is that it affords a much greater increase in the zygomatic area.

Incision, dissection, and bone exposure are the same as for the classic Le Fort I osteotomy. However, the bone must be exposed laterally for some distance beyond the maxillomalar suture toward the temporal process of the zygomatic bone. During this phase, the insertions of the masseter muscle must be carefully sectioned. In the retrotuberal area, too, more bone must be exposed upward, reaching the same area. Once the nasal plane has been prepared in the usual manner, a thin Lindemann bur or a thin, narrow oscillating saw is used to trace the osteotomy lines bilaterally. The line runs 2 to 3 mm below the infraorbital nerve and extends as far as possible laterally in the direction of the zygomatic arch, remaining 5 to 7 mm above the inferior border of the arch. The osteotomy is completed with a small vertical line as shown in Fig 7-18. These osteotomy lines as traced are then sectioned using thin osteotomes.

Using protected chisels, osteotomies of the nasal septum and the medial wall of the maxilla are made

in the usual way, as described for Le Fort I. The pterygomaxillary osteotomies, using a dedicated curved osteotome, must also be completed upward, but with great care due to the presence of the internal maxillary artery in this area. At this point, mobilization may be achieved with downward finger pressure. Once downfracture has been achieved, the maxilla is fully mobilized with the help of the Rowe forceps or with dedicated curved retrotuberal instruments, as was described for the classic Le Fort I osteotomy.

This type of osteotomy may entail a split into two segments along the median line or, better, along the paramedian line, as described in the section above. It may also be associated with superior repositioning (4 to 5 mm) and lateral translation to correct deviation of the dental midline. Rotary movements in the clockwise direction are also possible, using small posterior wedges, although the possible rotation is not large. Access to the nasal septum and, if necessary, to the turbinates, is similar to that described for Le Fort I.

With this type of osteotomy, fixation should preferably, though not necessarily, be achieved with four microplates, two anterior and two posterior (Fig 7-19). An excellent increase can be achieved in the zygomatic region, as already said, and hence this type of osteotomy stands as an alternative to maxillomalar osteotomy (described in the next section) in cases where this is contraindicated (see also chapter 9).

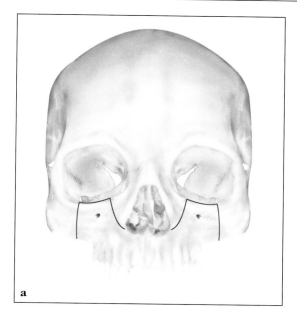

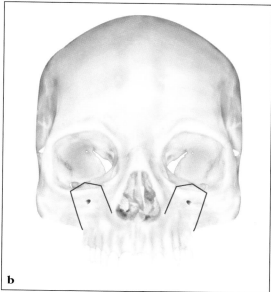

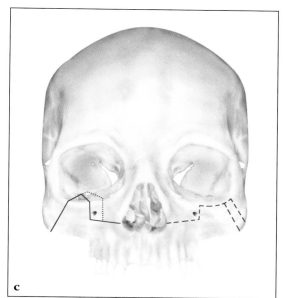

Fig 7-20 Maxillomalar osteotomy according to Keller and Sather (1990) *(a)* and Ferronato (1988) *(b)*, and the three tracings proposed by Brusati et al (1989) *(c)*.

Maxillomalar Osteotomy

Maxillomalar osteotomy, with advancement of the inferior rim of the orbit and of the zygomatic ridge, is indicated in patients with severe hypodevelopment of the middle third of the face who exhibit flattening of the suborbital area and the cheekbones.

The technique was introduced in 1969 by Obwegeser, and has since been used and described by Kufner (1970), Epker and Wolford (1975), Steinhaüser (1980), and Ferronato (1983), among others; it requires dual surgical access, ie, intraoral and extraoral subpalpebral access. Variants have been described, for example, by Keller and Sather (1990), Ferronato (1988), and Brusati et al (1989), for which intraoral access suffices, thus avoiding potential esthetic or functional complications (ectropion, entropion). A common denominator among the different techniques is the surgical approach, while osteotomy lines at the maxillomalar level differ (Fig 7-20).

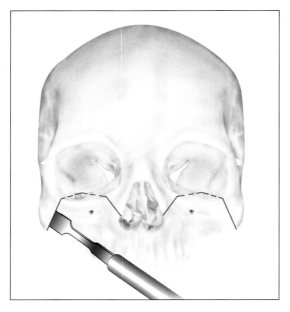

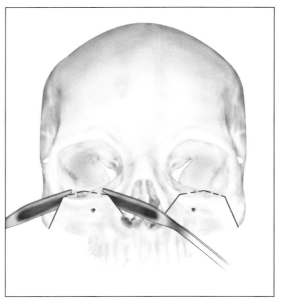

Fig 7-21 Inclination of the osteotomy is acute at the origin of the zygomatic process.

Fig 7-22 Osteotomy of the anterior part of the orbital floor, using special protected osteotomes.

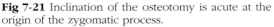

The procedure starts with the classic intraoral incision. The entire maxilla is exposed as described for the Bell high osteotomy. In this case, bone must be exposed as far laterally as possible toward the zygomatic arch to reach the zygomatic apophysis of the temporal bone. It is also necessary that the infraorbital nerve be very clearly exposed, and subperiosteal detachment must extend to the orbital floor. This phase may be facilitated using a slightly curved elevator; starting from the inferior orbital rim, the tissues are detached in the lateromedial direction and vice versa, exposing the part of the orbital floor necessary for the osteotomy (approximately 1 cm). This must always be done with maximum care to avoid damaging the infraorbital nerve or lacerating the periorbita.

The osteotomy lines are then traced. The lateral osteotomy line is traced starting from the inferior orbital rim, as far laterally as possible, moving inferiorly and posteriorly. The osteotomy is made at a considerable inclination; it is begun with a thin Lindemann bur and then completed with an oscillating saw and osteotome, maintaining the acute inclination (Fig 7-21). The advantage of this osteotomy line is that it enables the esthetic epicenter of the zygomatic area to be in-

cluded in the osteotomy segment to be advanced, with clear advantages with regard to the zygomatic ridge and a natural esthetic result. The inclination is important because the mobilized bone segment can be made to slide against the fixed part, which reduces stepping and facilitates fixation. In some cases fixation with only one or two bicortical screws may be adequate. It often prevents the need for bone grafts at the lateral osteotomy sites; if they are needed, their placement and fixation are facilitated.

A second osteotomy is made medially from the piriform rim to the medial portion of the inferior orbital rim. Once this phase is completed, osteotomy of the orbital floor is performed using two angled osteotomes especially designed for this step. These osteotomies reach the inferior orbital fissure, where they join (Fig 7-22).

Once these two osteotomy lines are completed, the operation proceeds with osteotomy of the lateral walls of the nose, detachment of the nasal septum, and pterygomaxillary disjunction. These procedures are as described for the classic Le Fort I, although additional care may be required in the pterygomaxillary osteotomy, which must be completed very carefully

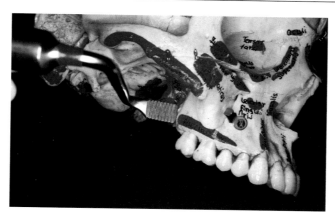

Fig 7-23 Complete mobilization of the maxillomalar complex is achieved using special retrotuberal instruments.

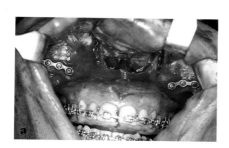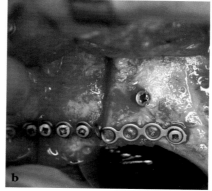

Fig 7-24 Fixation may be achieved with miniplates of 1-mm thickness *(a)*, or with miniplates of 0.5-mm thickness and 2-mm-diameter bicortical screws *(b)*.

both upward and mesially to facilitate mobilization of the maxillomalar complex.

Mobilization of the maxillomalar complex continues, including the inferior orbital rim and part of the orbital floor, using Rowe forceps. Once detachment is complete, retrotuberal instruments are used to mobilize the osteotomized segment, providing thrust behind the maxilla to displace it forward (Fig 7-23). If necessary, Rowe forceps can again be used to improve mobilization.

As was said above, in particular thanks to the inclination of the osteotomy lines, with this type of osteotomy, the mobilized maxillomalar complex has reasonable bone engagement, rather than leaving a gap,

making it quicker and easier to stabilize; this is done with miniplates or microplates and bicortical screws (Fig 7-24). For this type of osteotomy an intermediate splint must always be available (see chapter 10).

At the zygomatic level and, above all, at the medial level, bone grafts may be inserted and suitably fixed in place; these are useful to flatten any steps and to improve the naturalness of the esthetic outcome. Since mandibular setback osteotomy is often performed at the same time, the bone grafts may easily be obtained from the mandibular cortex at the proximal segment.

Surgical access is sutured as described for the classic Le Fort I osteotomy and concludes the procedure.

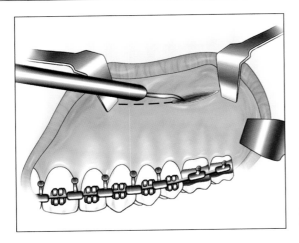

Fig 7-25 Incision for Schuchardt lateroposterior osteotomy.

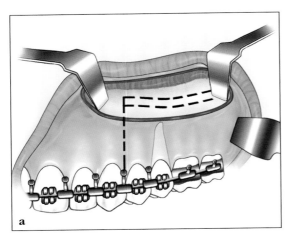

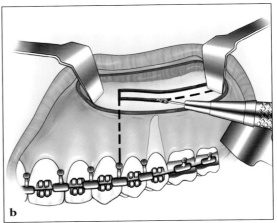

Fig 7-26 *(a and b)* Vertical and horizontal osteotomy lines.

Schuchardt Lateroposterior Segmental Osteotomy

This procedure was first described in 1942 by Schuchardt, who then better codified it in 1959. This type of osteotomy may be used to correct excessive extrusion of the posterior maxillary teeth (for example, in open bite or when antagonist teeth in the mandibular arch are missing) or to correct transverse maxillary defects, whether of deficit or excess. It may be used in association with a mandibular setback or advancement osteotomy.

Good orthodontic preparation is necessary for the outcome to be successful and must align the teeth and provide the space needed for the interdental osteotomies.

After a solution of anesthetic and vasoconstrictor diluted with physiologic solution (adrenaline 1:200,000 to 1:400,000) is infiltrated locally, an incision is made through the mucosa and periosteum at the level of the maxillary vestibular fornix unilaterally, with an incision similar to that made for the classic Le Fort I osteotomy (Fig 7-25).

The anterolateral wall of the maxilla is dissected subperiosteally, taking care to leave the mucosa adherent below the incision. The periosteum is dissected vertically downward at the point where the median vertical osteotomy will be made (generally between canine and premolar) (Fig 7-26).

The horizontal osteotomy follows, along the dentoalveolar segment to be mobilized. The osteotomy may be done with a bur or a saw, removing the appropriate amount of bone, if necessary, if the segment is to be repositioned superiorly. In regard to this repositioning, it must be taken into account that the osteotomized segment will fit in telescopically, and the ostectomy must be planned accordingly to avoid removing too much bone (see Fig 7-26).

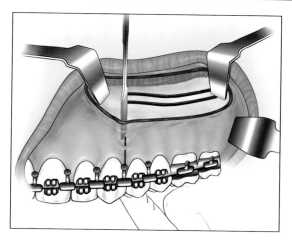

Fig 7-27 The interdental osteotomy is completed with a thin osteotome.

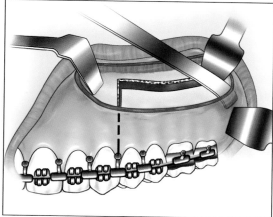

Fig 7-28 Pterygomaxillary disjunction using a curved osteotome.

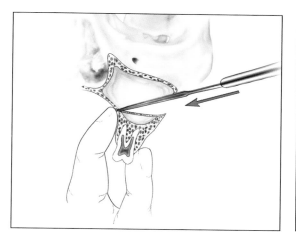

Fig 7-29 Palatal osteotomy with access through the vestibular ostectomy.

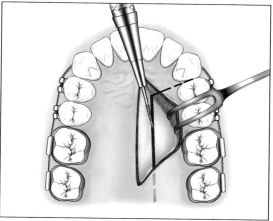

Fig 7-30 Osteotomy at the palatal level through direct access, as in the variant according to Perko (1972) and Bell and Proffit (1980).

The vertical osteotomies are now performed. Medially, the line extends as far as possible toward the alveolar process between the two teeth. The osteotomy is begun with a very thin bur or a microsaw and is completed with a flat, thin osteotome both at the level of the alveolar process and palatally, taking care not to lacerate the palatal mucosa. During this phase, the index finger should be placed palatally so that the tip of the osteotome will be felt when it has cut through the bone section (Fig 7-27). Posteriorly, pterygomaxillary disjunction is achieved with a curved osteotome, as in the Le Fort I osteotomy (Fig 7-28).

The operation now proceeds with osteotomy at the palatal level. If there has been an ostectomy, this delicate step may be performed by working through the horizontal slit while it is still open, inserting a flat scalpel through the maxillary sinus. The osteotomy is done by gently tapping the chisel and using the index finger placed palatally for reference (Fig 7-29). If there has been no vestibular ostectomy, it may be necessary to create palatal access to perform the osteotomy correctly (variation according to Perko [1972] and Bell and Proffit [1980]; Fig 7-30). In this case, a bur may also be used (Bell and Proffit 1980).

Once the segment has been mobilized, it is replaced in the planned position, based on the model surgery, with the help of an occlusal splint or a palatal resin plate, and held in place by rigid fixation with miniplates and screws. If a resin plate is used, this must be removed on completion of surgery to avoid compression and vascular complications (see chapter 12).

The procedure is concluded by suturing the surgical access.

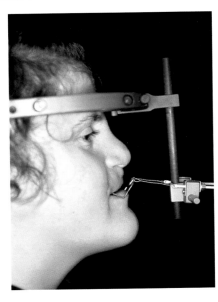

Fig 7-31 Example of maxillary distraction, in a classic case of severe hypoplasia secondary to cleft lip sequelae (Rigid External Distraction [RED] System [KLS Martin]).

Maxillary Distraction Osteogenesis

The success obtained with distraction osteogenesis techniques in the oral and maxillofacial area has inevitably led to the use of this method for treatment of hypodevelopment of the maxilla. The technique consists of an osteotomy of the classic Le Fort I type associated with extraoral posteroanterior traction, which is exercised by applying intraoral and extraoral distractors of varying complexities. Clearly, the principle is comparable to that of the Delaire mask. The advantages lie in the gradual traction that is exercised on the maxilla, with concomitant stretching of the soft tissues, and the possibility of achieving considerable advancement, even greater than 10 mm. Because of these characteristics, the technique appears to be indicated chiefly in cases with marked maxillary retrusion, for example, as in cleft lip sequelae, when scarring may also hinder advancement of the maxilla (Fig 7-31).

However, there is not always perfect control over the occlusal plane and occlusion, and thus frequent adjustments are required. The method is clearly contraindicated when mandibular osteotomy is also required. Hence, in the vast majority of cases, in normal orthodontic-surgical treatment of dentofacial anomalies, traditional techniques still appear to provide the most reliable approach.

Bibliography

Abubaker AO, Sotereanos GC. Modified Le Fort I (maxillary-zygomatic) osteotomy: Rationale, basis, and surgical technique. J Oral Maxillofac Surg 1991;49:1089–1097.

Bell WH. Revascularization and bone healing after anterior maxillary osteotomy: A study using adult rhesus monkeys. J Oral Surg 1969;27:249–255.

Bell WH, Proffit WR. Maxillary excess. In: Bell WH, Proffit WR, White RP Jr (eds). Surgical Correction of Dentofacial Deformities. Philadelphia: Saunders, 1980:341–343.

Bell WH, Mannai C, Luhr HG. Art and science of the Le Fort I downfracture. Int J Adult Orthodon Orthognath Surg 1988;1:23–52.

Benech A, Tarello F, Viterbo S. Segmental surgery of the maxilla: The long-term assessment of the dental-periodontal integrity of the osteotomized sites [in Italian]. Minerva Stomatol 1990;39:353–356.

Brusati R, Sesenna M, Raffaini M. On the feasibility of intraoral maxillo-malar osteotomy. J Craniomaxillofac Surg 1989; 17:110–115.

Champy M, Lodde JP, Wilk A. Thirty cases of intermediate transfacial osteotomies [in French]. Ann Chir Plast 1979; 24:351–357.

Dodson TB, Bays RA, Neuenschwander MC. Maxillary perfusion during Le Fort I osteotomy after ligation of the descending palatine artery. J Oral Maxillofac Surg 1997; 55:51–55.

Epker BN, Wolford LM. Middle-third osteotomies: Their use in the correction of acquired and developmental dentofacial and cranial deformities. J Oral Surg 1975;33:491–514.

Ferronato G. Approaches for extra- and intraoral surgical intervention in correcting dysgnathia with severe underdevelopment of the middle third of the face [in Italian]. Minerva Stomatol 1983;32:851–860.

Ferronato G. Intra-oral surgical approach for maxillo-malar advancement. Chir Testa Collo 1988;5:17–30.

Fox ME, Stephens WF, Wolford LM, El Deeb M. Effects of interdental osteotomies on the periodontal and osseous supporting tissues. Int J Adult Orthodon Orthognath Surg 1991;6:39–46.

Gotte P. Surgical interventions to the osseous bases and the alveolar processes before prosthetic rehabilitation [in Italian]. Riv Ital Stomatol 1978;47:17–35.

Herbosa EH, Rotskoff KS, Ramos BF, Ambrookian HS. Condylar position in superior maxillary repositioning and its effect on the temporomandibular joint. J Oral Maxillofac Surg 1990;48:690–696.

Ioannides C. "Quadrangular" Le Fort II osteotomy for hypoplasia of the midface [in French]. Ann Chir Plast Esthet 1991;36:101–107.

Keller EE, Sather AH. Intraoral quadrangular Le Fort II osteotomy. J Oral Maxillofac Surg 1987;45:223–232.

Keller EE, Sather AH. Quadrangular Le Fort I osteotomy: Surgical technique and review of 54 patients. J Oral Maxillofac Surg 1990;48:2–11.

Kufner J. Experience with a modified procedure for correction of open bite. In: Walker RV (ed). Transactions of the Third International Conference of Oral Surgery. London: Livingstone, 1970:18.

Kufner J. Four-year experience with major maxillary osteotomy for retrusion. J Oral Surg 1971;29:549–553.

Loh FC. A new technique of alar cinching following maxillary osteotomy. Int J Adult Orthodon Orthognath Surg 1993; 8:33–36.

Modica R, Benech A, Formengo B, Berrone S. Segmentation of the upper jaw in orthognathic surgery [in Italian]. Mondo Ortod 1988;5:11–24.

de Mol van Otterloo JJ, Tuinzing DB, Kostense P. Inferior positioning of the maxilla by a Le Fort I osteotomy: A review of 25 patients with vertical maxillary deficiency. J Craniomaxillofac Surg 1996;4:69–77.

Obwegeser HL. Surgical correction of small or retrodisplaced maxillae. The "dish-face" deformity. Plast Reconstr Surg 1969;43:351–365.

Perko M. Maxillary sinus and surgical movement of maxilla. Int J Oral Surg 1972;1:177–184.

Ronchi P, Chiapasco M, Frattini D. Modified intraoral maxillo-malar osteotomy: Long-term results in 16 consecutive cases. J Craniomaxillofac Surg 1997;25:46–50.

Schuchardt K. Ein beitrag zur chirurgischen kieferorthopädie unter berücksichtingung ihrer bedeutung für die behandlung angeborener und erworbener kieferdeformitäten bei soldaten. Dtsch Zahn Mund Kieferheilkd 1942;9:73.

Schuchardt K. Experience with the surgical treatment of deformities of the jaws: Prognathia, micrognathia and open bite. In: Wallace AG (ed). Second Congress of the International Society of Plastic Surgeons. London: Livingstone, 1959:73.

Schwestka-Polly R. Significance of the contour of the lateral surface of the maxilla for planning osteotomy lines in orthognathic surgery. Int J Adult Orthodon Orthognath Surg 1993;8:191–201.

Souyris F, Caravel JB, Reynaud JP. Intermediary osteotomies of the middle third of the face [in French]. Ann Chir Plast 1973;18:149–154.

Steinhäuser EW. Variations of Le Fort II osteotomies for correction of midfacial deformities. J Maxillofac Surg 1980; 8:258–265.

Stoelinga PJW, Brouns JJA. The quadrangular osteotomy revisited. J Craniomaxillofac Surg 2000;28:79–84.

Wagner S, Reyneke JP. The Le Fort I downsliding osteotomy: A study of long-term hard tissue stability. Int J Adult Orthodon Orthognath Surg 2000;15:37–49.

Wassmund M. Fracturen und luxationen des gesichtsschädels. Leipzig: Meusser, 1927.

West RA, Epker B. Posterior maxillary surgery: Its place in the treatment of dentofacial deformities. J Oral Surg 1972;30: 562–574.

Recommended reading

Bell WH, Proffit WR, White RP Jr (eds). Surgical Correction of Dentofacial Deformities. Philadelphia: Saunders, 1980.

Brusati R, Sesenna E. Chirurgia delle deformità mascellari. Milan: Masson, 1988.

Epker BN, Wolford LM. Dentofacial Deformities: Surgical-Orthodontic Correction. St Louis: Mosby, 1980.

Proffit WR, White RP Jr. Surgical-Orthodontic Treatment. St Louis: Mosby, 1991.

8

Soft Tissue Changes Following Maxillary and Mandibular Osteotomy

with Giorgio Novelli

- Nose and upper lip
- Zygomas and cheeks
- Lower lip and chin
- Considerations for double-jaw osteotomy

Nose and Upper Lip

The nose and upper lip undergo some significant changes, especially after osteotomy at the maxilla and middle third of the face, but also following mandibular osteotomy alone. It is therefore highly important to have an in-depth understanding of all these variables to select the most appropriate technique and manage surgery for the best possible result.

Although from the quantitative standpoint there is no strong correlation between upper lip changes and mandibular osteotomy, they should be considered at least from the qualitative standpoint, particularly in terms of the sagittal dimension. In general, in cases of mandibular setback, the upper lip may move backward by about 10% to 20% of the surgical displacement. In cases of mandibular advancement, the upper lip may advance by some 10% of the skeletal mandibular advancement. In general, mandibular setback usually produces a certain uncurling of the upper lip (Fig 8-1), whereas mandibular advancement tends to produce some curling of the upper lip (Fig 8-2).

Maxillary osteotomy logically produces much more significant changes to the tip of the nose, the upper lip, and the nasolabial angle. Many studies have reported on the relationship between maxillary osteotomy (particularly in cases of Le Fort I osteotomy) and changes in nasal esthetics and the shape of the upper lip. Typically these involve the width and shape of the alar base, the nasolabial angle, the position of the upper lip, and the projection of the tip of the nose and the supratip area. These changes are not only caused by the repositioning of the maxilla, but are also due to the extent of subperiosteal dissection and to the handling of muscles and mucosa when surgical access is closed.

Although the changes that may occur secondary to skeletal displacement of the maxilla cannot always be predicted precisely from the quantitative standpoint, they may be listed as follows (Fig 8-3).

- Advancement of the maxilla will move the tip of the nose forward and slightly upward, the alar base will tend to be enlarged, and the depression in the supratip area will be accentuated.
- Repositioning the maxilla superiorly will raise subnasale and labrale superior, and again the alar base will tend to widen; the nasolabial angle will become more acute with retraction of the columella.
- Repositioning the maxilla inferiorly will move both the alar base and the columella downward. Overlying tissues will become thinner, and the nasolabial angle will become more obtuse.
- Maxillary setback, which is very rare and could even be considered an exceptional operation, will decrease the projection of the tip of the nose and the upper lip.

Flaring of the alar base is generally an undesirable effect, although it may be an advantage in patients who have Class II occlusion with open bite and/or long face and in whom the base of the nose is particularly narrow. This enlargement of the alar base is, in reality, only partially due to the maxillary repositioning: The extension of the subperiosteal dissection and the disinsertion of the perioral and perinasal muscles appear to play an important role in producing this flaring. The amount of flaring ranges between 6% and 10% of the initial width, and some surgical strategies have been developed to reduce this undesirable effect, such as cinching the alar base and/or suturing to the anterior nasal spine (see chapter 7), although the results have not been entirely satisfactory and are often unpredictable. Thus some enlargement of the alar base is inevitable after Le Fort I osteotomy (Fig 8-4) and is often independent of the type of skeletal displacement.

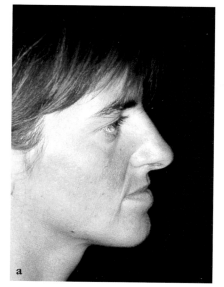
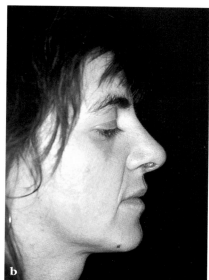

Fig 8-1 *(a and b)* Uncurling effect on the upper lip, consequent to mandibular setback osteotomy.

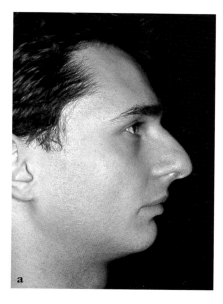
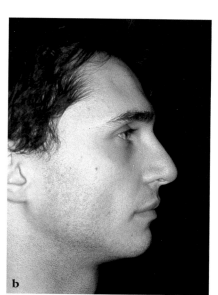

Fig 8-2 *(a and b)* Curling effect on the upper lip, consequent to mandibular advancement osteotomy; simultaneous rhinoplasty has no influence from this standpoint.

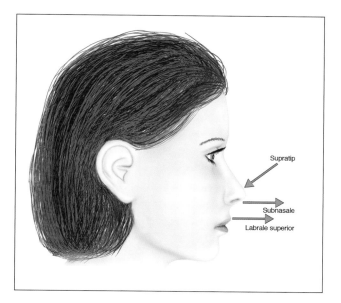

Fig 8-3 Points of the nose and upper lip that are altered consequent to a Le Fort I osteotomy.

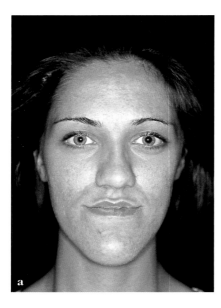

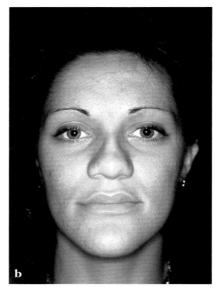

Fig 8-4 *(a and b)* Excessive enlargement of the alar base consequent to a Le Fort I osteotomy.

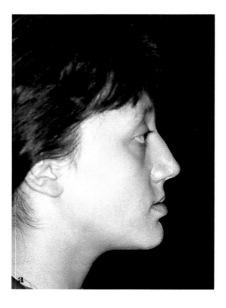

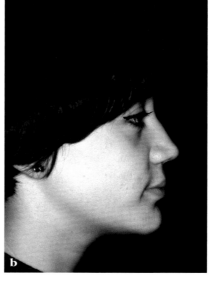

Fig 8-5 *(a and b)* The upper lip becomes more prominent after a Le Fort I advancement osteotomy.

Advancement of labrale superior after osteotomy to advance the maxilla depends in part on the advancement itself, but also to a great extent on the technique used to suture the intraoral surgical access. With adequate V-Y closure, or more precisely upturned Y (see chapter 7), an advancement of labrale superior that is between 70% and 90% of the skeletal displacement may be achieved, whereas these values range between 40% and 60% if that technique is not used. Hence a surgeon with experience with maxillary osteotomies can modulate the soft tissue outcome of maxillary osteotomy (position of labrale superior, exposure of prolabium, and prominence of the upper lip in general) by varying soft tissue management to meet esthetic requirements (Fig 8-5).

Subnasale will follow the direction of movement of the osteotomized maxilla. Jensen et al (1992) report an

average movement of subnasale of about 66% of the skeletal movement during horizontal advancement, whereas the value is 21% in superior repositioning. The increased depression of the supratip area is a direct consequence of the extent of displacement upward and forward of subnasale. In Le Fort I osteotomies to raise and advance the maxilla, the entire nose undergoes marked changes.

This consideration is very important because, simply by repositioning the maxilla, the nose may be recontoured, and, in some cases, this may be sufficient to completely eliminate a slight osteochondral hump (Fig 8-6). However, if the depression in the supratip area is too accentuated, this may be an undesirable side effect in patients with a globular tip of the nose that is already tilted upward (Fig 8-7).

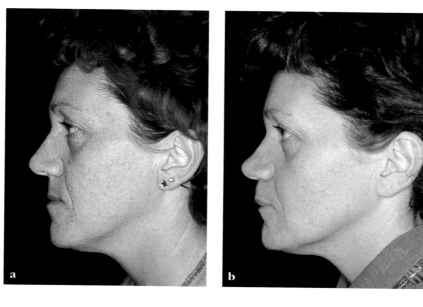

Fig 8-6 *(a and b)* Disappearance of a slight bone-cartilage hump after Le Fort I advancement osteotomy.

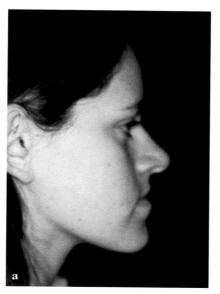
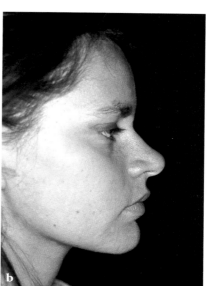

Fig 8-7 *(a and b)* Undesirable accentuation of the supratip area after a Le Fort I osteotomy for advancement and superior repositioning.

The nasolabial angle will become more acute if the maxilla is repositioned superiorly and advanced, whereas it will become more obtuse if the maxilla is set back and repositioned inferiorly, although quantitative data are not reported in the literature. Jensen et al (1992) report an average increase in this angle of 0.65 degrees per millimeter of maxillary advancement. In any case, since the differences vary widely (ranging between −7.9 and +9.7 degrees), the reliability of these data is debatable. The variability in reported data may partly be due to the fact that the nasolabial angle is closely linked to the inclination of the maxillary incisors (which provide lip support), and thus any changes in that angle are more a consequence of rotating the maxilla and/or the maxillary incisors than of movements in the horizontal or vertical planes. Thus, where considerable rotation of the maxilla is planned, changes to the paranasal and labial areas appear to be rather unpredictable. Preoperative planning of the inclination of the maxillary incisors is essential in these cases and should be based on the planned rotation. This is especially true in open bite cases (see chapter 4).

Based on all these considerations, in a good percentage of cases it is nevertheless possible to predict whether changes to the nose will have a positive or a negative effect on facial esthetics, and this can guide the surgeon concerning the appropriateness of performing simultaneous rhinoplasty (see chapter 9).

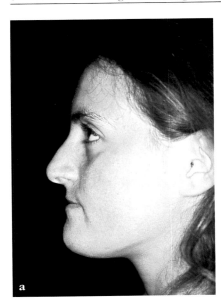
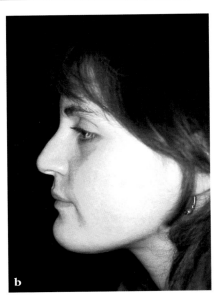

Fig 8-8 *(a and b)* Accentuation of the paranasal and zygomatic area after a Le Fort I advancement osteotomy.

Zygomas and Cheeks

Changes to the zygomas and cheeks chiefly occur after osteotomy of the maxilla or middle third of the face, but some changes may also occur after mandibular setback osteotomy alone. Changes to the zygomas and cheeks depend primarily on the thickness and tone of the soft tissues, as well as the patient's age. They are very difficult to predict, at least from the quantitative standpoint, compared to the changes occurring to the upper lip and nose. Furthermore, significant and reliable data are not available in the literature because of the difficulty of evaluating and measuring changes occurring in this area. It is obvious that changes will be more visible where soft tissues are thin, whereas they will be less evident in subjects with thick cheeks and abundant soft tissue. Furthermore, the ratio between highlights and shadow areas alters the subjective visual impression of a face, giving greater or lesser apparent importance to the cheekbones. Secondary changes to the cheeks and zygomas are, however, directly proportional to surgical advancement: the greater the surgical advancement, the greater the esthetic impact.

The type of osteotomy also clearly plays a significant role. In cases of classic Le Fort I maxillary osteotomy, there will be more filling out of the tissues in the cheek and paranasal areas, with a reduction in the nasogenial folds. Nevertheless, the play of highlights and shadows often appears to give prominence to the cheekbones that is more apparent than real, and in any case only involves the soft tissues (Fig 8-8).

With the Bell high osteotomy, there is a greater increase at the cheek area, since the skeletal structures have actually been advanced, and some increase in the width of the face (Fig 8-9). Even more marked variations occur after maxillomalar osteotomy, which advances the entire malar bone considerably, as well as the inferior orbital rim. Scleral exposure disappears, and there is a marked increase in the width of the face (Fig 8-10).

Osteotomy of the mandible alone, to correct Class III cases, also causes some changes to the cheeks. The increased thickness and change of shape, becoming more rounded, are obviously more noticeable in thin subjects. Furthermore, in these cases, again due to the play of highlights and shadows, the area of the cheekbones also appears more prominent even though no surgical intervention has taken place in this area (Fig 8-11). Nevertheless, especially in these cases, prediction of soft tissue changes will be more qualitative than quantitative.

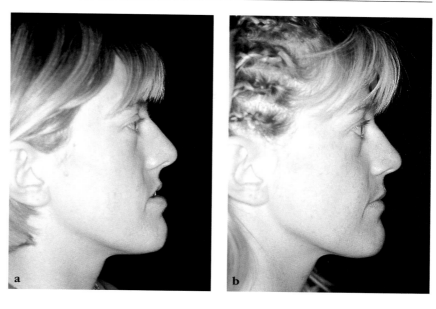

Fig 8-9 *(a and b)* Accentuation of the zygomatic eminence after a high Le Fort I maxillary advancement osteotomy.

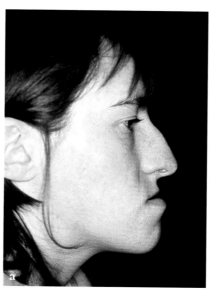

Fig 8-10 *(a and b)* Advancement of the zygomatic and orbital regions after a maxillomalar osteotomy.

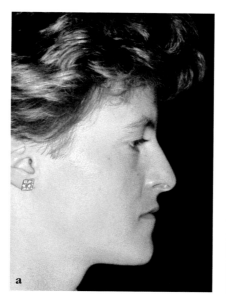
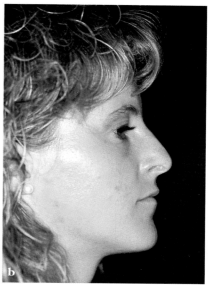

Fig 8-11 *(a and b)* The zygomatic region and cheeks are filled in after mandibular setback osteotomy alone.

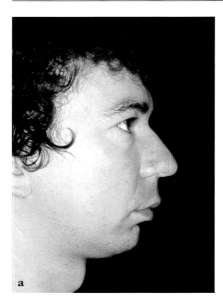 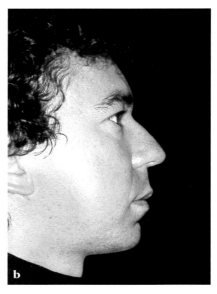

Fig 8-12 *(a and b)* In cases with decreased vertical dimension, mandibular osteotomy alone (in this case for advancement) produces some uncurling of the lower lip.

Lower Lip and Chin

Changes to the lower lip and chin are clearly more accentuated after mandibular osteotomy and genioplasty. However, some changes may also occur after maxillary osteotomy alone, for advancement or repositioning superiorly or inferiorly, with concomitant autorotation of the mandible.

With regard to mandibular osteotomy (Obwegeser–Dal Pont or Gotte), soft tissue pogonion and point B and the labiomental angle are virtually unchanged in shape, whereas the behavior of the lip and in particular prolabium is less predictable. From the sagittal standpoint, in cases of advancement osteotomy, soft tissue pogonion follows almost 100% of the surgical movement, whereas in cases of setback it follows 90% of the movement.

With regard to purely sagittal movements, the lower lip and prolabium follow these fairly closely; more significant changes occur where variations are also produced in the vertical dimension. This is chiefly due to the relationship with the upper lip and the maxillary incisors. In patients with an initial tendency to deep bite, once a new and normal vertical equilibrium has been achieved for both the lips and the incisors, there will be some uncurling of the lower lip, both in Class II and Class III cases (Fig 8-12). In patients with a tendency for slight open bite with increased vertical dimension and labial incompetence, once a normal labiodental seal has been achieved with labial competence, there will be some curling of the lower lip, both in Class II and Class III cases (Fig 8-13).

Similar considerations may be made with regard to the lower lip after osteotomy of the maxilla alone, for

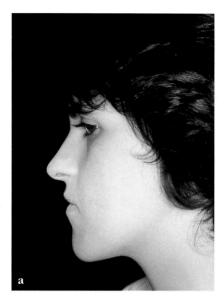 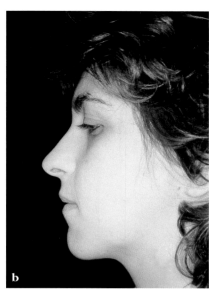

Fig 8-13 *(a and b)* In cases with increased vertical dimension, mandibular osteotomy alone (in this case setback) produces some curling of the lower lip.

advancement or to reposition it inferiorly or superiorly, with concomitant autorotation of the mandible. In these cases soft tissue pogonion clearly does not undergo any morphologic changes, but it passively follows the rotation of the mandible in the clockwise or counterclockwise direction. In these situations it becomes important, and also quite reliable, to make a cephalometric visual treatment objective (VTO) that includes the soft tissue (see chapter 10).

With regard to genioplasty, quantitative and qualitative changes involving the soft tissues of the chin are important and depend on the various possible configurations the genioplasty takes (see chapter 5). There are many studies in the literature on this subject, and the available data may be summed up thus: In genioplasty with advancement, the soft tissue pogonion will follow 80% to 90% of the surgical

movement. In genioplasty with vertical increase and clockwise rotation of the osteotomy fragment, the proportion is about 80%. In cases of genioplasty to reduce the vertical dimension, the proportion is 80% to 90%. Lastly, with genioplasty for reduction in the anteroposterior direction, the proportion may reach 90%; however, excess soft tissue may be left under the chin, the extent of which is neither predictable nor quantifiable, and the labiomental angle may undergo variations that are only qualitatively predictable and depend on the direction and extent of displacement of the osteotomy fragment.

Lastly, with regard to reduction genioplasty through grinding and bone contouring, the relationship between hard and soft tissues is approximately 50% in vertical reduction, whereas this drops to about 25% in the case of anteroposterior reduction.

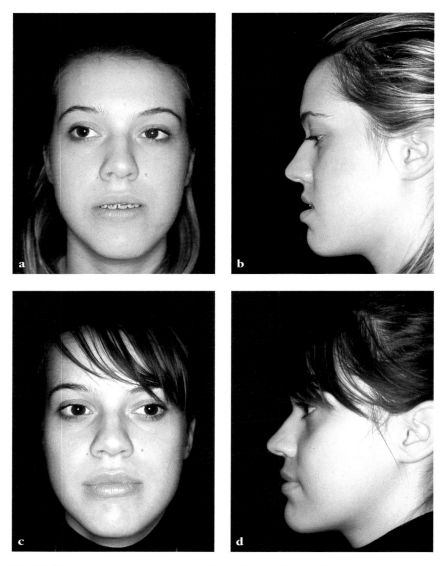

Fig 8-14 Double-jaw osteotomy in a Class III case *(a and b)* with final result *(c and d)* showing typically feminine characteristics (pronounced lip, protruding cheekbones).

Considerations for Double-Jaw Osteotomy

In cases of double-jaw osteotomy, changes produced in the soft tissues are only predictable from the qualitative standpoint, whereas quantitative prediction is more risky. Various reports have said that, in these cases, displacement of the soft tissues cannot be approximated by summing the values that would be predicted for the two individual operations. Furthermore, as we have already seen, all changes are greatly influenced by additional surgical procedures on the soft tis-

sues, in particular with regard to the middle third of the face (nose and upper lip). In practice, each surgeon should look at the results obtained personally and from this develop his or her own predictions relating to the various surgical procedures.

The possibility of performing a cephalometric and esthetic VTO is therefore subordinated to all these considerations (see chapter 10). These tools should only be considered as auxiliaries for the surgeon and orthodontist, and must not be depended on exclusively. All these considerations are, of course, truer in cases of combined osteotomies.

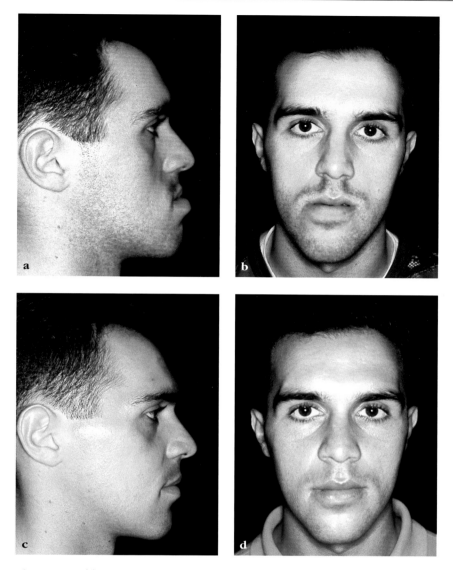

Fig 8-15 Double-jaw osteotomy in a similar Class III case *(a and b)* with final result *(c and d)* showing more masculine characteristics (less pronounced lip, larger nose, vertical increase of the lower third).

It is also important to produce and maintain feminine or masculine characteristics in a face, even though the same basic surgical procedures are used. Suitably modulated surgical techniques and adequate manipulation of the soft tissues will enable a surgeon with considerable experience to achieve the results that he or she has mentally decided upon. Figures 8-14 and 8-15 illustrate this concept: The same osteotomy procedure, with suitable strategies with regard to the soft tissues, may produce a typically feminine or masculine face.

133

Bibliography

de Assis A, Stark WJ, Epker BN. Cephalometric analysis of profile nasal esthetics. Part II. Patients with vertical maxillary excess. Int J Adult Orthodon Orthognath Surg 1996;11:205-210.

Betts NJ, Vig KWL, Vig P, Spalding P, Fonseca RJ. Changes in the nasal and labial soft tissues after surgical repositioning of the maxilla. Int J Adult Orthodon Orthognath Surg 1993;8:7-23.

Carlotti AE, Aschaffenburg PA, Schendel SA. Facial changes associated with surgical advancement of the lip and maxilla. J Oral Maxillofac Surg 1986;44:593-596.

Collins PC, Epker BN. The alar base cinch: A technique for prevention of alar base flaring secondary to maxillary surgery. Oral Surg Oral Med Oral Pathol 1982;53:549-553.

Ewing M, Ross RB. Soft tissue response to mandibular advancement and genioplasty. Am J Orthod Dentofacial Orthop 1993;7:18-24.

Hoffman GR, Staples G, Moloney FB. Cephalometric alterations following facial advancement surgery: 1. Statistical evalutation. J Craniomaxillofac Surg 1994;22:214-219.

Ingervall B, Thüer U, Vuillemin T. Stability and effect on the soft tissue profile of mandibular setback with sagittal split osteotomy and internal fixation. Int J Adult Orthodon Orthognath Surg 1995;10:15-25.

Jensen AC, Sinclair PM, Wolford LM. Soft tissue changes associated with double jaw surgery. Am J Orthod Dentofacial Orthop 1992;101:266-275.

Lee Y, Bailey J, Proffit WR. Soft tissue changes after superior repositioning of the maxilla with Le Fort I osteotomy: 5-year follow-up. Int J Adult Orthodon Orthognath Surg 1996;11:301-311.

Loh FC. A new technique of alar base cinching following maxillary osteotomy. Int J Adult Orthodon Orthognath Surg 1993;8:33-36.

Lundström A, Paulin G, Forsberg CM. Quantitative evaluation of the soft tissue profile in the planning of orthognathic surgery. Int J Adult Orthodon Orthognath Surg 1993;8:73-86.

Mommaerts MY, Lippens F, Abeloos JVS, Neyt LF. Nasal profile changes after maxillary impaction and advancement surgery. J Oral Maxillofac Surg 2000;58:470-475.

O'Ryan F, Schendel S. Nasal anatomy and maxillary surgery. I. Esthetic and anatomic principles. Int J Adult Orthognath Surg 1989;4:27-37.

Ronchi P, Chiapasco M. Simultaneous rhinoplasty and maxillomandibular osteotomies: Indications and contraindications. Int J Adult Orthodon Orthognath Surg 1998;13:153-161.

Rosenberg A, Muradin MSM, van der Bilt A. Nasolabial esthetics after Le Fort I osteotomy and V-Y closure: A statistical evaluation. Int J Adult Orthodon Orthognath Surg 2002;17:29-38.

Schendel SA, Eisenfeld JH, Bell WH, Epker BN. Superior repositioning of the maxilla: Stability and soft tissue osseous relations. Am J Orthod 1976;70:663-674.

Schendel SA, Carlotti AE. Nasal considerations in orthognathic surgery. Am J Adult Orthod Dentofacial Orthop 1991;100:197-208.

Stark WJ, Epker BN. Objective cephalometric evaluation of profile nasal esthetics. Part I. Method and normative data. Int J Adult Orthodon Orthognath Surg 1995;11:91-103.

Thüer U, Ingervall B, Vuillemin T. Stability and effect on the soft tissue profile of mandibular advancement with sagittal split osteotomy and rigid internal fixation. Int J Adult Orthodon Orthognath Surg 1994;9:175-185.

Recommended reading

Guyuron B. Genioplasty. Boston: Little, Brown, 1993.

9

Surgical Procedure Selection

- General principles
- Class III malocclusion
- Class II malocclusion
- Dentofacial asymmetry
- Open bite
- Double-jaw osteotomy and rhinoplasty

General Principles

The surgical correction of a dentofacial anomaly is generally done after completion of growth, and thus in adult patients. Only in rare cases of Class II malocclusion or dentofacial asymmetry may surgery in adolescent subjects be considered, as discussed below.

The final decision concerning the type of osteotomy or osteotomies to employ for surgical correction of a dentofacial anomaly must be made upon completion of preoperative orthodontic treatment and based on the evaluation of morphology, esthetics, and, to a lesser extent, cephalometry. Naturally, right from the start of orthodontic treatment it should already be clear what type of operation will most likely be required. However, in some cases preoperative orthodontic treatment may bring about changes that, within certain limits, may alter the planned surgery.

As well as deciding the type of osteotomy to be adopted (maxillary alone, mandibular alone, or double-jaw), it is also appropriate to decide whether supplementary surgical procedures will be required (genioplasty, rhinoplasty, or correction of zygomas or mandibular angle) and whether such procedures can or should be performed at the same time as the primary osteotomy or be postponed for some months. From the purely theoretical standpoint, such ancillary procedures should always be postponed until the result has stabilized, especially with regard to soft tissue adaptation to the new skeletal configuration. However, such an approach is often at odds with reality since the patient, having corrected the primary skeletal anomaly and therefore having achieved most of his or her goals (both esthetic and functional) is unlikely to agree to further "lesser" surgery. As a general rule,

ancillary procedures should be postponed in cases of severe dentofacial asymmetry, as will be explained in detail below. In other cases with skeletal displacement that is principally in only two directions (sagittal and vertical) ancillary procedures can, and in some cases should, be performed at the same time. The nose is a separate matter and is dealt with in the final section of this chapter.

The clinical, morphologic, esthetic, and functional approach that should guide the choice of surgical procedure varies with the type of anomaly. Class III and Class II malocclusion, dentofacial asymmetries, and open bite will therefore be considered separately. In a high percentage of cases esthetic considerations will dominate, and cephalometric factors will be less important.

Naturally, in planning any osteotomy, an in-depth evaluation of the changes that the soft tissues will undergo is indispensable (see chapter 8). The possibility of performing a cephalometric and esthetic visual treatment objective (VTO) will be discussed in full in chapter 10.

It should always be remembered that all procedures that entail advancing skeletal structures have a so-called lifting effect on the soft tissues, and therefore tend to produce some facial rejuvenation. This occurs chiefly with osteotomy of the middle third of the face. The opposite can occur with osteotomies that involve setting skeletal structures back, in particular with regard to the mandible and the soft tissue beneath the chin. If mandibular setback is too marked, this may bring about a facial aging effect, especially in older patients.

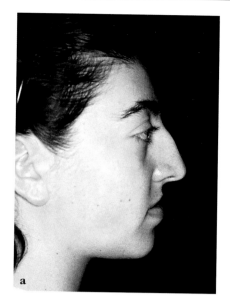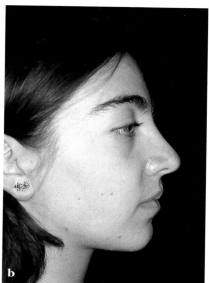

Fig 9-1 Example of a Class III case with indication to advance the maxilla by Le Fort I osteotomy. Preoperative view *(a)* and postoperative view, with rhinoplasty *(b)*.

Class III Malocclusion

The choice of surgical procedure to correct Class III malocclusions essentially takes into account esthetic evaluation in the three planes of space: sagittal, vertical, and transverse. It must answer the following question: Which is more appropriate, a mandibular osteotomy, a maxillary osteotomy, or a double-jaw operation? Cephalometric analysis of skeletal structures takes second place after esthetic considerations; if skeletal values are in agreement with the surgical approach selected on esthetic grounds, so much the better; if not, then esthetic evaluation should always dominate.

Furthermore, surgical correction of Class III malocclusions must always be postponed until growth is completed and thus, in general terms, not performed in women younger than 18 years and men younger than 19 or 20 years. Surgical correction that is done too early can easily lead to a relapse because of residual mandibular growth.

From the sagittal standpoint, the parameters that indicate advancement of the maxilla with Le Fort I osteotomy are flattening of the paranasal areas, accentuated nasogenial fold, moderate flattening of the cheekbones, obtuse nasolabial angle, slight evidence of maxillary prolabium, and prominent nose with some degree of hump and tip tilted downward (Fig 9-1). Where a larger increase at the middle third is necessary, a Bell high osteotomy may be considered because it provides greater fullness at the cheekbones (Fig 9-2). In cases of severe hypoplasia of the middle third of the face with flattening of the inferior orbital rim and scle-

ral exposure, a maxillomalar osteotomy may be employed (Fig 9-3). However, this type of osteotomy (see chapter 7) only affords limited vertical or transverse movement and thus indications are specific: anomaly that is solely anteroposterior, normal or decreased vertical dimension, and maxillary dental midline coinciding with the median axis of symmetry or at most deviated by 2 mm. In other cases, where this type of osteotomy cannot be adopted, the best alternative is the classic Le Fort I osteotomy associated with implantation of alloplastic material in the suborbital area; the materials that are currently most widely used and most reliable are porous polyethylene (Medpor [Porex]; Fig 9-4) and Gore-Tex (W. L. Gore).

The extent of advancement may reach 8 to 10 mm with the classic Le Fort I osteotomy or with the Bell high osteotomy. Slightly less advancement is possible with maxillomalar osteotomy (up to 6 to 7 mm). In general, osteotomy of the maxilla alone may suffice to correct negative overjet of 3 to 4 mm (considering that the advancement required is always 2 to 3 mm more than the existing negative overjet). Naturally, the essential condition is that the position of the mandible is esthetically acceptable and that the mandibular dental midline coincides with the facial midline axis (a compromise of up to 1 mm may be admissible). For larger amounts of initial overjet it may be preferable to consider double-jaw osteotomy in order to avoid excessive bimaxillary protrusion.

With regard to mandibular osteotomy, the preferable types are the Obwegeser–Dal Pont and Gotte osteotomies, if necessary associated with a median osteotomy in selected cases. Correction of Class III mal-

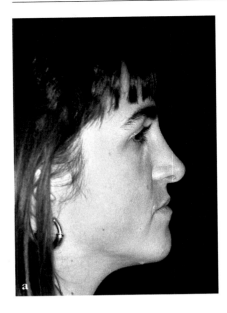

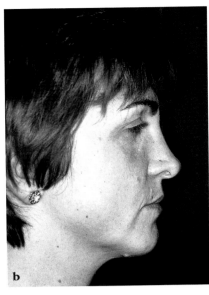

Fig 9-2 Example of a Class III case with indication for a Bell high osteotomy of the maxilla. Preoperative view (a) and postoperative view (b).

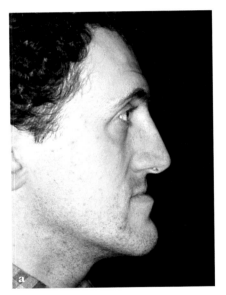

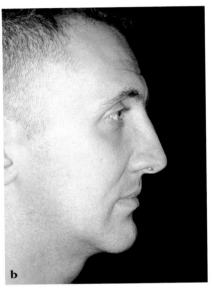

Fig 9-3 Typical orbital-zygomatic retrusion in which a maxillomalar osteotomy is indicated (double-jaw surgery). Preoperative view (a) and postoperative view (b).

occlusion through mandibular osteotomy alone is possible if the middle third is esthetically acceptable and if the maxillary dental midline coincides with the facial midline axis (Fig 9-5). In this case, too, a tolerance of 1 mm is acceptable. With regard to the extent of setback, from the purely surgical standpoint this may even exceed 10 mm. However, correction of Class III cases with mandibular osteotomy alone should be limited to clinical situations with a negative overjet not more than 5 to 6 mm. Double-jaw osteotomy should otherwise be preferred because it guarantees greater skeletal and muscular stability in these cases, as excessive stretching of the pterygomasseteric sling is avoided (see also chapter 13). Furthermore, marked mandibular setback may produce excess soft tissue beneath the chin, which

is unsatisfactory from the esthetic standpoint. It should be remembered that the necessary setback is always 2 to 3 mm more than the preoperative negative overjet, and it is important to take into account that soft tissue pogonion will be retruded by approximately 90% of the surgical setback.

The position of pogonion on the anteroposterior plane may be further modified by genioplasty. It is important that, especially in cases with concomitant open bite or vertical excess with clockwise rotation of the mandible, soft tissue pogonion is often slightly accentuated with a decrease in the labiomental angle. In these patients, although there is Class III malocclusion, advancement genioplasty will be necessary (Fig 9-6).

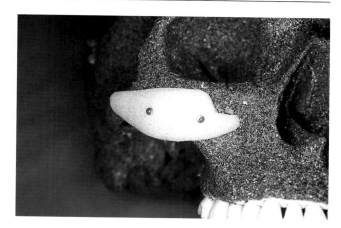

Fig 9-4 Zygomatic implants in porous polyethylene (Medpor).

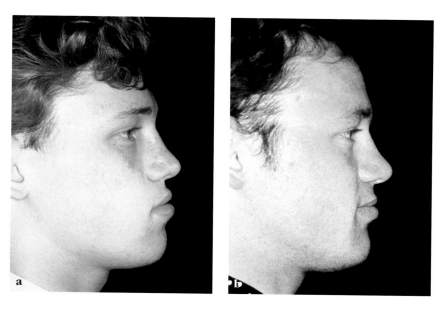

Fig 9-5 Classic example of skeletal Class III malocclusion with indication for simple mandibular setback osteotomy. Preoperative view *(a)* and postoperative view *(b)*.

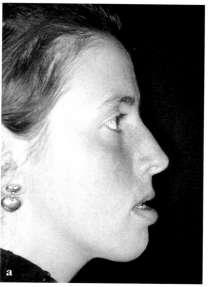
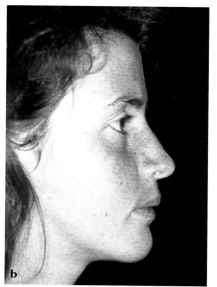

Fig 9-6 Class III malocclusion with clockwise rotation of the mandible; there is also an indication for advancement genioplasty in association with double-jaw surgery. Preoperative view *(a)* and postoperative view *(b)*.

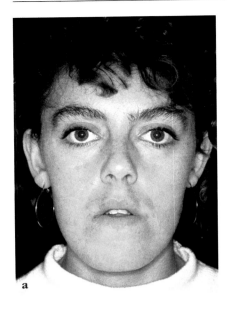

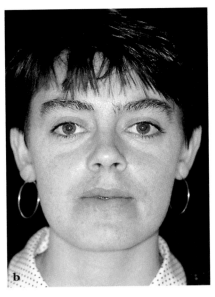

Fig 9-7 Class III malocclusion with vertical excess: indication for double-jaw surgery with superior repositioning of the maxilla. Preoperative view *(a)* and postoperative view *(b)*.

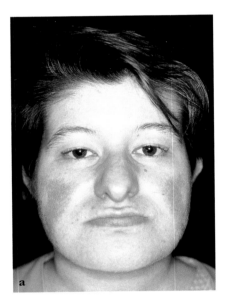

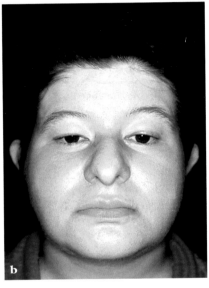

Fig 9-8 Class III malocclusion with vertical hypodevelopment: indication for double-jaw surgery with inferior repositioning of the maxilla. Preoperative view *(a)* and postoperative view *(b)*.

With regard to the vertical dimension, the fundamental parameters to take into consideration are the relationship between lips and teeth, gummy smile if present, labial competence or incompetence, and the ratio between middle and lower thirds of the face. A vertical excess of the maxilla with labial incompetence, gummy smile, and excessive tooth exposure tends to indicate repositioning of the maxilla superiorly (Fig 9-7). Repositioning can be considerable, as much as 10 mm, and in these cases it may be useful to reduce the turbinates surgically (see chapter 7). On the other hand, in a small percentage of cases characterized by little vertical de-

velopment and insufficient tooth exposure (short face), repositioning the maxilla downward is indicated (Fig 9-8). If, however, the vertical excess is exclusively in the lower third, genioplasty with vertical reduction will be required (Fig 9-9) (see chapter 5).

With regard to transverse dimensions, these concern both the occlusal relationship and esthetic parameters. From the occlusal standpoint, transverse discrepancy should be corrected during preoperative orthodontic treatment (see chapter 4). Only in particular cases may segmental maxillary osteotomy, in two or more pieces, or, alternatively median osteotomy of

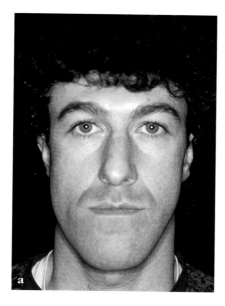 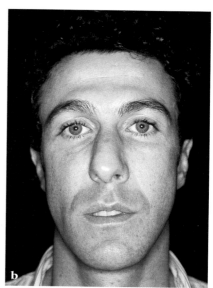

Fig 9-9 Class III malocclusion with vertical excess of the lower third: indication for vertical reduction with genioplasty, associated with double-jaw surgery. Preoperative view *(a)* and postoperative view *(b)*.

the mandible, be considered (see chapters 5 and 7). However, the transverse changes that can be obtained with these types of osteotomy are fairly limited: 3 to 4 mm with maxillary expansion, and the same with the changes that can be produced in mandibular intermolar width, whether by means of reduction or, in rare cases, expansion. This limitation is due, on one hand, to the fact that the palatine fibromucosa is not elastic and, on the other hand, to the action of the pterygoid, masseter, and mylohyoid muscles. With regard to esthetics, the fundamental parameter in the transverse dimension is the ratio between the bizygomatic and the bigonial widths (see chapter 2). In Class III cases there is usually a reduced bizygomatic width, and various methods exist to achieve an increase in this measurement. First, a Bell high osteotomy or a maxillomalar osteotomy may help to increase this width. Alternatively, other surgical methods may be used, such as implantation of alloplastic material (as mentioned above) or a "greenstick" osteotomy of the zygomatic area according to Mommaerts et al (1995 and 1999) (Fig 9-10). These ancillary surgical procedures can be performed concomitantly with a classic Le Fort I osteotomy or be postponed by at least 6 months, depending on clinical indications (where osteotomy is solely for advancement, they may be done simultaneously; in cases where there is also significant vertical movement or rotation of the maxilla, it is preferable to wait several months because of the unpredictability of

soft tissue changes consequent to maxillary rotation; see chapter 8). Lastly, the bigonial width may be slightly reduced, if necessary, by reducing the mandibular angles or by associating a median osteotomy in particular selected cases (see chapter 5). Correction of the mandibular angles may be done quite easily intraorally by reduction with a pear-shaped bur (Fig 9-11a) or through osteotomy and resection with an angled saw (Fig 9-11b).

A final consideration that is no less important concerns the nose: Changes that it will undergo spontaneously must be evaluated (see chapter 8) together with the appropriateness of rhinoplasty, associated or postponed (see the section on rhinoplasty below).

Lastly, there are some lesser procedures that, if performed at an early age, can help to guide growth in a favorable direction and that, in some borderline cases, may reduce the tendency for a skeletal Class III malocclusion to develop. Chapter 1 explained that low tongue posture may be a cause of Class III malocclusion. In some cases this is due to the presence of a short lingual frenulum, and in these situations early lingual frenulectomy may change the posture of the tongue and thus guide the growth pattern in a more favorable physiologic direction. Furthermore, in some patients with a tendency for hypodevelopment of the maxilla, postponing upper lip frenulectomy may help to guide growth more favorably, facilitating early orthodontic and orthopedic treatment.

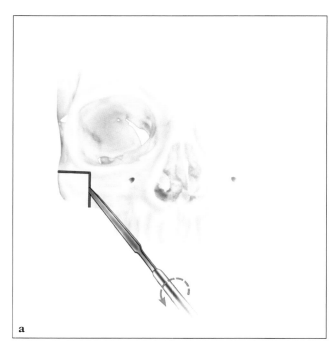
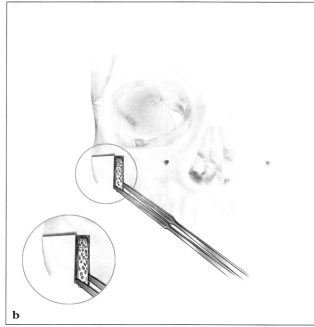

Fig 9-10 Diagram of the Mommaerts technique for zygomatic increase: After the osteotomy lines are made, a greenstick fracture is made with the osteotome *(a)* followed by interposition of autologous bone or alloplastic material *(b)*. The method is performed intraorally.

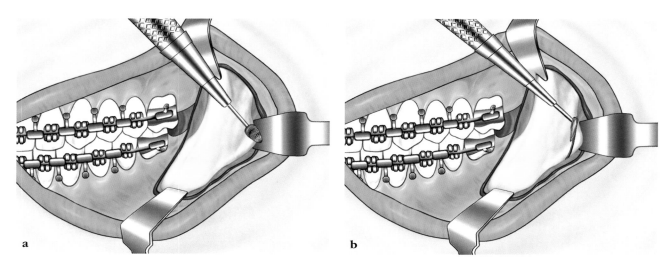

Fig 9-11 Diagram for reduction and/or contouring of the mandibular angles (intraorally) using a bur *(a)* or an angled saw *(b)*.

Class II Malocclusion

In Class II cases, the surgical procedure must also essentially be planned following esthetic rather than cephalometric indications and, again, must take into consideration the three dimensions of space: sagittal, vertical, and transverse.

The esthetic parameters that must be considered have already been mentioned in chapter 1. They concern the nose; the nasolabial angle; the shape and characteristics of the upper lip, including its relationship with the maxillary incisors; the presence or absence of an accentuated nasogenial fold; exposure of tooth and gingiva at rest and when smiling; labial competence or incompetence; tone and shape of the lower lip; position and characteristics of soft tissue pogonion; the labiomental angle; shape and characteristics of the mandibular angles; the suprahyoid muscles; and in general all the soft tissue in this area.

An important initial consideration is that, within Class II cases, in the great majority there is a common clinical feature: mandibular hypodevelopment of both the positional and the structural type. Furthermore, in a very high percentage of cases the maxilla is in the normal position or even retruded. True skeletal maxillary protrusion is an exceptional case.

The apparent initial maxillary protrusion is usually due to a flaring of the maxillary incisors, almost as though in an attempt to compensate naturally for skeletal hypodevelopment and to provide adequate support for the upper lip. Preoperative orthodontic treatment, by repositioning the teeth in their correct inclination, eliminates this compensation and clarifies the maxillary skeletal retrusion, if any. Clinical findings in this situation are supported by cephalometric data (Ellis et al 1985; Lawrence et al 1985; McNamara 1981), although, as already stated, cephalometric values are always less important than clinical and esthetic data. However, correspondence between clinical and cephalometric data obviously helps to strengthen these interpretive concepts of Class II malocclusion (see also chapters 1 and 2).

Thus, in the great majority of cases, correction of a skeletal Class II situation requires a mandibular osteotomy for advancement, generally with the Obwegeser–Dal Pont method. The variant according to Gotte may be used only for fairly limited advancement because it provides less engagement between the two bone segments.

Once the concept has been accepted that mandibular advancement will be necessary (except in particular cases addressed below), two questions must be answered: Can mandibular osteotomy alone fully resolve the esthetic and occlusal problems, or must it be associated with other surgical procedures? Should surgery await completion of growth, or may it be anticipated in patients who are still growing? With regard to the first question, the cephalometric VTO may be of some help (see chapter 10), but the experience and intuition of the surgeon and orthodontist play a fundamental role. Obviously, the answer to this question must concern all three directions in space: sagittal, vertical, and transverse. First and foremost, it is clear that the possibility of correcting a Class II case with mandibular osteotomy alone requires that there be perfect coincidence between the maxillary dental midline and the facial midline axis (again, tolerance is 1 mm) and the presence of a maxillary occlusal plane parallel to the bipupillary line. Esthetic evaluations are also naturally very important.

From the sagittal standpoint, because a structural hypodevelopment of the mandible coexists in a high percentage of cases, advancement genioplasty may also be indicated (Fig 9-12). A Le Fort I maxillary advancement osteotomy (and thus a double-jaw advancement) may also be indicated in patients with a large and prominent nose, thin and retruded upper lip with slight visibility of the prolabium, obtuse nasolabial angle, and accentuated nasogenial fold (Fig 9-13). Moreover, double-jaw advancement may also be considered, independently of cephalometric values, in cases of severe mandibular hypodevelopment in which, for dental and/or periodontal reasons, optimal orthodontic decompensation cannot be achieved, and in which there is a need for the maximum possible advancement of the lower third of the face (Fig 9-14).

From the vertical standpoint, the parameters to consider are the same as those listed above: relationship between lips and teeth, interlabial relationship, gummy smile, and the ratio between the middle and lower thirds of the face. Thus repositioning of the maxilla superiorly may be indicated (Fig 9-15) or, more rarely in cases of a so-called short face, repositioning it inferiorly; both can be achieved with the classic Le Fort I osteotomy. With regard to the lower third of the face, there may be an indication for genioplasty for vertical increase (Fig 9-16). In patients with increased vertical dimension, open bite, and condylar resorption (almost always young women), the procedure must be planned to avoid any skeletal movement that might produce compression at the mandibular condyles.

With regard to transverse parameters, obviously occlusal discrepancies must be resolved during the preparatory orthodontic treatment, as already seen, both through purely orthodontic movements and by

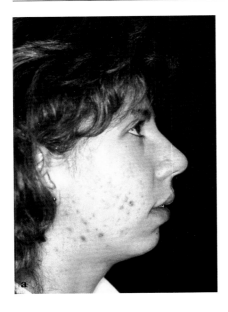

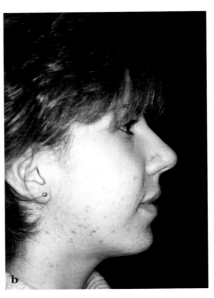

Fig 9-12 Class II case with elective indication for mandibular advancement osteotomy, associated with advancement genioplasty. Preoperative view *(a)* and postoperative view *(b)*.

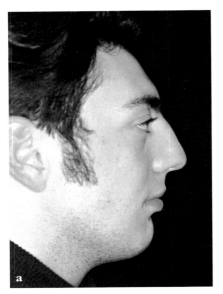

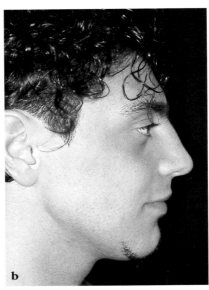

Fig 9-13 Class II case with indication for double-jaw advancement: large nose and thin, retruded upper lip. Preoperative view *(a)* and postoperative view *(b)*.

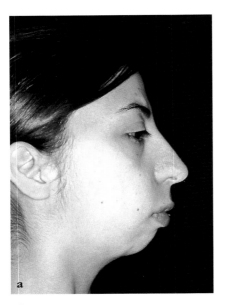

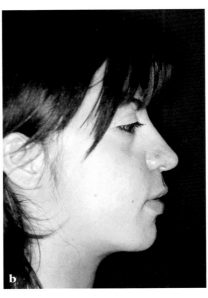

Fig 9-14 Class II case with marked mandibular hypodevelopment and retrusion and insufficient preoperative orthodontic decompensation: indication for double-jaw advancement with advancement genioplasty. Preoperative view *(a)* and postoperative view *(b)*.

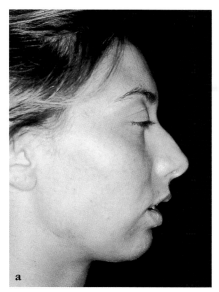
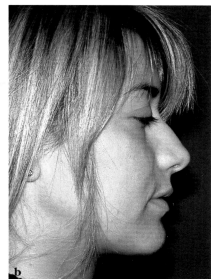

Fig 9-15 Class II case with vertical excess: indication for double-jaw surgery, with superior repositioning of the maxilla and advancement of the mandible. Preoperative view *(a)* and postoperative view *(b)*.

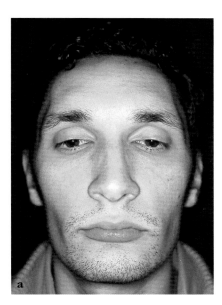
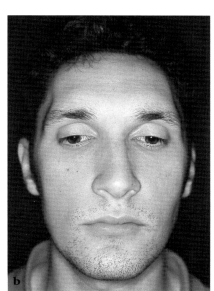

Fig 9-16 Class II case with reduced vertical dimension of the lower third: indication for genioplasty with vertical increase, associated with mandibular advancement osteotomy. Preoperative view *(a)* and postoperative view *(b)*.

combined procedures (see chapter 4). From the esthetic point of view, the transverse diameter at the zygomatic level rarely requires correction. It is more frequent for there to be indications for ancillary surgery at the mandibular angles. In some Class II, division 2 cases, surgical reduction of the mandibular angles may be indicated, with one of the two methods described in Fig 9-11 (Fig 9-17), whereas in patients with severe mandibular hypodevelopment, preformed implants of alloplastic material (Medpor) may be used to accentuate the mandibular angles (Fig 9-18).

Any conditions indicating the need for simultaneous or delayed rhinoplasty must be evaluated (see below). Mandibular distraction osteogenesis may also be indicated as an auxiliary treatment (see chapter 5).

There are a small number of Class II cases that do not require mandibular osteotomy. These patients have a vertical excess of the maxilla, with consequent clockwise rotation of the mandible and moderate dental overjet. In these situations, correction may be achieved by repositioning the maxilla upward, again with a Le Fort I osteotomy, with the corresponding concomitant counterclockwise autorotation of the mandible, which will correct the overjet and advance soft tissue pogonion (Fig 9-19). This procedure must be carefully planned by means of a precise cephalometric VTO (see chapter 10). Opinions differ with regard to timing of the surgical procedure. A favorable effect on growth has been reported to occur following surgical advancement of the mandible in growing subjects (Snow et al 1991; Vig and Turvey 1989), whereas others have found the contrary, with severe relapse (Huang and Ross 1981). The study by Snow et al on 12 patients subjected to surgical advance-

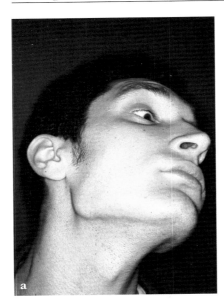
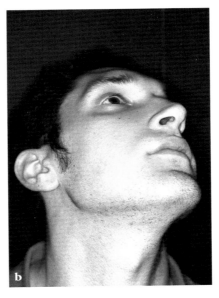

Fig 9-17 Class II, division 2 case with accentuation of the mandibular angles: indication for contouring of the mandibular angles, associated with mandibular advancement osteotomy. Preoperative view *(a)* and postoperative view *(b)*.

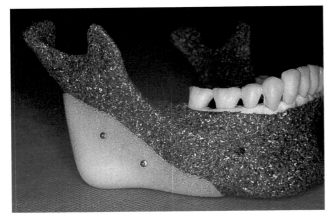

Fig 9-18 Implants for mandibular angles in porous polyethylene (Medpor).

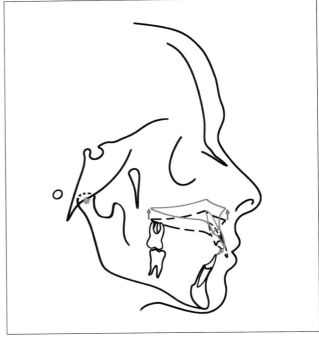

Fig 9-19 Diagram of maxillary superior repositioning and concomitant autorotation of the mandible to correct a slight Class II malocclusion with vertical excess.

ment during growth (mean age at surgery, 14.2 years) reported residual sagittal and vertical mandibular growth in 10 patients. This growth, however, was compensated by vertical growth of the maxilla, so that the anteroposterior position of pogonion did not change. We may, therefore, reasonably suppose that surgery for mandibular advancement alone, in the absence of maxillary or vertical problems, may be performed before the end of adolescence, provided that

the growth peak is concluded, which means at least 6 to 12 months after the onset of menarche in girls. For boys the timing is obviously more difficult to evaluate, and an acceptable age for early surgery might be around 14 to 15 years. In all other patients, in whom vertical problems coexist or double-jaw surgery is indicated, it is more prudent to await the end of adolescence: 18 years for girls and 19 to 20 years for boys.

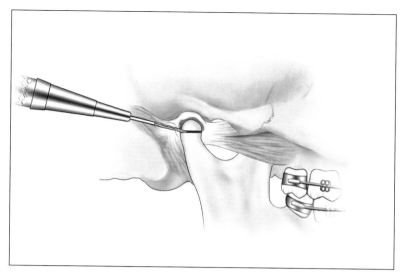

Fig 9-20 Diagram of high condylectomy, indicated in cases of active condylar hyperplasia.

Dentofacial Asymmetry

The principal aim in this type of anomaly is naturally to achieve as symmetric a result as possible, although perfect and absolute symmetry cannot always be achieved. Indeed there is always some degree of asymmetry between the two halves of any face, however attractive the appearance. As discussed in chapter 2, symmetry is inseparable from the concept of harmonious proportions and attractiveness, and thus increasing symmetry will inevitably improve esthetics.

In planning surgery to treat dentofacial asymmetries, there are two fundamental aspects to consider, and the following questions must be answered: Is there any pathologic condylar growth still in the active phase? Will maxillary osteotomy be required to achieve symmetry? Is surgery indicated at an early stage of growth, or is it always preferable to wait until the period of adolescence is over?

With regard to condylar growth, if active pathologic growth is suspected, it can be investigated and demonstrated by bone scintigraphy with technetium 99 (see chapter 1). Unfortunately, though, false negatives may occur with this imaging method. It is important to keep this in mind since active pathologic growth may cause long-term relapses that cannot otherwise be explained.

Where severe pathologic condylar growth has been ascertained through scintigraphy and is in continual and rapid evolution but has not yet caused significant

compensatory inclination of the maxilla (this situation usually occurs immediately after the peak of growth at puberty), early surgical treatment by high condylectomy on the affected side may be considered. The access route is preauricular, as described by Brusati and Sesenna (1988) (Fig 9-20), and the procedure should be accompanied on the healthy side by vertical osteotomy of the mandibular ramus performed intraorally. This approach should enable self-correction of the malformation to occur by modification of the unfavorable growth pattern and prevention of the maxilla from becoming involved in the malformation process (West 1994). It is obviously necessary to provide suitable postoperative orthodontic treatment for these patients, as well as particularly careful follow-up. However, opinions are not in complete agreement about this method, others (Klaassen and Steinhäuser 1994) being of the opinion that scintigraphy is not very reliable; Klaassen and Steinhäuser also report a marked increase in functional joint disorders in patients subjected to condylectomy during growth. In all other cases, in which there is already evident deviation of the maxilla, it is more prudent to postpone surgical correction until the end of adolescence.

In adults in whom growth is completed, both the position of the maxilla and the characteristics of the condyles must be taken into account. Where there is no significant demonstrable pathologic condylar growth and no alterations of the maxilla in any of the three dimensions in space, evaluated both clinically and cephalometrically (in this case, posteroanterior

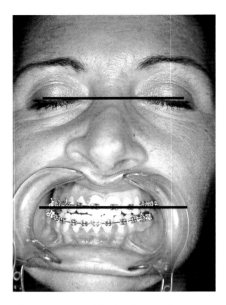 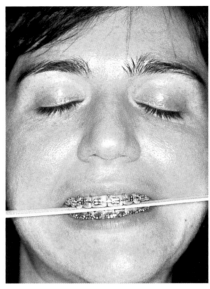 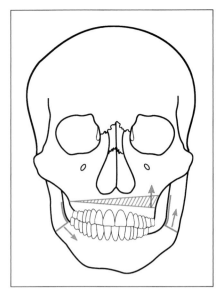

Fig 9-21 Mandibular laterodeviation (hemimandibular elongation): The favorable position of the maxilla and maxillary dental midline indicate mandibular osteotomy alone.

Fig 9-22 Dentofacial asymmetry with inclination of the maxilla: Double-jaw surgery is indicated.

Fig 9-23 Diagram of the osteotomy lines in dentofacial asymmetry with canting of the occlusal plane.

cephalometry may be important), mandibular surgery may suffice for correction (Fig 9-21). The most indicated types of osteotomy are classic bilateral osteotomy according to Obwegeser–Dal Pont or, even better, the variant according to Gotte, which carries a lower risk of distorting or dislocating the condyles (see chapter 6). In some cases, an Obwegeser–Dal Pont or Gotte osteotomy may be performed on the side where the mandible is advanced, associated with vertical osteotomy of the ramus on the side where the mandible is retruded. Naturally, in this situation, a period of maxillomandibular fixation will be needed.

If the position of the maxilla is altered, even if in only one direction of space, double-jaw osteotomy will be required. In these patients, clinical examination of the maxilla, as described in chapter 1, is very important, and the occlusal plane, the dental midline, and the position of the canines must be evaluated. Cephalometric data also has its own importance, especially on the diagram in posteroanterior projection. The exact position of the maxilla is of fundamental importance in patients with dentofacial asymmetry (Fig 9-22). Although planning methods have recently been proposed that start with mandibular repositioning as the focus of surgery (Raffaini and Brevi 1994), the au-

thor believes that the classic and most frequently reported sequence, which starts from the perfect repositioning of the maxilla and continues with correction of the mandible, is still the most reliable (Fig 9-23). Problems relating to model surgery and the use of intermediate splints are addressed in chapter 10.

For adult patients who have definitely completed growth but in whom scintigraphy is positive for residual condylar growth, the problem arises of whether it is necessary to intervene on the affected condyle at the same time the other osteotomies are performed, or whether it is better to wait until scintigraphy normalizes and provides certainty that growth is complete here too. In these patients, a positive finding from scintigraphy might also indicate condylar growth as the consequence of asymmetric malformations rather than their cause; condylar growth would be a functional response by the condyle to an altered anatomic conformation. In this case, surgical correction with classic osteotomies would produce condylar normalization. However, there is no generalized agreement surrounding this problem. To wait for scintigraphy to normalize may be the correct approach in patients aged 18 or 20 years. The extent of the positive value provided by scintigraphy may offer some help in decision making. Where

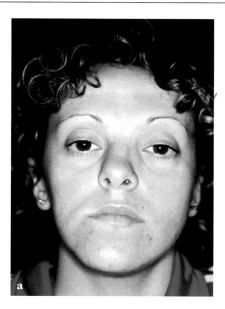 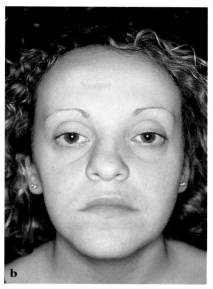

Fig 9-24 Dentofacial asymmetry with compensatory deviation of the nose *(a)*; after correction of the dentofacial asymmetry, the deviation of the nose is more evident *(b)*.

the value is markedly elevated and is supported by computerized tomography examination, simultaneous condylectomy is indicated. In less clear-cut cases it is reasonable to wait for some months and repeat the test. If the scintigraphy value has decreased, or in any case has not further increased, then classic osteotomy surgery may follow.

On the contrary, if a simultaneous condylectomy is indicated, the surgical sequence is as follows: Where mandibular repositioning is sufficient, high condylectomy is first performed on the affected side, followed by compensatory contralateral osteotomy, which may be done according to the technique of Obwegeser–Dal Pont or that of Gotte. In cases of double-jaw osteotomy, the maxilla is first repositioned (with or without an intermediate splint; see chapter 10), and then high condylectomy is performed on the affected side followed by osteotomy according to Obwegeser–Dal Pont or Gotte on the same side. On the contralateral side one of these two osteotomy techniques, or alternatively simple vertical osteotomy of the ramus, may be adopted.

Lastly, ancillary procedures are of fundamental importance in providing complete treatment for dentofacial asymmetries. In many cases, ancillary surgical procedures are required at the chin, outline and corners of the mandible, or nose. There is substantial agreement that it is preferable to postpone these procedures for at least 6 months because three-dimensional adaptation of the soft tissues to the new skeletal configuration may mask or accentuate other residual imperfections or slight asymmetries. Genioplasty may be performed in one of the different configurations described in chapter 5. In some cases hemigenioplasty may be indicated, as described by Raffaini et al (1994) (see chapter 5). To correct the mandibular outline and/or angles, contouring techniques may be used (see Fig 9-11) or alloplastic material (Medpor) may be grafted or implanted (see Fig 9-18). Structural hypodevelopment can often only be corrected in this way: Apposition bone grafts frequently undergo marked and unpredictable resorption.

Particular attention must be paid to the nose: Deviation of the nose often occurs as a compensatory mechanism for the dentofacial malformation, and this may become apparent or more noticeable once the underlying asymmetry has been corrected. Rhinoplasty will be necessary in these cases but should always be postponed to a subsequent phase (Fig 9-24).

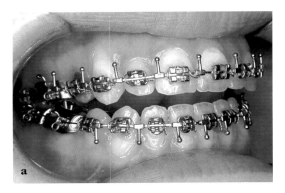

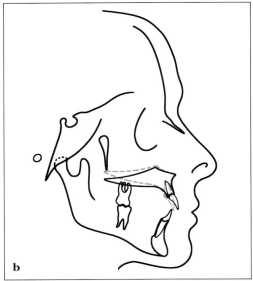

Fig 9-25 Example of open bite *(a)* that can be corrected by maxillary osteotomy and mandibular autorotation *(b)*.

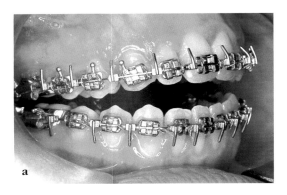

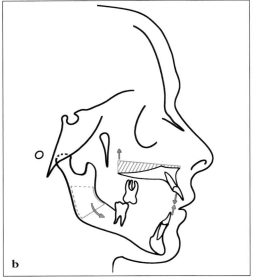

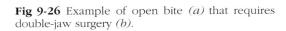

Fig 9-26 Example of open bite *(a)* that requires double-jaw surgery *(b)*.

Open Bite

Open bite is the dentofacial anomaly for which, in the author's opinion, cephalometric data take on determinant importance, often even dominating esthetic considerations. In total open bite there is always a vertical alteration of the maxilla, in excess, accompanied by a reduction in the craniospinal angle, which may even take on a negative value. This is accompanied by a concomitant clockwise autorotation of the mandible, in some cases aggravated by an increase in the gonial angle. Normalization of the craniospinal angle thus becomes the necessary and irreplaceable cornerstone for correcting open bite.

In these situations, the elective intervention consists of Le Fort I maxillary osteotomy; the maxilla is repositioned superiorly, the extent of this repositioning being much more marked in the posterior part (thanks to the use of a posterior cuneiform osteotomy). In less severe cases (anterior open bite of 2 to 3 mm), the bite can be closed with simple concomitant autorotation of the mandible (Fig 9-25). In cases with greater vertical discrepancy (maxillary anterior dental open bite more than 3 mm), a mandibular Obwegeser–Dal Pont or Gotte osteotomy will need to be associated with the maxillary osteotomy. In these cases the bite cannot be closed simply by raising and rotating the maxilla in association with concomitant autorotation of the mandible (Fig 9-26).

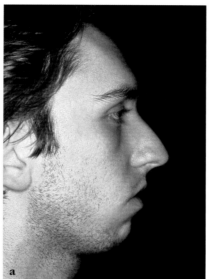
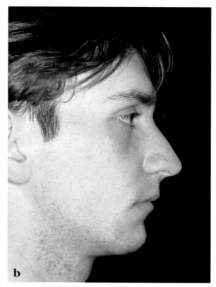
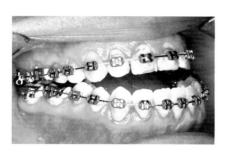

Fig 9-27 Example of severe anterior open bite that requires three-piece maxillary osteotomy and mandibular Kole anterior subapical osteotomy (accentuation of the maxillary curvature and inversion of the curve of Spee).

Fig 9-28 Open bite with deficient mental symphysis; indication for advancement genioplasty associated with double-jaw surgery. Preoperative view *(a)* and postoperative view *(b)*.

An old concept that should be discredited in treating open bite is that the gonial angle is inviolable. Thanks partly to the adoption of rigid fixation, the gonial angle may be reduced, obviously in those cases with angular values above the normal range (130 ± 7 degrees; see chapter 2). Nevertheless, some manipulation of the gonial angle may be accepted even in cases with values within the normal range: Since this range is a full 14 degrees, a decrease may usually be achieved while remaining within it. For variations of this magnitude, the musculature adapts relatively quickly to the new situation. To obtain adequate correction of the gonial angle, Gotte bilateral osteotomy of the mandibular angle is, in the author's opinion, more indicated than the traditional Obwegeser–Dal Pont osteotomy because it acts directly on the angle of the mandible (see chapter 5).

Naturally, in planning surgical displacement in open bite cases, great care must always be taken with the pterygomasseteric sling. Stretching or applying excessive stress to these muscles will inevitably cause relapse, and it is therefore of determinant importance to evaluate cephalometric data at this level very carefully.

In anterior open bite cases, as already mentioned in chapter 4, a three-piece maxillary osteotomy may

be indicated, with clockwise rotation of the anterior segment. Generally, since the anterior open bite also involves the mandibular arch, it will be necessary to employ a mandibular Gotte osteotomy and/or a Kole anterior subapical osteotomy (Fig 9-27).

Although particular attention must be paid to some cephalometric details (craniospinal angle, gonial angle, anterior and posterior vertical height) and to some functional aspects (maxillary curvature and curve of Spee), this does not mean that esthetic problems are of secondary importance. We can act on facial esthetics by suitably modulating the displacement of the two jaws on the sagittal plane. Correction of vertical problems proceeds in conjunction with correction of the dental open bite, and the chin also plays a very important role in these patients. There is frequently a vertical excess associated with some anteroposterior retrusion, and appropriate genioplasty to advance the chin, combined with vertical reduction, will be required to solve these problems adequately (Fig 9-28).

It must also be decided whether simultaneous or delayed rhinoplasty should be performed, as will be examined in more detail in the next section.

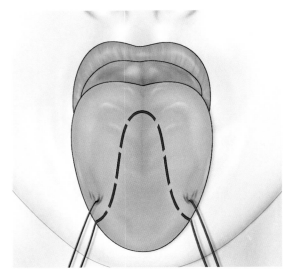

Fig 9-29 Diagram of incision for partial glossectomy according to Kole (Capozzi et al 1969).

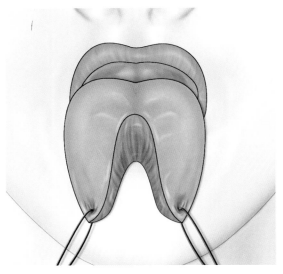

Fig 9-30 Full-thickness resection in the area of the tip and partial thickness resection in the central area.

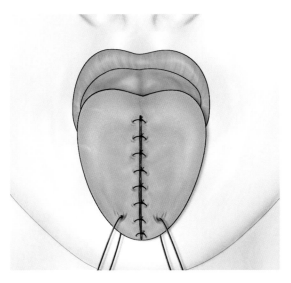

Fig 9-31 Suturing.

One last consideration must be made with regard to the tongue. As seen in chapter 1, the tongue can play a role in causing open bite. In most cases, the problem concerns tongue posture and thus should be corrected with osteotomies, suitably planned from the cephalometric standpoint, and, most importantly, associated with adequate preoperative and postoperative reeducation physiotherapy, if necessary under the guide of a speech specialist.

Nevertheless, there are rare cases of true macroglossia (see chapter 1). In these cases, and only when the diagnosis is certain, partial glossectomy should be performed either at the same time as the osteotomy or, if maxillomandibular fixation is planned, 1 week earlier. The most widely used technique to reduce the size of the tongue both longitudinally and transversely is that proposed by Kole (Capozzi et al 1969), shown in Figs 9-29 to 9-31.

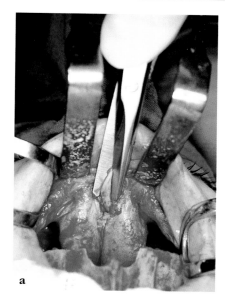
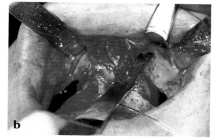
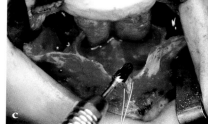

Fig 9-32 Resection of the base of the septum *(a)*, basal osteotomies *(b)*, and contouring of the anterior nasal spine and the piriform apertures *(c)*.

Double-Jaw Osteotomy and Rhinoplasty

The introduction of rigid fixation has enabled the surgeon to make all the necessary corrections, including rhinoplasty, in a single operation, and without doubt this is an interesting possibility. However, some considerations concerning the suitability of this combined procedure are necessary: First and foremost, as discussed in chapter 8, spontaneous changes occur to the nose following maxillary osteotomy. These may be favorable or unfavorable, and their implications must be clearly understood.

The philosophy that can and must guide the surgeon in deciding whether rhinoplasty should be done simultaneously is a dual one: to take advantage of correcting all anomalies in a single operation, exploiting the favorable effects of maxillary osteotomy to the full, and to eliminate all unfavorable effects.

If the favorable effects are emphasized and exploited to the best, in some cases a limited rhinoplasty may suffice, with minimal resection of the hump and alar cartilage. This is often the case in patients with a narrow nose, some degree of hump, and the tip tilted downward. Current trends on the principles of rhinoplasty adapt well to these situations. It is also important to remember that some maneuvers, such as correcting the septum, basal osteotomies, and contouring of the nasal spine and piriform apertures, can be performed at the time of surgery under direct visual control, once the maxilla has been mobilized and before definitive fixation is completed (Fig 9-32).

The unfavorable effects, which substantially consist of a widening of the alar base and an increased depression in the supratip area, may be eliminated through some relatively simple techniques, such as making a full-thickness reduction of the nasal alae and grafting a fragment of cartilage, which can quite easily be taken from the nasal septum after mobilization of the maxilla, onto the dorsum of the nose.

Notes on surgical technique. The operation begins with nasotracheal intubation, which must be put in place in a particularly atraumatic and gentle fashion by an anesthetist who is properly trained in this type of maneuver. The maxillary or double-jaw osteotomy is then performed according to the planned technique. Particular care must be taken during all surgical maneuvers, which must be extremely gentle to minimize intraoperative and postoperative edema. For this purpose, intraoperative methylprednisolone may also be administered. Great care is needed when detaching the floor of the nose to avoid laceration. When indicated, resection of the base of the septum is performed after the downfracture. In this way, a preexisting deviation may easily be corrected and cartilage may be harvested for later use. Rigid fixation is then applied and the occlusion obtained is very carefully checked. If the occlusion is perfect and stable, osteotomy of the nasal bone is then performed, in open surgery, before the mucosa is sutured but without completion of the fracture upward. The alar base is then cinched and/or sutured to the anterior nasal spine, and the mucosa of the superior fornix is closed. These two phases are of great importance and must be very precise to obtain the best possible control over the width of the base of the nose and the projection of the upper lip. Intubation is then switched from nasotracheal to orotracheal. The operative field is then regained, and rhinoplasty is completed by making marginal and/or intercartilage incisions and, depending on requirements, resecting the hump, contouring the alar cartilage, completing the nasal base osteotomies, placing cartilage grafts on the dorsum if indicated, and, if necessary, making a further reduction of the alar base.

From the above considerations, it is clear that indications for simultaneous rhinoplasty and double-jaw osteotomy are as follows:

- A narrow nose with narrow alar base, pronounced hump, and tip tilted downward is the elective indication for a combined operation, because small retouching can be done and the favorable effects of maxillary osteotomy can be exploited in full. This applies to Class III and Class II cases, as well as cases of slight open bite (Fig 9-33).
- In patients with a narrow nose with a small hump and tip pointing slightly downward, the favorable

spontaneous changes induced by maxillary osteotomy are generally sufficient to obtain an excellent esthetic result without rhinoplasty. If necessary, the final results can be further optimized by suitably modulating the displacement of the maxilla and carefully and appropriately managing soft tissue closure, as described in chapters 7 and 8 (Fig 9-34).
- In patients with a globular tip and/or one that tilts upward, and in whom maxillary osteotomy is indicated for sagittal, vertical, or transverse correction, rhinoplasty may be indicated, primarily to eliminate the unfavorable effects at the level of the supratip, with reduction and contouring of the alar cartilage and cartilage graft at the dorsum of the nose (Fig 9-35).

Naturally, especially when double-jaw osteotomy and simultaneous rhinoplasty are planned, in male subjects it will be necessary to maintain a typically male profile and shape, and to leave a somewhat larger nose, while avoiding an excessive upward tilt at the tip. A slight hump may be preferable rather than an excessively thin tip that is tilted too far upward (Fig 9-36).

In patients in whom significant rotation of the maxilla is planned, for example, as in moderate-to-severe open bite, simultaneous rhinoplasty is contraindicated because of the difficulty or impossibility of predicting the spontaneous changes to the nose and soft tissues consequent to such rotation (see chapter 8).

Furthermore, simultaneous rhinoplasty is severely contraindicated in all cases of dentofacial asymmetry, in which, as seen in the previous sections, cosmetic correction should be postponed by at least 6 months. Lastly, for cases in which rather complex rhinoplasty will be necessary and/or open surgery will be needed (very large noses, complete deviation, tip asymmetry, cleft lip sequelae), it is preferable to postpone the rhinoplasty until bone and soft tissues have had time to stabilize.

A last consideration concerning the association of rhinoplasty with mandibular osteotomy alone: In these cases there is normally no particular contraindication to combining the two operations, thanks to the predictability of the skeletal and soft tissue outcome (Fig 9-37), except in cases with significant mandibular laterodeviation, as seen above.

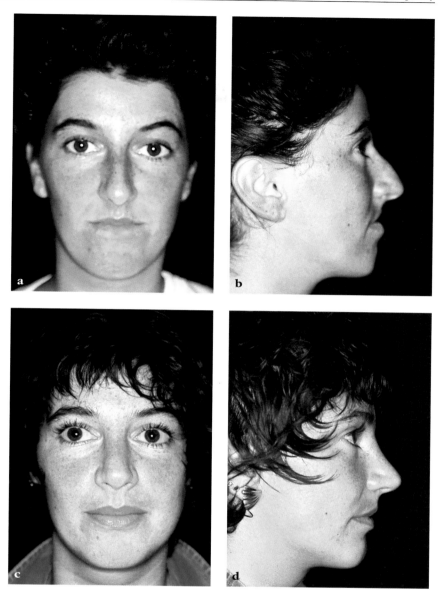

Fig 9-33 Skeletal Class III case with typical indication for double-jaw surgery and simultaneous rhinoplasty. Preoperative views *(a and b)* and postoperative views *(c and d).*

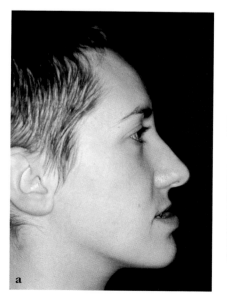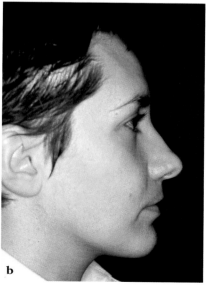

Fig 9-34 Class III case with indication for double-jaw surgery: In this case the spontaneous and predictable changes to the nose mean that rhinoplasty is not required. Preoperative view *(a)* and postoperative view *(b).*

155

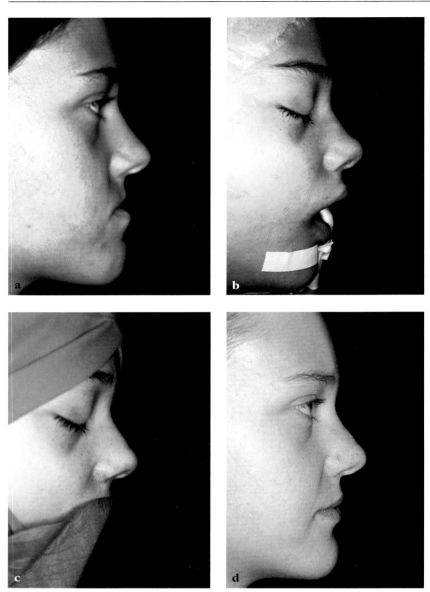

Fig 9-35 Class III case requiring double-jaw surgery (a); the configuration of the nose after the osteotomies (b); the profile after rhinoplasty with cartilage graft (c); and the long-term result (d).

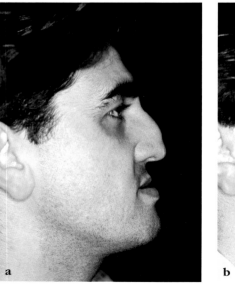
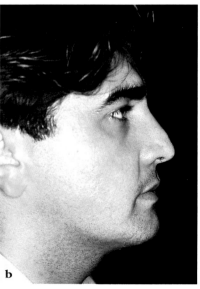

Fig 9-36 Class III case with indication for double-jaw surgery and rhinoplasty; in male patients the reduction of the nose should not be excessive. Preoperative view (a) and postoperative view (b).

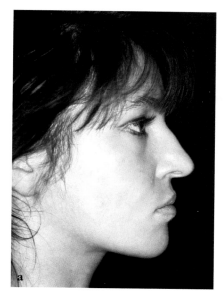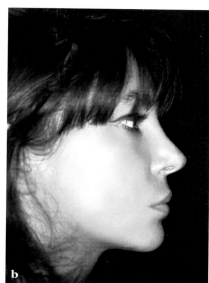

Fig 9-37 Class III case with indication for mandibular setback osteotomy alone: Association of rhinoplasty is not particularly problematic. Preoperative view *(a)* and postoperative view *(b)*.

To conclude, the association of rhinoplasty with single- or double-jaw osteotomy makes it possible, during a single operation, to correct significant esthetic and functional problems, with the undoubted advantage of patient satisfaction. However, this method should be used with caution and only after gaining an indepth knowledge of the spontaneous changes that occur to the soft tissues following osteotomy. Furthermore, rigid fixation must be employed and thus absolutely perfect orthodontic preparation is needed. Lastly, collaboration of the anesthetist and intraoperative and postoperative control of edema are of fundamental importance.

Bibliography

Ayoub AF, Stirrups DR, Moos KF. Stability of sagittal split advancement osteotomy: Single- versus double-jaw surgery. Int J Adult Orthodon Orthognath Surg 1995;10:181–192.

Becelli R, Renzi G, Carboni A, Cerulli G, Perugini M. Evaluation of the esthetic results of a 40-patient group treated surgically for dentoskeletal Class III malocclusion. Int J Adult Orthodon Orthognath Surg 2002;17:171–179.

Benech A, Oria A, Fornengo B, Modica R. An evaluation of the postoperative stability of the dental arches following interventions for segmental osteotomy [in Italian]. Minerva Stomatol 1991;40:15–22.

Brusati R, Sesenna E. Chirurgia delle deformità mascellari. Milan: Masson, 1988.

Busby BR, Bailey LJ, Proffit WR, Phillis C, White RP Jr. Long-term stability of surgical Class III treatment: A study of 5-year postsurgical results. Int J Adult Orthodon Orthognath Surg 2002;17:159–170.

Capozzi L, Kole H, Rossi G, Perko M, Miclavez N. Chirurgia ortognatodontica. Venice: S. Nicolò, 1969:97–103.

Carlotti AE, Aschaffenburg PA, Schendel SA. Facial changes associated with surgical advancement of the lip and maxilla. J Oral Maxillofac Surg 1986;44:593–596.

Cottrell DA, Wolford LM. Factors influencing combined orthognathic and rhinoplastic surgery. Int J Adult Orthodon Orthognath Surg 1993;8:265–276.

Ellis E 3rd, McNamara JA Jr, Lawrence T. Components of adult Class II open bite malocclusion. J Oral Maxillofac Surg 1985;43:92–105.

Fini G, Govoni FA, Migliano E, Liberatore GM. La settorinoplastica in chirurgia ortognatica. Riv Ital Chir Maxillofac 1994;5:17–25.

Fridrich L, Casko JS. Genioplasty strategies for anterior facial vertical dysplasias. Int J Adult Orthodon Orthognath Surg 1997;12:35–41.

Hoffman GR, Moloney FB, Effeney DJ. The stability of facial advancement surgery (in the management of combined mid and lower dento-facial deficiency). J Craniomaxillofac Surg 1994;22:86–94.

Huang CS, Ross PB. Surgical advancement of the mandible in growing children. Am J Orthod 1981;82:89–98.

Jensen AC, Sinclair PM, Wolford LM. Soft tissue changes associated with double jaw surgery. Am J Orthod Dentofacial Orthop 1992;101:266–275.

Kahnberg KE. Correction of maxillofacial asymmetry using orthognathic surgical methods. J Craniomaxillofac Surg 1997;25:254–260.

Kawamoto HK Jr. Discussion of reduction mentoplasty. Plast Reconstr Surg 1982;70:151–167.

Klaassen PPJO, Steinhäuser EW. Long-term treatment evaluation of hemimandibular hyperplasia. J Craniomaxillofac Surg 1994;22:16–17.

Kwon TG, Mori Y, Minami K, Lee SH, Sakuda M. Stability of simultaneous maxillary and mandibular osteotomy for treatment of Class III malocclusion: An analysis of three-dimensional cephalograms. J Craniomaxillofac Surg 2000; 28:272–277.

Lawrence T, Ellis E 3rd, McNamara JA Jr. The frequency and distribution of skeletal and dental components in Class II orthognathic surgery patients. J Oral Maxillofac Surg 1985;43:24–34.

Lugstein A, Mossbock R. Correction of open bite by mandibular surgery. Int J Adult Orthodon Orthognath Surg 1990; 5:125–132.

Marchetti C, Cocchi R, Gentile L, Bianchi A, Bassi M. Ruolo della condilectomia nell'hemimandibular hyperplasia. Riv Ital Chir Maxillofac 1997;8:21–29.

McNamara JA Jr. Components of Class II in children 8-10 years of age. Angle Orthod 1981;51:177–202.

Mobarak KA, Krogstad O, Espeland L, Lyberg T. Long-term stability of mandibular setback surgery: A follow-up of 80 bilateral sagittal split osteotomy patients. Int J Adult Orthodon Orthognath Surg 2000;15:83–95.

Mommaerts MY, Abeloos JV, De Clerq CA, Neyt LF. The "sandwich" zygomatic osteotomy: Technique, indications and clinical results. J Craniomaxillofac Surg 1995;23:12–19.

Mommaerts MY, Nadjmi N, Abeloos JV, Neyt LF. Six year's experiences with the zygomatic "sandwich" osteotomy for correction of malar deficiency. J Oral Maxillofac Surg 1999;57:8–13.

Müller-Schelken H. Esthetic corrections in cases of orthognathic surgery. Int J Adult Orthodon Orthognath Surg 1989;4:229–237.

Obwegeser HL, Makek MS. Hemimandibular hyperplasia—Hemimandibular elongation. J Maxillofac Surg 1986;14: 183–208.

Oliveira JAGP, Bloomquist DS. The stability of the use of bilateral sagittal split osteotomy in the closure of anterior open bite. Int J Adult Orthodon Orthognath Surg 1997;12: 101–108.

O'Ryan F, Schendel S. Nasal anatomy and maxillary surgery. I. Esthetic and anatomic principles. Int J Adult Orthodon Orthognath Surg 1989a;4:27–37.

O'Ryan F, Schendel S. Nasal anatomy and maxillary surgery. II. Unfavorable nasolabial esthetics following Le Fort I osteotomy. Int J Adult Orthodon Orthognath Surg 1989b;4:75–84.

O'Ryan F, Schendel S, Carlotti A. Nasal anatomy and maxillary surgery. III. Surgical techniques for correction of nasal deformities in patients undergoing maxillary surgery. Int J Adult Orthodon Orthognath Surg 1989;4:157–174.

Proffit WR, Phillips C, Tulloch JFC, Medland PH. Surgical versus orthodontic correction of skeletal Class II malocclusion in adolescents: Effects and indications. Int J Adult Orthodon Orthognath Surg 1992;7:209–220.

Raffaini M, Brevi B. Una proposta di razionalizzazione nel trattamento delle asimmetrie mandibolo-facciali dell'adulto. Ortognatodonzia Ital 1994;3:513–541.

Raffaini M, Monteverdi R, Sesenna E. L'emimentoplastica: Una tecnica per correggere le asimmetrie del mento. Riv Ital Chir Maxillofac 1994;5:9–11.

Reynolds S, Ellis E 3rd, Carlson D. Adaptation of the suprahyoid muscle complex to large mandibular advancements. J Oral Maxillofac Surg 1988;46:1077–1085.

Robiony M, Costa F, Demitri V, Politi M. Iperplasia emimandibolare e allungamento emimandibolare: Ruolo della scintigrafia ossea. Riv Ital Chir Maxillofac 1997;3;17–21.

Ronchi P, Moncada R, Frattini D, Marinoni M. La rinoplastica associata alle osteotomie maxillo-mandibolari: Possibilità e indicazioni. Riv Ital Chir Maxillofac 1995;6;33–40.

Ronchi P, Chiapasco M. Simultaneous rhinoplasty and maxillomandibular osteotomies: Indications and contraindications. Int J Adult Orthodon Orthognath Surg 1998;13: 153–161.

Schendel SA, Eisenfeld JH, Bell WH, Epker BN. Superior repositioning of the maxilla: Stability and soft tissue osseous relations. Am J Orthod 1976;70:663–674.

Schendel SA, Carlotti AE. Nasal considerations in orthognathic surgery. Am J Orthod Dentofacial Orthop 1991;100: 197–208.

Severt TR, Proffit WR. Postsurgical stability following correction of severe facial asymmetry. Int J Adult Orthodon Orthognath Surg 1997;12:251–261.

Simmons KE, Turvey TA, Phillips C, Proffit WR. Surgical-orthodontic correction of mandibular deficiency: Five-year follow-up. Int J Adult Orthodon Orthognath Surg 1992;7: 67–79.

Snow MD, Turvey TA, Walker D, Proffit WR. Surgical mandibular advancement in adolescents: Postsurgical growth related to stability. Int J Adult Orthodon Orthognath Surg 1991;6:143–154.

Vig KWL, Turvey TA. Surgical correction of vertical maxillary excess during adolescence. Int J Adult Orthodon Orthognath Surg 1989;4:119–128.

West R. Hemimandibular hyperplasia and elongation. J Craniomaxillofac Surg 1994;22:10–11.

Wolford LM. The sagittal split ramus osteotomy as the preferred treatment for mandibular prognathism. J Oral Maxillofac Surg 2000;58:310–312.

Recommended reading

Proffit WR, White RP Jr. Surgical-Orthodontic Treatment. St Louis: Mosby, 1991.

10

Surgical Planning and Simulation

with Luigi Colombo

- Surgical feasibility criteria
- Cephalometric visual treatment objective
- Esthetic visual treatment objective
- Orthodontic-surgical clinical record
- Model surgery and intermediate splint
- Preparation of final splint

Surgical Feasibility Criteria

Surgical feasibility means that the planned osteotomy, be it a single- or double-jaw operation, is technically possible and will achieve a postoperative occlusion (the so-called surgical occlusion) that is sufficiently stable and will provide good stability in the immediate postoperative period. Hence surgical feasibility must be evaluated primarily, if not exclusively, through study cast analysis.

The main criteria that must be taken into account for the final occlusion are as follows: the canine relationship must be a perfect Class I; the dental midlines must be centered; the anterior overbite must be approximately 1 to 2 mm (3 mm in cases of open bite); the overjet must be 1 to 2 mm (preferably 2 mm in Class III cases and 1 mm in Class II cases); and the molar relationship must be correct, depending on the initial planning (Class I, II, or III, depending on any planned extraction of premolars; see chapter 4).

The casts are evaluated manually by placing them in the planned occlusion following the molar class; the occlusion is checked to ensure that there are no deviating premature contacts (Fig 10-1). In some cases, selective grinding at the cusps or, preferably, the fossae of some premolars or molars may be necessary and is permissible. The required amount of grinding should be limited; otherwise it will be necessary to make further orthodontic correction.

As a general rule it is always preferable to perform all orthodontic correction in the preoperative phase to achieve a surgical occlusion as near ideal as possible. This makes it possible to accelerate the period of postoperative physiotherapy (see chapter 11), with undoubted advantages both from the functional standpoint and with regard to medium- and long-term

stability. If necessary, some fairly simple maneuvers may be postponed until the postoperative phase, such as closure of any diastemas and slight lateral open bite at the premolars. In the surgical occlusion, a moderate crossbite limited to one or two premolars or molars may even be tolerated (dental and not skeletal). This may easily and quickly be corrected in the postoperative phase.

Only when specific orthodontic movements are not possible initially is an incomplete surgical occlusion acceptable, but this will require the use of particular splints in the postoperative period, as well as an even more careful management of the patient during this phase. This is most likely to occur in Class II, division 2 cases with a very accentuated curve of Spee. In these cases, complete leveling of the curve of Spee, with extrusion of the premolars, can be done more easily after surgery. Only anterior contacts and those at the molar level are maintained with the splint (Fig 10-2).

In light of the above, it is inevitable that impressions must be taken and casts made from them very frequently, especially during the last phases of preoperative orthodontic treatment, when they are required on the occasion of nearly every checkup. Obviously, these impressions are taken without the archwires in place, and the plaster casts must be of excellent quality (Fig 10-3).

Once full surgical feasibility has been ascertained, the rectangular arches are prepared with the related surgical brackets (Fig 10-4). In particular, it must be remembered that it is indispensable to band the mandibular second molars, while a direct bonded bracket is sufficient for the mandibular first molars. In addition, if maxillary osteotomy is to be performed, the maxillary first and second molars must be banded (direct bonded brackets should not be used; see chapter 4).

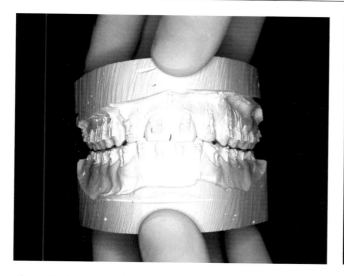

Fig 10-1 Testing surgical feasibility.

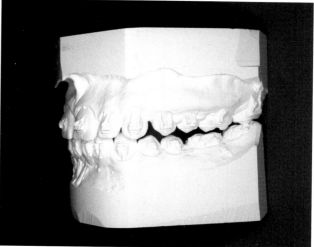

Fig 10-2 Preparation of the dental arches in a Class II, division 2 case; the curve of Spee will be leveled during the postoperative phase.

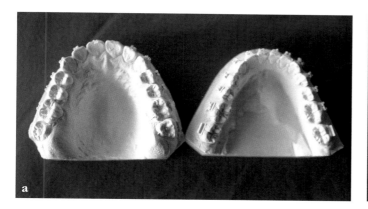
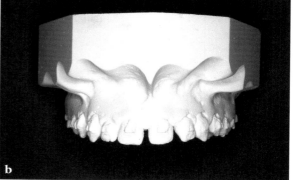

Fig 10-3 (a and b) The plaster casts must, at all stages, be of excellent quality.

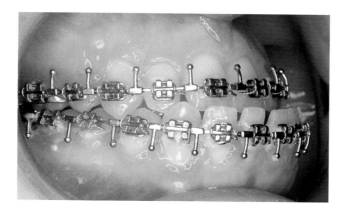

Fig 10-4 Surgical brackets in place.

Cephalometric Visual Treatment Objective

The first step in preparing a visual treatment objective (VTO) is to make the prediction tracing on a lateral cephalometric radiograph. The sagittal and vertical displacement that is planned for each jaw will be evaluated on this tracing. The surgical displacement is planned on the basis of clinical and esthetic indications and, to a lesser extent, cephalometric indications (see chapter 9). Clearly, the data that are obtained only concern skeletal displacement, although, with some approximation and depending on the specific structures involved (nose, upper lip, lower lip, soft tissue pogonion), it is possible to extrapolate from the skeletal displacement some indications concerning the soft tissue profile.

From the operative standpoint, the starting point is the cephalometric analysis made on completion of presurgical orthodontic preparation.

The operations that can be simulated are Le Fort I maxillary osteotomy, mandibular advancement or setback osteotomy, genioplasty, or the combination of two or more of these methods. The simplest situation is that of mandibular advancement or setback osteotomy alone. In these cases the cephalometric VTO is drawn by simply repositioning the mandible graphically in its new position and in correct relation to the maxilla, and retracing it on a clean sheet of acetate. New cephalometric values can then be obtained, together with indications for an associated genioplasty if needed. It should be remembered that, in the case of sagittal mandibular osteotomy, soft tissue pogonion follows almost 100% of the skeletal surgical movement (see chapter 8). With regard to simulating genioplasty on the VTO, the osteotomy is traced in one of the configurations described in chapter 5, and the displacement on the VTO coincides exactly with the surgical displacement, at least as far as the skeletal movement is concerned (for soft tissue considerations, see chapter 8).

In cases in which a maxillary osteotomy alone is planned for advancement and/or superior repositioning, or in some cases of inferior repositioning, it is clear that the mandible will have to adapt itself to the new spatial configuration by autorotation, the geometric center of rotation being the center of the condyle. This autorotation is naturally more accentuated as vertical movements of the maxilla increase. In these situations, the maxilla should first be repositioned graphically on the tracing in the correct occlusal relationship with the mandible; the planned vertical displacement is then made on the tracing, rotating the entire maxillomandibular complex around the condyles as the center of rotation. In this way, the new skeletal cephalometric values can also be measured, and indications may be gained concerning the need for genioplasty. This procedure is particularly important in slight Class II cases with vertical excess of the maxilla, which must be corrected by Le Fort I osteotomy for superior repositioning, with concomitant autorotation of the mandible (see chapter 9).

With regard to the upper lip and nose, on the contrary, the prediction is linked to several different factors, including surgical ones, as was explained in detail in chapter 8. Based on the skeletal displacements and the expected soft tissue handling, the new profile can be extrapolated. However, its new configuration on the VTO is rather subjective and thus also to some extent arbitrary, although naturally it does retain some indicative value (see also the section on the esthetic VTO below).

In cases of double-jaw surgery, since the cornerstone is again the maxilla, this must be displaced first on the tracing: In practice, on a clean sheet of acetate, the maxilla is traced in the planned spatial position (sagittal, vertical, or rotational movements) in relation to fixed structures of the cranial base (sella-nasion plane). At this point, with the same tracing procedure on a third sheet, the mandibular surgery is simulated, maintaining the condyles and rami in their starting position and displacing the body of the mandible, taking care to ensure correct repositioning in terms of occlusion (molar and canine class, overjet, overbite). The definitive tracing may now be made, and a fresh cephalometric analysis can be done to confirm the validity of the planning or reveal the need for modifications. In these cases, too, alongside the basic maxillary and mandibular movements, genioplasty may also be simulated, following the method described, and may indicate surgical movement from the qualitative and quantitative standpoints.

Naturally, with regard to the soft tissues, here too the new profile is only indicative in these cases and has no absolute value, both because of the subjective nature of the changes and because of the possibility that the soft tissue position will be influenced in various ways by surgery. It is also important to remember that the cephalometric VTO has no absolute value because, as has already been stressed, in a large percentage of cases esthetic and morphologic criteria rather than cephalometric data dictate the choice of surgical operation.

One further point must be added: Numerous cephalometric software programs have now come onto the market, including for the VTO. However, the authors believe it is possible to obtain comparable accuracy and precision using the classic method of working

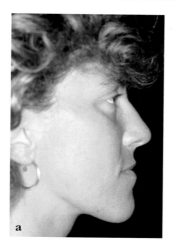
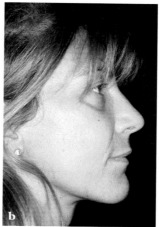
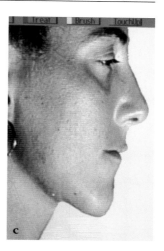

Fig 10-5 Esthetic VTO in a Class III case (maxillary advancement and mandibular setback): *(a)* preoperative view; *(b)* the result actually achieved; *(c)* computerized esthetic VTO.

on sheets of acetate, provided that the simulation is done by the surgeon personally: He or she is better able to outline the changes that will occur to the soft tissues, based on the surgical displacement, on the manipulation of soft tissues during closure, and, not least, on his or her surgical and clinical experience.

Esthetic Visual Treatment Objective

As a complement to the cephalometric VTO, in some circumstances the patient may request a full esthetic preview of the predictable outcome. This prediction may also be of use to the surgeon in guiding surgical choices or strategies (see also chapters 8 and 9). Some computerized programs have been marketed relatively recently for this purpose, using as their starting point a photograph of the patient taken in profile with a video camera. This may undoubtedly facilitate communication between surgeon and patient; however, two questions must be asked: How reliable are these programs? Is it appropriate to show the patient such preview images, presenting them as reliable and true?

With regard to this last point, which is of medicolegal relevance, in the authors' opinion it is extremely risky to show the patient these pictures, because to do so may raise expectations that cannot easily or with any certainty be achieved through surgery.

The authors instead believe that a long and in-depth discussion with the patient is more useful to understand his or her needs and expectations, to ex-

plain the problems and concrete possibilities of surgery, and to develop together the most appropriate surgical strategy. Similar cases may sometimes be examined with the patient, analyzing the results that were obtained and discussing possibilities and predictable outcome in the patient's case.

We have some reservations with regard to the reliability of these software programs. First and foremost, the esthetic VTO, in the great majority of programs, is only taken in profile. Furthermore, in the transition from the image photographed by the video camera to the video representation, there is an error in either direction of 0.5 mm due to "discreetization" (transformation of the image into a numeric code). The manipulation involved in superimposition introduces a further error of up to 1 mm for each point displaced along the x-axis. In practice, actual measurements may present an error of up to 0.94 mm in the horizontal plane and up to 1.28 mm in the vertical plane. Hence, for example, in operations on the maxilla, whether for advancement or superior repositioning, the preview is not very reliable.

Furthermore, changes to the soft tissues after surgery may vary in different ways (see chapter 8). This is why whenever there is significant involvement of the middle third of the face, the esthetic VTO loses most of its reliability (Fig 10-5).

Programs for mandibular surgery alone are more reliable, particularly in Class II cases (Fig 10-6). In these cases the esthetic VTO may also be of some use when deciding whether to incorporate surgical improvement to the chin and/or the labiomental fold.

However, computerized VTO is less reliable with regard to mandibular setback. There are two facial types: long, oval, thin faces with not very pronounced cheeks

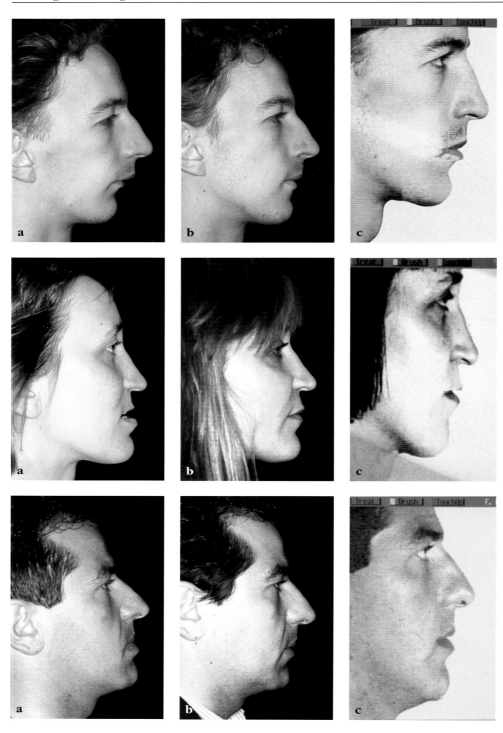

Fig 10-6 Esthetic VTO in a Class II case (mandibular advancement): *(a)* preoperative view; *(b)* the result actually achieved; *(c)* computerized esthetic VTO.

Fig 10-7 Esthetic VTO in a Class III case (mandibular setback): *(a)* preoperative view; *(b)* the result actually achieved; *(c)* computerized esthetic VTO.

Fig 10-8 Esthetic VTO in a Class III case (mandibular setback): *(a)* preoperative view; *(b)* the result actually achieved; *(c)* computerized esthetic VTO.

(these are the more frequent type), and rounded faces with marked cheeks and buccal fat pads. In the first case, as seen in chapter 8, mandibular setback produces fuller soft tissues in the cheeks, causing some rounding of the face. In these situations the computerized esthetic VTO is often unreliable at predicting the result at the cheeks (Fig 10-7). We have found better reliability in cases with thick cheeks and more rounded faces (Fig 10-8). However, these cases are relatively rare.

In light of all these considerations, we do not recommend such methods for use in discussion with the patient. Furthermore, from the standpoint of their usefulness for the surgeon, we feel that the cost of such procedures is not fully justified. In most cases, a careful cephalometric VTO and an in-depth discussion with the patient are sufficient for planning surgery that is appropriate for the desired esthetic goals.

SURGICAL PLAN

PREOPERATIVE ORTHODONTIC TREATMENT _____

    DURATION _____

    TECHNIQUE _____

    OPTIMAL GOALS REACHED _____

    ORTHODONTIST _____

MAXILLARY REPOSITIONING _____

    ADVANCEMENT _____

    SETBACK _____

    SUPERIOR _____ R _____ L _____

    INFERIOR _____ R _____ L _____

    POSTERIOR CUNEIFORM _____

    ANTERIOR CUNEIFORM _____

    VERSUS MANDIBULAR INCISORS _____

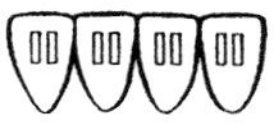

MANDIBULAR OSTEOTOMY _____

GENIOPLASTY _____

OBSERVATIONS _____

_____

Fig 10-9 Proposed orthodontic-surgical clinical record (to complete the initial record, see chapter 1).

Orthodontic-Surgical Clinical Record

Once the type of osteotomy or osteotomies and the extent of skeletal displacement in millimeters in the three planes of space have been established, based on the considerations discussed in chapter 9 and in the above paragraphs, these decisions are entered into the last part of the clinical record, which concerns surgical planning.

Figure 10-9 shows a proposed clinical record form; it is the last part of the general orthodontic-surgical record. An evaluation of the preoperative orthodontic treatment should also be entered into this record, including duration, technique used, and goals achieved. Since the crucial point of the entire three-dimensional skeletal restructuring of the face relies on the position of the maxilla, it is extremely important to mark the displacements, in millimeters, that are planned in the three dimensions of space, as well as any cuneiform ostectomies. The new position of the maxillary dental midline as it relates to the mandibular dental midline must also be carefully recorded. This is very important both for model surgery and in cases in which such a procedure is not performed (see the next section).

Lastly, the type of mandibular osteotomy that will be employed, the type of fixation, the need for genioplasty, and the number of millimeters of displacement that are planned must be established.

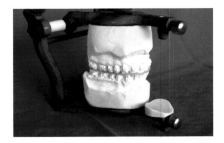

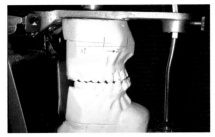

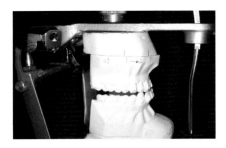

Fig 10-10 Casts and final splint mounted on the occluder for a single-jaw operation.

Fig 10-11 Casts mounted in the articulator at average values and the programmed repositioning for the maxilla.

Fig 10-12 Model surgery performed on the maxilla and occlusal relationship for making the intermediate splint.

Model Surgery and Intermediate Splint

Simulation of the surgical operation on plaster casts is an essential stage in designing and planning the operation. If the planned operation involves a single jaw, mandibular or maxillary osteotomy alone, the cast need not be mounted in the articulator. Casts may be mounted in a simple occluder in the planned final occlusion. It is always helpful to prepare a final splint (Fig 10-10; see also the next section), which will be very useful both during the operation and, especially, for managing the immediate postoperative period in cases requiring immediate finalization and postoperative physiotherapy (see chapter 11).

In cases of double-jaw surgery, the casts are first mounted in the articulator at average values, as a preliminary to what is known as model surgery. The plaster casts must be able to slide; reference points must be marked on the maxillary cast according to the clinically planned displacement (Fig 10-11). The maxillary cast is then relieved or sectioned to enable it to be repositioned in the articulator. In this way the new interarch relationship that will be achieved after maxillary osteotomy is reproduced exactly. At this point, to make it easier to find this relationship on the operating table, it has been suggested that an interocclusal splint, known as an intermediate splint, should be used to guide repositioning and fixation of the maxilla (Fig 10-12).

This procedure requires several steps, both clinical and laboratory: the facebow recording, making the interocclusal wax impression, transferring it to the articulator at average values, sectioning the maxillary cast, repositioning and fixing it, and preparing the interme-

diate splint. At each step an error or a slight imperfection may be introduced. The sum of slight imperfections throughout these steps may result in a different position than that planned, in some cases significantly different. All these procedures take the surgeon considerable time, and this phase of model surgery cannot and must not be delegated to anyone else, least of all to the laboratory technician. With any case, it frequently happens that at the moment of fixing the maxilla after removal of the temporary maxillomandibular fixation and the intermediate splint, the position achieved differs from the position planned clinically in relation to the reference landmarks used (bipupillary line, inner canthi, facial midline axis, mandibular dental midline). When this happens, it is obviously necessary to make appropriate changes in order to achieve the desired position, and only then proceed with fixation.

To avoid all these problems, it has been suggested that the intermediate splint be replaced with rigorous clinical planning and equally careful control over of the position of the maxilla during surgery (Lapp 1999; Perkins et al 1992; Renzi et al 2002). This may be achieved by using different landmarks: some suggest temporarily inserting a screw in the glabella region, others use graduated helmets or masks. In our opinion, with good positioning of the head on the operating table and equally careful preparation of the operating field (see chapter 7), the center of the palpebral fissure and the inner canthi are valid landmarks to check the position and vertical dimension of the maxilla (Fig 10-13). To further increase control, an instrument derived from the Fox plane (used in fabrication of complete dentures) may be used (Fig 10-14). The position of the maxillary dental midline may be checked in relation to the mandibular dental midline (obviously be-

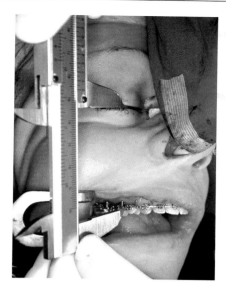

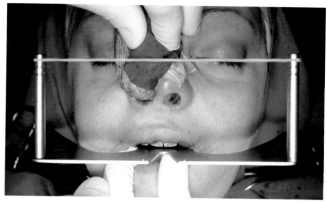

Fig 10-13 Verifying that the maxilla is vertical on the operating table. The landmarks used are the inner canthi and the palpebral fissures.

Fig 10-14 Verifying the horizontal position of the maxilla using an instrument derived from the Fox plane.

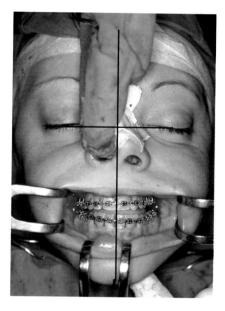

Fig 10-15 The maxillary dental midline may also be checked intraoperatively in relation to the facial midline axis, evaluated from the inner canthi.

fore osteotomy of the mandible) and/or the facial midline axis, which may be evaluated by examining the patient from above and behind and carefully evaluating the midpoint between the two inner canthi (Fig 10-15).

There are, however, some cases in which the intermediate splint is truly necessary: The procedure is essential whenever the maxilla is to be repositioned inferiorly, whether unilaterally or bilaterally, and also in maxillomalar osteotomies. In the former case, the lack of bone contact, and thus of points of reference and stabilization between the two osteotomized surfaces, obviously requires a stable occlusal relationship, which only an intermediate splint can provide. In maxillomalar osteotomies, the osteotomy surfaces in practice only make contact at the level of the orbit floor, the maxillomalar ridges, and the rising branches of the

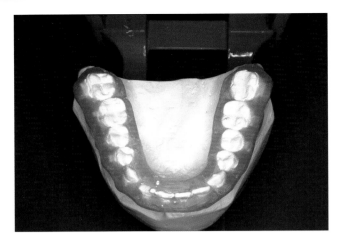

Fig 10-16 Preparation of the final splint.

maxilla, and are not sufficient to guarantee landmarks and provide proper stability. In these cases, too, temporary maxillomandibular fixation will be required, the position being determined by the intermediate splint.

Moreover, in cases in which surgical displacement of the maxilla is fairly complex and concerns all three planes of space (this essentially occurs in the more severe forms of dentofacial asymmetry), an intermediate splint may be of great help to the surgeon while repositioning the maxilla. However, as was said above, the position designated by the intermediate splint cannot and must not be considered dogmatically correct. Rather, the three-dimensional position of the maxilla must be evaluated carefully, critically, and fully on termination of the procedure, and if necessary the position must be changed and corrected if the result is not perfectly centered with regard to the anatomic landmarks mentioned above.

Lastly, in practice an intermediate splint is also necessary when the maxilla is subjected to segmental osteotomy (see chapter 7).

Preparation of Final Splint

To prepare the final splint, plaster casts of excellent quality are needed. Those on which model surgery was done can be used, mounted in the occluder or articulator at average values, depending on the situation; alternatively, duplicates can be used.

Occlusion must be evaluated overall, particularly with regard to stability. If there are any destabilizing

contacts, selective grinding may be done, taking care to mark the points that are relieved with a colored pencil so that the same corrections can be made directly on the patient's teeth when trying the splint in the mouth.

For the splint to be thick enough to avoid the risk of its breakage during surgical maneuvers, the occlusion is raised by 1 mm, creating a slight gap between the two arches. Subsequently, with sticks of wax, the teeth are bordered on both the buccal and lingual sides, and any parts that might interfere with occlusion are removed (Fig 10-16). Self-hardening acrylic resin is prepared and, during the wait for hardening to begin, all parts of the tooth arch that will come into contact with the resin are carefully treated with separating solution. When the resin begins to thicken, it is shaped into a small roll and placed on the occlusal surface of the mandibular cast. The occluder or articulator is then gently closed, taking care not to put pressure on the anterior part to avoid reducing the slight interarch gap that is indispensable for the splint to achieve adequate thickness.

Once the resin has hardened, the finishing phase follows. With the use of burs and laboratory micromotors, all parts that might interfere with occlusion and those that can create disturbance or problems in the mouth are relieved (Fig 10-17).

As mentioned above, it is indispensable to test the splint in the mouth before the day of surgery, obviously on two separate occasions for the two arches. If necessary, points that create instability can be relieved, again using products that act as occlusion markers. It is also equally clear that if a split and/or dentoalveolar

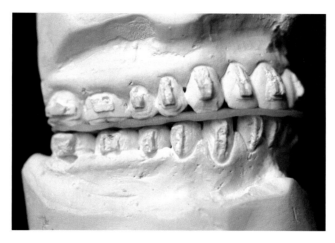

Fig 10-17 Completed final splint.

osteotomy is planned, it will not be possible to test the splints in the mouth before surgery. In these cases it may be advisable to make two splints on different casts, but sectioned and prepared in the same way, to avoid any unpleasant surprises in the operating room.

Bibliography

Aharon PA, Eisig S, Cisneros GJ. Surgical prediction reliability: A comparison of two computer software systems. Int J Adult Orthodon Orthognath Surg 1997;12:65–78.

Eales EA, Newton C, Jones ML, Sugar A. The accuracy of computerized prediction of the soft tissue profile: A study of 25 patients treated by means of the Le Fort I osteotomy. Int J Adult Orthodon Orthognath Surg 1994;9:141–152.

Ehmer U, Rohling J, Dorr K, Becker R. Calibrated double split cast simulations for orthognathic surgery. Int J Adult Orthodon Orthognath Surg 1989;4:223–227.

Ellis E 3rd. Bimaxillary surgery using an intermediate splint to position the maxilla. J Oral Maxillofac Surg 1999;57:53–56.

Ferguson JW, Luyk NH. Control of vertical dimension during maxillary orthognathic surgery. J Craniomaxillofac Surg 1992;20:333–336.

Gerbo LR, Poulton DR, Covell DA, Russel CA. A comparison of a computer-based orthognathic surgery prediction system to postsurgical results. Int J Adult Orthodon Orthognath Surg 1997;12:55–63.

Giangreco TA, Forbes DP, Jacobson RS, Kallal RH, Moretti RJ, Marshall SD. Subjective evaluation of profile prediction using video imaging. Int J Adult Orthodon Orthognath Surg 1995;10:211–217.

Johnson DG. Intraoperative measurement of maxillary repositioning: An ancillary technique. Oral Surg Oral Med Oral Pathol 1985;60:266–268.

Kolokitha OG, Athanasiou AE, Tunkay OC. Validity of computerized predictions of dentoskeletal and soft tissue profile changes after mandibular setback and maxillary impaction osteotomies. Int J Adult Orthodon Orthognath Surg 1996;11:137–154.

Lapp TH. Bimaxillary surgery without the use of an intermediate splint to position the maxilla. J Oral Maxillofac Surg 1999;57:57–60.

Perkins SJ, Newhouse RF, Bach DE. A modified Boley gauge for accurate measurement during maxillary osteotomies. J Oral Maxillofac Surg 1992;50:1018–1019.

Phillips C, Bailey LT, Kiyac HA, Bloomquist D. Effects of a computerized treatment simulation on patient expectations for orthognathic surgery. Int J Adult Orthodon Orthognath Surg 2001;16:87–98.

Renzi G, Carboni A, Perugini M, Becelli R. Intraoperative measurement of maxillary repositioning in a series of 30 patients with maxillomandibular vertical asymmetries. Int J Adult Orthodon Orthognath Surg 2002;17:111–115.

Ronchi P, Frattini D, Colombo L, Marinoni M, Giorgi M. Il V.T.O. chirurgico ed estetico nelle dismorfie dento-maxillo-facciali con il software della Rx Data Design. Riv Ital Chir Plastica 1994;26:85–94.

Sarver DM, Johnston MW. Video imaging: Techniques for superimposition of cephalometric radiography and profile images. Int J Adult Orthodon Orthognath Surg 1990;5:241–248.

Scarbrough FE, Ghali GE, Smith BR. Anatomic guidelines for placement of external references for maxillary repositioning. Oral Surg Oral Med Oral Pathol Oral Radiol Endod 1997;84:465–468.

Schwestka R, Engelke D, Kubein-Meesenburg D, Luhr HG. Control of vertical position of the maxilla in orthognathic surgery: Clinical application of the sandwich splint. Int J Adult Orthodon Orthognath Surg 1990;5:133–136.

Speculand B, Jackson M. A halo-caliper guidance system for bimaxillary (dual arch) orthognathic surgery. J Maxillofac Surg 1983;11:87–91.

Takahashi I, Takahashi T, Kawamoto T, et al. Application of video surgery to orthodontic diagnosis. Int J Adult Orthodon Orthognath Surg 1989;4:219–222.

Van Sickels JE, Larsen AJ, Triplett RG. Predictability of maxillary surgery: A comparison of internal and external reference marks. Oral Surg Oral Med Oral Pathol 1986;61:542–545.

Wood DP, Korne PH. Estimated and true hinge axis: A comparison of condylar displacements. Angle Orthod 1992;62:167–175.

11

Postoperative Treatment

with Luigi Colombo

- Immediate postoperative treatment
- Active and passive postoperative physiotherapy
- Orthodontic finishing treatment
- Retention

Immediate Postoperative Treatment

The patient leaves the operating room after surgery with elastics placed interocclusally as a guide; these are generally vertical, from canine to canine. When maxillomandibular fixation is in place, the patient must return to full consciousness in a dedicated environment, preferably within the operating suite (the patient must be under continual observation for at least 1 hour before being sent to the ward). High-dose antiemetic and cortisone administration is advisable to prevent postoperative vomiting and edema. (The authors generally use 125 mg of methylprednisolone every 8 hours on day 1, subsequently reducing the dose.)

The nasogastric tube is removed after several hours, when all danger of vomiting has passed. Sufficient aspiration and proper cleansing of the oral cavity are important. Perioperative antibiotic prophylaxis generally ends within 8 hours after the completion of surgery. The diet on day 1 is limited to water and cold tea.

Active and Passive Postoperative Physiotherapy

In most patients who have been treated with rigid internal fixation, postoperative physiotherapy begins on day 1. The patient is invited to make gentle mouth opening and closing movements guided by the elastics and the interocclusal splint (Fig 11-1). In practice, this type of therapy must ensure adequate functional recovery of mandibular movements or, more correctly, mandibular dynamics as a whole.

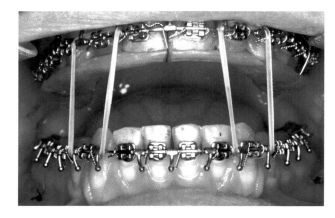

Fig 11-1 Postoperative physiotherapy starts immediately after the operation and is guided by the elastics and the splint.

Condylar remodeling, which always occurs during the postoperative phase, in this way occurs under the influence of the functional stimuli produced by the new mandibular dynamics, laying the foundations for good stability, even in the long term. It thus seems clear that this phase is an extremely important and delicate step within the orthodontic-surgical treatment plan.

In the immediate postsurgery period, the patient must be checked daily, taking care to recognize any small imperfections in occlusal relationship, which may be corrected easily by modulating the intensity and direction of the elastic traction. Already on day 2 or 3, opening and closing movements are combined with gentle lateral and protrusive movements. The elastics must be changed daily by the patient and worn 24 hours a day. The diet must be strictly liquid, and, for the first 7 days, oral hygiene must be limited to chlorhexidine mouth rinses. Use of a toothbrush or oral irrigator (eg, Waterpik [Waterpik Technologies]) is permitted 1 week after surgery.

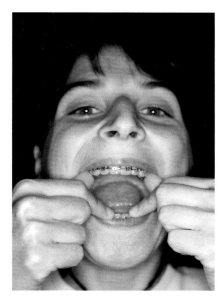

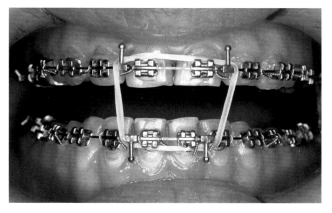

Fig 11-2 Gentle passive mobilization exercises performed by the patient.

Fig 11-3 In some open bite cases an anterior box elastic technique may be useful.

Active mandibular movements, again guided by the elastics and the occlusal splint, are gradually increased day by day, both in extent and in direction. During this phase the patient should be checked every 3 or 4 days. In the authors' opinion it is important that patient management, at least for the duration of postoperative physiotherapy, be in the hands of the surgical team.

Normally, over a 2-week period, the patient achieves a substantial degree of mandibular opening, about 3.0 to 3.5 cm, and lateral movements. At this point the occlusal splint may be removed, but the functional therapy must not be changed substantially and the use of the elastics should continue 24 hours a day.

During this phase the patient continues to make increasingly wide active opening, protrusive, and lateral movements of the mandible, until progressive functional recovery is complete. These exercises should be done several times a day, in general at meal times, when the patient temporarily removes the interocclusal elastics while eating and performing oral hygiene. Meanwhile, the diet becomes increasingly solid, returning to normal 4 weeks after surgery. By this time, full functional recovery of all movements has usually been achieved. In patients with hypomobility tendencies, some gentle passive manual mobilization exercises may be suggested to the patient (Fig 11-2).

After this period, occlusal stability and range of mandibular movements have reached levels of relative safety, so that the time for which the interocclusal elastics are worn can be gradually reduced until they are only worn during the night. However, the patient must diligently continue mandibular exercises. Postoperative physiotherapy is generally complete at about 4 to 6 weeks after surgery. At that point the patient may begin orthodontic finishing treatment.

There are certain cases, however, in which, in order to avoid pain, some muscle groups, particularly the internal pterygoid, masseter, and geniohyoid muscles, will adapt into a posture that results in some degree of mandibular retrusion with a slight anterior open bite. This usually occurs in cases of surgery to correct Class II malocclusion with open bite, in which the maxilla has been repositioned superiorly and/or rotated in combination with advancement or autorotation of the mandible, frequently associated with genioplasty. In these cases, slightly stronger Class II elastic traction (approximately 100 g) may be applied, using the anterior box elastic technique (Fig 11-3). In some patients with severe skeletal open bite and a large change in vertical dimension, a short period of maxillomandibular fixation may be indicated (not to exceed 3 to 4 days) to be applied on day 2 or 3 postsurgery. Subsequently, functional recovery is not substantially different from the above in terms of methods and time frame.

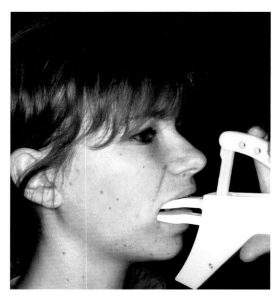

Fig 11-4 More vigorous passive mobilization exercises done by the patient with the help of a mandibular mobilizer (TheraBite, Atos Medical).

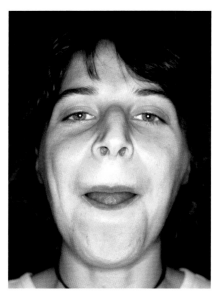

Fig 11-5 Lip physiotherapy exercises to stretch the musculature.

For patients treated with wire osteosynthesis and 4-week maxillomandibular fixation, physiotherapy begins immediately after the fixation has been removed. At first these patients will have more difficulty in making opening, lateral, and protrusive movements because of the extended period of functional muscle and joint inactivity. It is important to achieve normal values for mandibular range of motion as quickly as possible. Sometimes it may be necessary to persevere with passive mobilization exercises of the mandible in the days after the maxillomandibular fixation has been removed, also using particular devices or mobilizers if necessary (Fig 11-4). Within 3 or 4 weeks of removal of maxillomandibular fixation, occlusal stability is generally achieved (with reduction in the use of interocclusal elastics), as is satisfactory functional recovery of mandibular range of motion.

Another important aspect of postoperative physiotherapy is lingual and labial reeducation. In patients with open bite and/or atypical swallowing and interposition of the tongue, lingual reeducation gymnastics is of great importance. Frequently the long-term success of orthodontic-surgical treatment may partly depend on an adequate physiotherapy program. It may sometimes be helpful to have the cooperation of a speech therapist; in some cases such reeducation may begin in the preoperative phase.

Postoperative reeducation is also important for the labial musculature; this is especially true for patients with hypotonic orbicularis oris muscles and labial incompetence. In these cases, the exercises involve stretching and strengthening of the labial musculature and should be begun 4 or 5 days after surgery, once edema is resolved, and then continued for at least 6 or 8 weeks (Fig 11-5).

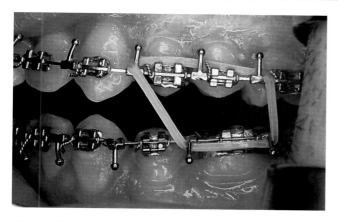

Fig 11-6 Use of lateroposterior vertical elastics to level the curve of Spee in a Class II, division 2 case.

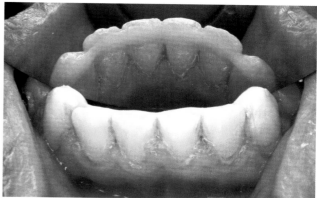

Fig 11-7 Fixed mandibular dental retention using a bonded resin retainer.

Orthodontic Finishing Treatment

After the physiotherapy phase is completed, at most 4 to 6 weeks after surgery, the patient may begin the final orthodontic treatment. The goal is to achieve ideal occlusal relationships in terms of canine class, molar class (which, as defined in chapter 4, cannot be Class I if therapeutic extractions of premolars are limited to one arch), and coincidence of the dental midlines. In practice, in this phase some simple orthodontic maneuvers will suffice, such as closing any small residual diastemata, correcting a slight lateral crossbite, perfecting intercuspation, optimizing overjet and overbite depending on the initial dentoskeletal type (see chapters 3 and 10), and conserving any edentulous spaces (as determined during the presurgical planning phase) in expectation of prosthetic rehabilitation.

Obviously the duration of the final orthodontic phase depends on the degree of preparation achieved during presurgical treatment. In most cases, however, 2 or 3 months will suffice. In particular cases, the orthodontic work needed may be more than mere finishing touches, as for example in some Class II cases, in which the curve of Spee could not be adequately corrected before surgery. In these patients progressive extrusion of the molar and premolar segments will be necessary, using vertical elastics together with the occlusal splint that was used for surgery as a guide, after suitably relieving the distal segments, until complete closure of the lateral open bite and flattening of the curve of Spee have been achieved (Fig 11-6).

Lastly, it is important to remember that the interocclusal elastics used as a guide during postoperative physiotherapy may also be used in the early phases of the final orthodontic treatment, until they are gradually and completely abandoned.

Retention

Retention in orthodontic-surgical treatment serves the dual purpose of stabilizing tooth relationships and contributing to skeletal stability, although in our opinion this latter point depends to a greater extent on other factors, such as condylar position and condition of the musculature, as has already been said. It is, however, important to stress that good dental retention contributes to maintaining the final occlusion that was achieved surgically, guaranteeing occlusal stability, which will surely have positive effects on the final stability in the broadest sense. In general, the methods used for retention are those used in traditional orthodontics rather than in surgical treatment.

Fixed retainers are normally preferred, applied to the mandibular and maxillary anterior segments in cases in which there is high risk of dental relapse in these areas (resolution of tooth crowding without extraction or decompensation) (Fig 11-7). In some cases, especially at the maxillary arch, it may be indicated to use removable retainers of various types, for example to be worn at night, partly to guarantee stability of orthodontically and orthopedically corrected transverse relations (Fig 11-8).

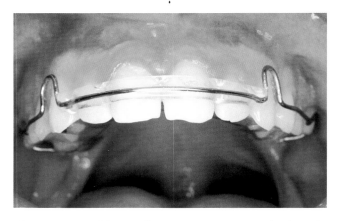

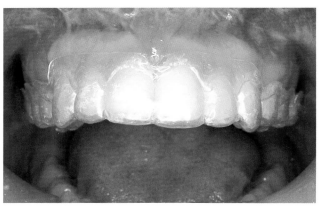

Fig 11-8 Removable maxillary retention using a palatal acrylic retainer.

Fig 11-9 Removable maxillary retention using the esthetic Essix retainer.

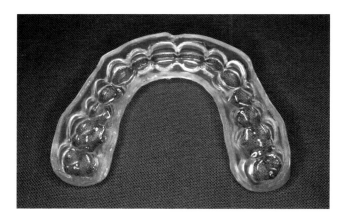

Fig 11-10 The Osamu maxillary retention device.

Transverse retention is of particular importance in cases of orthodontic and/or surgical expansion of the maxillary arch to ensure better control over relapse (see chapter 13).

The Essix retainer (Essix Raintree), a type of maxillary retention that is esthetically acceptable and generally well tolerated by the patient and which may therefore also be used during the day, is shown in Fig 11-9. However, this method is not recommended in cases of maxillary arch expansion. A similar device, which is slightly more rigid and thus slightly more effective, is the Osamu retainer (Scheu-Dental) (Fig 11-10).

In any case, it is fundamental that all teeth be present in the arch. Edentulous spaces of varying widths that were maintained during previous phases (in some cases using temporary removable surgical prosthetic devices during the operation) must be properly replaced as soon as possible with prosthetic implants, fixed partial dentures, or removable or fixed prostheses, not the least to guarantee proper stability.

Bibliography

Aragon SB, Van Sickels JE, Dolwick MF, Flanary CM. The effects of orthognathic surgery on mandibular range of motion. J Oral Maxillofac Surg 1985;43:938–943.

Athanasiou AE, Mavreas D. Tomographic assessment of alterations of the temporomandibular joint after surgical correction of mandibular prognathism. Int J Adult Orthodon Orthognath Surg 1991;6:105–112.

Boyd SB, Karas ND, Sinn DP. Recovery of mandibular mobility following orthognathic surgery. J Oral Maxillofac Surg 1991;49:924–931.

Ellis E 3rd, Carlson DS. The effects of mandibular immobilization on the masticatory system. A review. Clin Plast Surg 1989;16:133–146.

Nagamine T, Kobayashi T, Nakajima T, Hanada K. The effects of surgical-orthodonthic correction of skeletal class III malocclusion on mandibular movement. J Oral Maxillofac Surg 1993;51:385–389.

Proffit WR, Phillips C. Adaptations in lip posture and pressure following orthognathic surgery. Am J Orthod Dentofacial Orthop 1988;93:294–302.

12

Specific Class I Dentofacial Anomalies

- Lateral crossbite
- Skeletal deep bite
- Long face syndrome

Chapter 1 examined those types of dentofacial anomaly that, based on clinical experience and epidemiology, are of most interest for clinician, surgeon, and orthodontist, namely Class II and Class III malocclusion, open bite, and dentofacial asymmetry. Other occlusal and/or skeletal alterations (although less frequent from the statistical standpoint) occur with Class I dental malocclusion, or even normal occlusion, that can only be corrected fully and stably, from both the functional and the esthetic standpoints, through surgery. This is particularly the case of lateral crossbite, skeletal deep bite, and pure long face syndrome.

Lateral Crossbite

Lateral crossbite in skeletal Class I patients without any other vertical problems is not rare. This type of alteration involves almost exclusively the dental system, with no repercussions on facial esthetics. In patients still in the growth phase, the problem can easily be solved with the usual orthodontic-orthopedic treatment aimed at achieving an expansion of the maxillary arch. However, in adult patients, when the extent of crossbite is such that it cannot be resolved orthodontically (maxillary expansion arches, buccolingual torque applied to the mandibular arch, crossed elastic bands), surgery will be necessary.

An exact clinical and instrumental diagnosis is fundamental to planning treatment correctly. In almost all cases the problem consists of a transverse contraction of the maxilla. It is essential to evaluate whether there are any deflecting premature contacts, specifically at the canine level, conditioning a positional (but not a structural) mandibular deviation that apparently aggravates the extent of crossbite, and whether the contraction is symmetric or asymmetric. To make this deter-

mination, clinical examination and study of the casts are both very important. Clinically, the evaluation should be made with the patient relaxed and in centric occlusion; diagnosis is completed through a geometric study of the casts, comparing the two hemiarches. Frequently what appears to be a unilateral problem is in reality due to a bilateral and symmetric contraction of the maxilla, with deflecting premature contacts that deviate the mandible to one side (Fig 12-1).

Cases with true asymmetric contraction of the maxilla are less frequent, and for the most part are due to unilateral agenesis of the premolars or to the prior unilateral extraction of molars or premolars during the growth phase.

Where crossbite is due to prevalently symmetric contraction of the maxilla, treatment will take the form of the classic surgical-orthodontic disjunction of the maxilla, already described in detail in chapter 4. In these cases, surgery is the first phase of treatment; after 3 or 4 months of stabilization (a hypercorrection of 15% to 20% is always necessary) the orthodontic phase can begin; the most appropriate approach and orthodontic techniques for the specific clinical case should be selected.

In cases with asymmetric unilateral contraction, in which diagnosis is certain both clinically and from the geometry of the casts, there are two possible surgical approaches. The first entails a Schuchardt lateroposterior osteotomy of the maxilla (see chapter 7). In this case, the anterior interdental osteotomy line must be drawn taking into account the extent of the crossbite (generally between lateral incisor and canine, or between canine and first premolar). The osteodental segment must be completely and carefully mobilized. Fixation will be in the usual manner with microplates and/or a resin palatal plate fixed to the maxillary arch with interdental wire. The necessary postoperative orthodontic work will complete the case.

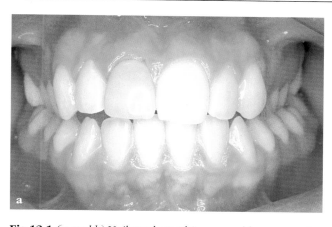
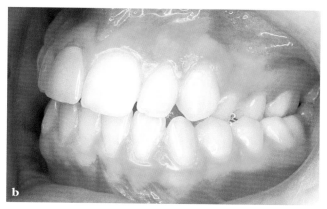

Fig 12-1 *(a and b)* Unilateral crossbite, caused by symmetric contraction of the maxilla.

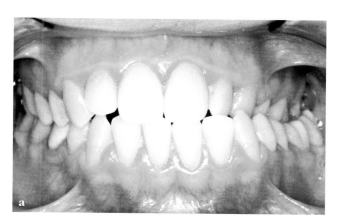
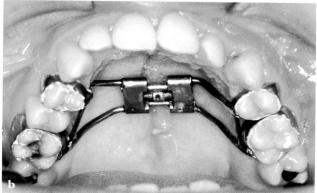
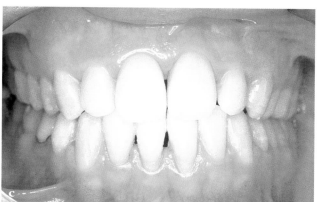

Fig 12-2 Unilateral crossbite caused by asymmetric contraction of the maxilla, due to the absence of one premolar *(a)*; treatment with surgical-orthodontic asymmetric expansion using Schuchardt osteotomy lines *(b)*; final result *(c)*.

An alternative to purely surgical mobilization entails drawing the osteotomy lines as above and, with the help of an expansion appliance cemented to premolars and molars, achieving gradual and asymmetric expansion (Fig 12-2). In this case, too, hypercorrection of 15% to 20% will be necessary and, after the usual stabilization period of 3 to 4 months, postoperative orthodontic finishing treatment can begin.

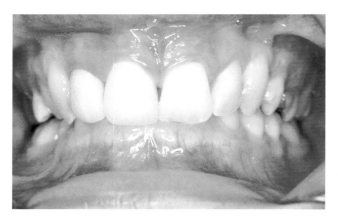

Fig 12-3 Skeletal deep bite in Class I malocclusion.

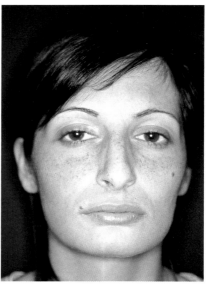

Fig 12-4 Clinical and morphologic characteristics of skeletal deep bite: evident vertical reduction of both the middle and lower thirds of the face.

Skeletal Deep Bite

As seen in chapters 1 and 9 there are some alterations in Class III or Class II malocclusions with considerable reduction of the vertical height and thus with skeletal deep bite that, from both sagittal and vertical standpoints, require appropriate orthodontic-surgical treatment. As was said for open bite in Class I cases, in skeletal deep bite with sagittal relation that is clearly Class I there may be indications for surgery, since the skeletal vertical deficiency is such that orthodontic correction alone cannot provide adequate stability nor, even more clearly, an acceptable esthetic outcome. These cases are quite rare compared to the sagittal and/or vertical dentofacial anomalies that were considered in previous chapters; however, they are worth separate consideration.

Skeletal deep bite, a dentofacial alteration that is infrequently found, is characterized by deep bite, molar and canine Class I occlusion, marked reduction of the vertical dimension of both the middle and the lower thirds of the face, frequently with skeletal bimaxillary retrusion. This anomaly has sometimes been classified as *short face* (in contrast to long face, which will be examined in the following section) based on the skeletal and facial components. It must not be confused with Class II, division 2 malocclu-

sion, with which it may have some morphologic and esthetic characteristics in common (see chapter 1). It is also necessary to remember that some Class II, division 2 cases are only apparently such, because once the anterior segment consisting of the maxillary incisors has been "unlocked," the mandible can spontaneously and stably reposition itself in Class I malocclusion. These cases should really be classified as skeletal deep bite.

Another important clinical characteristic of patients with skeletal deep bite is that they have particularly strong and well-developed muscles, especially the masseter muscles and, to a lesser extent, the temporal muscles, which strongly condition the anomaly and also limit the possibility of correction by orthodontics alone.

The problems connected with this alteration are occlusal and esthetic. From the occlusal standpoint the deep bite is particularly accentuated and is essentially due to the lingualization and extrusion of the maxillary incisors and, to a lesser extent, the mandibular incisors (Fig 12-3). From the clinical and esthetic standpoints these patients exhibit a significant reduction in the vertical dimension, often with insufficient development of the mental symphysis and accentuation of the labiomental fold (Fig 12-4), as well as insufficient or no tooth exposure, both at rest and when smiling. In some cases there is also bi-maxillary retrusion.

From the treatment standpoint, since malocclusion is Class I, the approach is initially orthodontic. Orthodontic management of these patients, however, is not simple because of the muscular problems mentioned above. It often may be indicated to begin with a lingual appliance on the mandibular arch and a buccal appliance on the maxillary arch. Dental deep bite can be corrected in part by extrusion of the posterior teeth (however, these tooth movements may be strongly contrasted by the musculature) and in part by intrusion and slight vestibularization of the anterior teeth, both maxillary and mandibular. In the final phase of treatment, a buccal appliance may also be applied to the mandibular arch.

From the surgical standpoint, correction of skeletal deep bite requires that the maxilla be repositioned inferiorly and frequently slightly advanced, with simultaneous mandibular osteotomy to reposition the mandible inferiorly and advance it. Frequently, in cases of hypodevelopment of the chin, genioplasty to lower the chin will also be necessary (see chapter 5).

The maxillary osteotomy should be a classic Le Fort I (see chapter 7). Given the strong tendency for vertical relapse, the inferior repositioning of the maxilla must be overcorrected by about 20% of the initial requirement. The fundamental parameter in this evaluation is the labiodental relationship, rather than cephalometric or anthropometric measurements. It is essential with this type of repositioning to use an intermediate splint (see chapter 10) and always to place an autologous bone graft at the osteotomy sites. Given the size of the bone gap (sometimes the inferior repositioning is as much as 7 to 8 mm), the harvesting site is almost always the iliac crest. Fixation must always be with four microplates, two anterior and two posterior.

With regard to the mandible, the most indicated type of osteotomy for these patients is the classic Obwegeser–Dal Pont osteotomy (see chapter 5) with rigid fixation using miniplates. Reduction of the mandibular angles may also be indicated, since they are frequently excessively pronounced and square in patients with deep bite.

In some cases, the most difficult ones to treat, it is not possible to correct the dental deep bite completely before surgery because of opposition by the muscles. In this situation surgery must be planned at an earlier phase, and a surgical occlusion must be provided, with anterior contacts and posterior lateral crossbite, that may be closed more easily during postoperative orthodontic treatment with guided extrusion of molars and premolars. This procedure also appears to provide better stability of the vertical relationship that is achieved.

Retention is a big problem with these patients. In the author's opinion, the best guarantee for stability of the final outcome is that provided by surgical overcorrection of the concomitant skeletal alteration: This may reasonably be considered a significant contributing cause of the dental deep bite. However, this does not mean that all methods that may improve long-term tooth retention should not be used (see chapter 11).

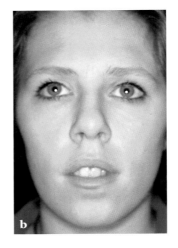
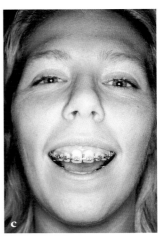

Fig 12-5 Dental *(a)* and clinical and morphologic characteristics *(b)* of pure long face syndrome; note the gummy smile during preoperative orthodontic alignment *(c)*.

Long Face Syndrome

Vertical problems in excess may be a significant component in all types of anomaly, sagittal or asymmetric (Class III or Class II malocclusion, asymmetries, open bite). However, there are some cases in which skeletal vertical excess is the sole alteration, in the presence of a valid and acceptable Class I occlusion. Such an anomaly is called *pure long face syndrome*, and it should not be confused with all the other forms of long face associated with varying degrees of malocclusion (Class I, II, or III).

This particular form of dentofacial anomaly, which is not found frequently, is distinguished by a Class I malocclusion with correct molar, canine, and incisal relationships, both in terms of overjet and overbite, but with a skeletal vertical excess of the maxilla that produces a noticeable gummy smile, often associated with some degree of labial incompetence. These are the primary or indeed the only problems existing in these patients, and thus the clinical and therapeutic implications are exclusively esthetic (Fig 12-5).

However, it is important to remember that in some cases a clockwise rotation of the mandible is associated with vertical excess of the maxilla, and this creates conditions for a slight Class II malocclusion to develop. The two situations should therefore be carefully

distinguished (see chapters 9 and 10 for more information about treatment for patients with Class II malocclusion and vertical excess). However, although rare, cases of pure long face syndrome in Class I malocclusion do exist and are thus worth a specific mention. Furthermore, in some cases the orthodontist may be faced with this situation at the conclusion of orthodontic treatment that was begun, and correctly performed, during growth for a Class I or Class II dental malocclusion. On completion of orthodontic treatment the outcome may be, in patients with excessive vertical growth, a gummy smile that requires specific surgical treatment.

The chief problems, as stated, are gummy smile and, in some cases, labial incompetence (occlusion generally does not of itself require any type of treatment; at the most, simple tooth alignment to correct slight crowding or some tooth rotation may be necessary). Some surgical methods have been described to treat gummy smile (Miskinyar 1983); however, the results are not always satisfactory nor predictable. Moreover, in cases with true vertical skeletal excess of the maxilla, these methods appear to be completely inadequate and do not have any influence on the associated labial incompetence. Therefore, the best solution, from the etiopathogenic standpoint, is vertical reduction of the maxilla by means of a Le Fort I osteotomy for superior repositioning, with concomitant autorotation of the mandible. The operation is exactly the same as that used to correct some cases of slight Class II malocclusion with vertical excess (see chapters 9 and 10). The extent of superior repositioning must be evaluated on the basis of clinical and esthetic considerations alone, essentially the labiodental relationship, gingival exposure, and interlabial relationship.

In some cases orthodontic treatment is neither necessary nor required. Bands or attachments are applied in these cases for the sole purpose of using surgical arches in the intraoperative phase and immediately postsurgery during the early physiotherapy phase. Indeed, in the author's opinion it is preferable to use orthodontic appliances in place of bars because the latter may cause gingival or periodontal problems that can be quite severe.

Bibliography

Bays RA, Grego JM. Surgically assisted rapid palatal expansion: An outpatient technique with long-term stability. J Oral Maxillofac Surg 1992;50:110-113.

Bell WH, Proffit WR. Maxillary excess. In: Bell WH, Proffit WR, White RP Jr (eds). Surgical Correction of Dentofacial Deformities. Philadelphia: Saunders, 1980:341-343.

Bittner C, Pancherz H. Facial morphology and malocclusions. Am J Orthod Dentofacial Orthop 1990;5:372-380.

Costa F, Robiony M, Politi M. Stability of Le Fort I osteotomy in maxillary inferior repositioning: Review of the literature. Int J Adult Orthodon Orthognath Surg 2000;15:197-204.

De Mol van Otterloo JJ, Tuinzing DB, Kostense P. Inferior positioning of the maxilla by a Le Fort I osteotomy: A review of 25 patients with vertical maxillary deficiency. J Craniomaxillofac Surg 1996;24:69-77.

Freihofer HP. Surgical treatment of the short face syndrome. J Oral Surg 1981;39:907-911.

Hoffman GR, Moloney FB, Effeney DJ. The stability of facial advancement surgery (in the management of combined mid and lower dento-facial deficiency). J Craniomaxillofac Surg 1994;22:86-94.

Huggins DG, McBride LJ. The influence of incisor position on soft tissue facial profile. Br J Orthod 1975;2:141-146.

Kraut RA. Surgically assisted rapid maxillary expansion by opening the midpalatal suture. J Oral Maxillofac Surg 1984;42:651-655.

Major PW, Philippson GE, Glover KE, Grace MGA. Stability of maxilla downgrafting after rigid or wire fixation. J Oral Maxillofac Surg 1996;54:1287-1291.

Miskinyar SA. A new method for correcting a gummy smile. Plast Reconstr Surg 1983;72:397-400.

Opdebeeck H, Bell WH. The short face syndrome. Am J Orthod 1978;73:499-511.

Phillips C, Medland WH, Fields HW Jr, Proffit WR, White RP Jr. Stability of surgical maxillary expansion. Int J Adult Orthodon Orthognath Surg 1992;7:139-146.

Pogrel MA, Kaban LB, Vargervikì K, Baumrind S. Surgically assisted rapid maxillary expansion in adults. Int J Adult Orthodon Orthognath Surg 1992;7:37-41.

Quejada JC, Bell WH, Kawamura H, Zang X. Skeletal stability after inferior maxillary repositioning. Int J Adult Orthodon Orthognath Surg 1987;2:67-74.

Schendel SA, Eisenfeld JH, Bell WH, Epker BN. Superior repositioning of the maxilla: Stability and soft tissue osseous relations. Am J Orthod 1976;70:663-674.

Shetty V, Mendoca J, Caputo AA, Chaconas SJ. Biomechanical rationale for surgical-orthodontic expansion of the adult maxilla. J Oral Maxillofac Surg 1994;52:742-749.

Stromberg C, Holm J. Surgically assisted, rapid maxillary expansion in adults. A retrospective long-term follow-up study. J Craniomaxillofac Surg 1995;23:222-227.

13

Complications and Common Errors

with Stefano Panigatti

- Preoperative orthodontic complications
- Intraoperative complications
- Early postoperative complications
- Neurosensory disorders
- Late postoperative complications

Preoperative Orthodontic Complications

During preoperative orthodontic treatment, the orthodontic biomechanics applied are those normally used in traditional treatment. Hence possible complications do not differ from those that may occur during any tooth displacement and essentially consist of root resorption and periodontal problems. It is clear that there is a higher risk of such complications where tooth movement is more extensive, both in the sense of bodily tooth movement and of changes in inclination. The importance of drawing up a complete plan right from the start is therefore also essential to reduce the incidence of complications. Indeed, by applying the philosophy of "everything in its right place," the act of repositioning the teeth in their correct places in relation to the alveolar process and the underlying bone substantially contributes to preventing the possible periodontal complications that may be caused by tooth movement itself because all such movements tend to increase the natural physiologic harmony.

In some cases, presurgical orthodontic treatment may produce a generalized resorption of the root apexes as a complication at the end of treatment. The etiopathogenesis of this disease, generally known as *rhizolysis*, is not yet fully understood, and although several studies suggest the significance of genetic factors, it is also clear that orthodontic forces are a significant mechanical factor in its genesis. In consideration of the fact that rhizolysis is increasingly frequent in adult patients and directly proportional to the duration of treatment, it may easily be deduced that patients tend to be exposed to a higher risk presurgery. In fact, it is significant that some of these patients have already undergone orthodontic treatment during growth or, even worse, after completion of growth, for the (futile)

purpose of compensating or masking an esthetic or skeletal problem simply by moving the teeth (Fig 13-1). In any case, slight resorption after preoperative and/or postoperative orthodontic treatment does not compromise either tooth stability or the stability of the result as a whole.

Along with complications linked to the biomechanics of tooth movement, there are other equally significant complications caused by actual strategic errors consequent to inadequate planning or loss of control over tooth movement. One of the most frequent errors, typical of orthodontists with less experience in the field of orthodontic-surgical treatment, is that of producing an excessive expansion of the maxillary arch in Class III cases. This tends to occur if surgical feasibility is not tested on the plaster casts methodically and continually (see chapters 4 and 10) and if the orthodontist's attention is concentrated on intraoral examination. This may lead to hyperexpansion of the maxillary arch, in some cases reaching a truly abnormal extent, such that it could properly be considered a pseudo–Brodie syndrome of iatrogenic origin. In this situation, the tooth movement needed to correct the transverse anomaly involves an increased incidence of complications, such as root resorption and gingival recession. Furthermore, in some cases the hyperexpansion obtained becomes so stabilized and accentuated that it requires additional surgical correction. The case shown in Fig 13-2 is indicative of this relationship, and a Perko-Bell osteotomy (see chapter 7) with simultaneous mandibular osteotomy was needed.

Another relatively frequent error that can occur in treating Class III cases is loss of control over the inclination of the maxillary incisors, with excessive vestibularization of these teeth. This may be due to loss of posterior anchorage, but may also be caused by adopting orthodontic mechanics that are unsuitable for preoperative treatment. From this standpoint, in the au-

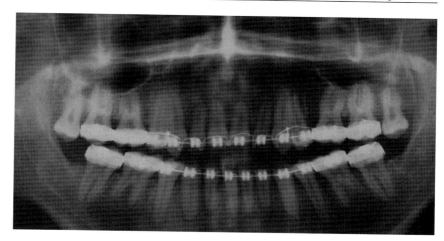

Fig 13-1 Evident rhizolysis in orthodontic-surgical treatment.

Fig 13-2 *(a)* Skeletal Class III case with asymmetric hyperexpansion of the maxillary arch. *(b)* The test of surgical feasibility reveals the lack of transverse coordination. *(c)* Orthodontic preparation for lateroposterior osteotomy according to Perko (1972) and Bell (Bell and Proffit 1980). *(d)* Segmental osteotomy performed in association with mandibular osteotomy. *(e)* Final result.

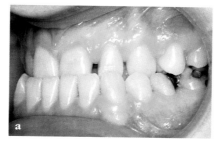
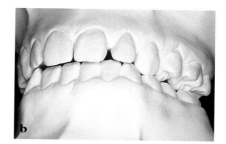
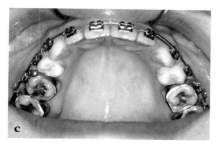
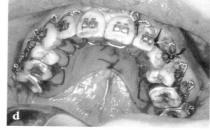
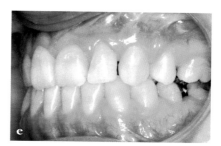

thors' opinion the most suitable techniques are the classic edgewise technique or the two-dimensional technique; the bioprogressive technique and the straight-wire technique, if used in inexperienced hands, may be more risky. Excessive vestibularization of the maxillary incisors inevitably reduces the space available for surgical displacement of the maxilla, especially in the sagittal sense. In these cases, the necessary secondary orthodontic correction of the axis of the maxillary incisors may cause significant root resorption or quite severe periodontal complications. Surgical correction may be needed to compensate for this planning error or an inappropriate choice of or-

thodontic techniques. Figure 13-3 is significant from this standpoint, and shows a possible surgical solution to the iatrogenic problem.

A loss of control over the inclination of the mandibular incisors may also occur, along with excessive vestibularization, particularly in Class II, division 1 cases. The orthodontic method applied is also essential in these cases. It is the authors' opinion that the traditional edgewise technique or the two-dimensional technique provides better control over inclination of the mandibular incisors. When excessive linguovestibular inclination has been produced, orthodontic correction is not practicable given the lack of periodontal and

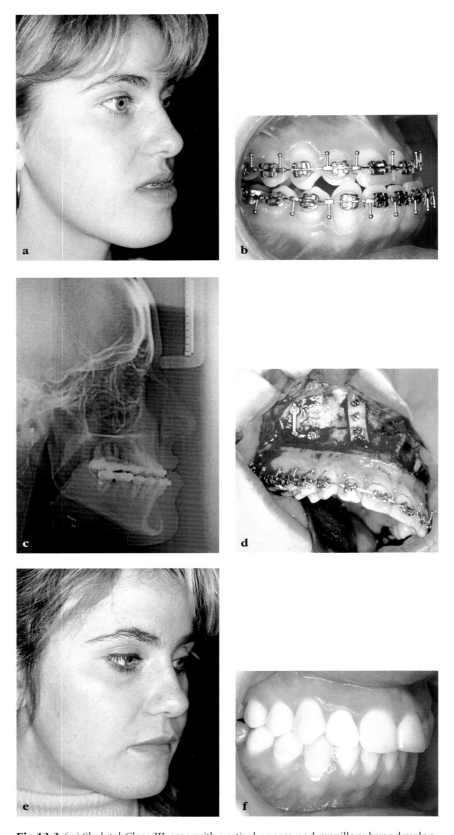

Fig 13-3 (*a*) Skeletal Class III case with vertical excess and maxillary hypodevelopment. (*b*) The occlusion shows a lack of decompensation at the maxillary incisors. (*c*) The lateral radiograph shows marked vestibularization of the maxillary incisors. (*d*) Le Fort I osteotomy is performed to correct the vertical problem, and at the same time the flattening of the paranasal areas is corrected using a bone graft taken from the mandibular cortex as a "biologic plate." Final esthetic (*e*) and occlusal results (*f*).

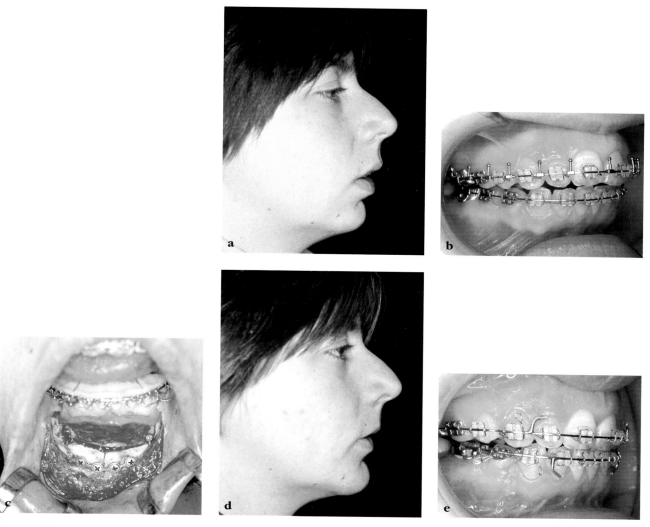

Fig 13-4 *(a)* Evident Class II malocclusion due to mandibular retrusion. *(b)* Orthodontic preparation did not decompensate the mandibular incisors, which are excessively vestibularized even on clinical examination, and the overjet is insufficient to achieve a good esthetic result with mandibular advancement osteotomy alone. *(c)* A Kole anterior subapical osteotomy to correct the mandibular incisal axis, and genioplasty, are thus performed. Final esthetic *(d)* and occlusal results *(e)*.

bone support present in the mental symphysis region. In these situations, the extent of possible surgical advancement of the mandible will be curtailed, and the esthetic impact may be almost insignificant. To solve this problem it may become necessary to perform ancillary advancement genioplasty or even to consider double-jaw advancement in selected cases. Lastly, there are some situations in which the only way that the excessive vestibularization of the mandibular incisors can properly be solved is through a Kole subapical osteotomy (see chapter 5) combined with a mandibular advancement osteotomy (Fig 13-4).

Intraoperative Complications

Intraoperative complications vary depending on the specific type of surgery. There are numerous reports in the literature, and each surgical team acquires more experience over the years. Complications for each type of surgical operation are described below, and more detailed consideration is given to those that, based on the literature and our own experience, we believe to be the most significant.

Obwegeser–Dal Pont or Gotte bilateral split mandibular osteotomy

Possible complications with these types of osteotomy are vascular or nervous lesions, undesired fractures, and condylar dislocation. Problems relating to condylar dislocation are discussed in detail in chapter 6, and readers are referred to that chapter for details.

Vascular lesions may occur to the various branches of the facial artery and the internal carotid artery. In practice, lesions to the internal carotid artery are an exceptional occurrence because proper subperiosteal dissection on the medial side of the mandibular ramus and good protection of the soft tissues with an appropriate retractor should safeguard the artery. Nevertheless, indirect lesions, such as postoperative thrombosis or arterovenous fistulas, have been reported (Lanigan 1988; Lanigan et al 1991).

Lesions of the facial artery or its terminal branches are more frequent, especially when a bur is used to make the osteotomy groove on the buccal side. However, here, too, if proper care is taken to keep the dissection subperiosteal, and provide adequate protection for the soft tissues, this occurrence should be avoided. In any case, any lesions that occur to terminal branches may easily be controlled by electrocoagulation. In the authors' experience of more than 20 years of surgery and approximately 1,000 osteotomies, they have never had vascular complications to the facial artery.

Undesired fractures of the mandibular ramus are reported in the literature with an incidence around 1% or 2%. The authors have personally seen this complication on three occasions, and in each case the problem was solved relatively easily by stabilizing the fracture with miniplates.

The nerve lesions as described in the literature may involve the facial nerve and, classically, the inferior alveolar nerve. Lesions to the facial nerve may be due to compression by the retractor on the medial and deep side of the mandibular ramus. The rare cases described in the literature (frequency being around 0.1% to 0.3%) all resolved spontaneously within a few weeks (Jones and Van Sickels 1991; Stajcic and Roncevic 1990; Taher 1988). The authors had one case of partial deficit of the facial nerve (superior and medial branch) that was fully resolved in 15 days.

Complication with the inferior alveolar nerve may be due to a partial or total traumatic lesion that occurs while performing the osteotomy, or else to stretching or compression by the different retractors. Stretching may also be caused by the mandibular advancement required to correct severe Class II cases. The occurrence of a partial or total intraoperative traumatic lesion of the vascular-nervous bundle during osteotomy is reported in the literature with a variable incidence, in some reports as high as 12% (Leira and Gilhuus-Moe 1991), and may be correlated with the thickness of the external cortex and the relationship between this cortex and the nerve itself. In some cases the nerve runs very close to the external cortex, and special care must be taken and particular surgical strategies used when performing the osteotomy (as demonstrated on the DVD accompanying this book). In the case of traumatic lesions, the authors do not think that neurosuture is indicated because it is extremely difficult to perform and has a very low success rate. It may, however, be useful simply to bring the two ends close together, holding them in place with fibrin glue (Tissucol [Baxter]). Lesions due to compression or stretching are much more frequent and are a main cause of long-term neurosensory disorders. To reduce this risk, it is essential when using rigid fixation with miniplates to use only monocortical screws. Other factors, such as the association of genioplasty, age, general health, and postoperative edema, may also influence this outcome. This significant problem is dealt with in more detail below.

Vertical osteotomy of the mandibular ramus

Complications associated with this type of osteotomy include accidental hemorrhage, lesions of the vascular-nervous bundle, undesired fractures, condylar malposition, and, in general, malposition of the proximal segment.

Hemorrhagic complications occur with the same frequency reported for bilateral split osteotomy. However, if the hemorrhage occurs at the medial side of the ramus while performing the osteotomy, it is more difficult to control because of the limited room to maneuver. This may cause immediate or medium-term consequences, such as hematoma and osteomyelitis, in some cases severe, as reported by Quinn and Wedell (1988). Lesions of the vascular-nervous bundle are decidedly less frequent than in bilateral split osteotomy; however, they are more difficult to deal with because of the lack of visibility.

Undesired fractures may occur if the osteotomy line is incomplete and may involve both the inferior border of the mandible and the proximal or distal segment; furthermore, if the oscillating saw is used without due care, including for small rotary movements (like an osteotome), the blade may break and be extremely difficult to recover.

The complication with the highest incidence with this type of osteotomy is that of condylar dislocation and, in general, dislocation of the entire proximal segment. This is due to the very nature of the osteotomy, which does not involve any type of fixation. In this circumstance, muscular traction may be particularly intense or irregular and may cause significant distraction of the proximal segment. This may result in problems such as delayed or failed consolidation or postoperative malocclusion of varying severity.

Median and Kole anterior subapical mandibular osteotomy

Complications linked to this type of osteotomy are essentially due to the need to make interdental osteotomy sections, and are therefore mainly of an endodontic and/or periodontic nature (Dorfman and Turvey 1979; Schultes et al 1998). To minimize the risk of these complications, it is appropriate to create small diastemata during preoperative orthodontic treatment (above all deviating roots and apexes). Furthermore, it is important to use a saw with a very fine blade while performing the osteotomy. Lastly, it is preferable to complete the osteotomy manually at the level of the neck of the teeth, using very thin osteotomes (see chapter 5).

Genioplasty

The most frequent complications due to genioplasty are neurosensory disorders. Although traumatic lesion of the mentalis nerve at the level of the foramen where it emerges is an exceptional event (indeed, it can easily be avoided by providing adequate protection for the nerve and thus may properly be considered as due to faulty surgical technique), the same may not be said for lesions caused by stretching and/or compression, which may sometimes not be fully reversible. All the neurosensory problems consequent to mandibular surgery are discussed below.

Other types of complications, such as undesired fractures or unfavorable osteotomy lines, may be easily avoided with proper use of the oscillating or recip-

rocal saw, reducing the use of osteotomes to a minimum. The authors have never experienced problems of this type.

Lastly, bleeding from the arterioles of the buccal floor may occur but is easily controlled by electrocoagulation after the osteotomy is complete and the symphysis fragment mobilized.

Le Fort I maxillary osteotomy and Bell high osteotomy

Intraoperative complications due to these two types of osteotomy, if performed correctly, are relatively infrequent and easily controlled. During 20 years of activity, the authors have never had any particular difficulty, and certainly none that could not easily be managed.

One of the most frequent occurrences, as also reported in the literature, is bleeding from the pterygoid plexus of veins or the descending palatine artery. Rigorous and careful subperiosteal dissection when exposing the maxilla protects against bleeding of the pterygoid plexus. In any case, venous bleeding in this area can be halted relatively easily by proper tamponade (in this regard, controlled hypotension is always recommended and reduces all risk of hemorrhage).

Lesions to the palatine artery may occur during disjunction of the pterygoid from the maxilla if the osteotome is directed too high or too deep. However, bleeding can easily be stopped by ligation or electrocoagulation of the artery after the downfracture is completed and the maxilla mobilized. It should be said that studies by Bell (1969), Bell et al (1975), and later by Dodson et al (1997) have clearly shown that the integrity of the two descending palatine arteries is not essential for the maxilla to remain vascularized, provided that the vascularization of the palatine fibromucosa and the mucoperiosteal pedicles is maintained (as it always is with these types of osteotomy).

Damage to the internal structures of the maxilla during disjunction of the pterygoid and maxilla must be considered as resulting from incorrect orientation of the osteotome. However, this too can easily be controlled after mobilization of the maxilla is complete (significantly, in this regard, it is recommended that the retrotuberal osteotomy be done as the last step before the definitive downfracture). Direct or indirect trauma to the internal maxillary or internal carotid arteries, with risk of postoperative hemorrhage or thrombosis, may come about as a result of unfavorable fracture of the pterygoid processes, possibly with irradiation to the base of the skull (Lanigan 1988); fortunately, though, such occurrences are very rare.

Lacerations to the nasal mucosa plane (see chapter 7) should not be considered a complication and

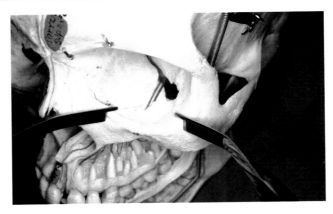

Fig 13-5 Correct use of protected osteotomes makes it possible to avoid damaging the periorbital area and the infraorbital nerve.

may easily be repaired before performing fixation of the maxilla.

With regard to the teeth, if the osteotomy line is rigorously maintained at least 4 to 5 mm from the apexes, all dental damage will be avoided.

Lesions resulting from stretching of the infraorbital nerves are always possible, but usually regress spontaneously within a few days, or at most 2 to 3 weeks.

Lastly, with regard to the innervation and vitality of the teeth, the surgical technique inevitably involves sectioning the small vascular-nervous branches of the pulp; however, several studies have shown that tooth vitality is regained within a few months. However, specific and more sophisticated tests may reveal some long-term, and possibly permanent, loss of tooth sensitivity. However, it is necessary here to distinguish closely between tooth sensitivity in the true sense and tooth vitality. The latter, as already said, is always conserved.

Multiple-piece Le Fort I osteotomy

In this type of osteotomy, the most dangerous complication is the risk of partial or total necrosis of the maxilla, mainly of vascular origin. There are a number of reports of vascular disorders in the literature. However, in a large percentage of these cases the complication results from an error in planning, in performing the mucosal incisions, or in the surgical technique itself. It is, however, clear that in all these cases the integrity of the descending palatine arteries and the mucoperiosteal pedicles must be absolutely respected. In this regard, it is once again essential to point out that palatal plates must only be used for the time when it is strictly necessary to reposition and fix the mobilized osteodental segments, and no longer (see also chapter 7).

Another type of complication that may occur during a two-piece median osteotomy is that of lacerating the palatine fibromucosa, which is particularly thin in the posterior two thirds, with consequent danger of oronasal fistula. To guard against this complication, which is a significant one, it is important not to make the entire median line section using the bur, but to complete it with a thin and delicate osteotome, making small rocking movements.

Lastly, dental and periodontal problems are undoubtedly possible complications of the interdental osteotomy. Lesions to the roots and loss of bone and/or gingival support have been reported (Dorfman and Turvey 1979; Schultes et al 1998). In these cases, as mentioned above (see also chapter 4), proper orthodontic preparation is necessary and must create adequate interdental diastemata. Furthermore, an appropriate and gentle surgical technique is fundamental, using very fine oscillating saws and very thin osteotomes, to complete separation of the osteodental fragments.

Maxillomalar osteotomy

The specific complications described in the literature for this type of osteotomy comprise lesions of the infraorbital nerves, the orbital floor or the periorbital region, and undesired fractures at the anterior wall of the maxilla.

In the authors' experience with 30 osteotomies performed according to the particular technique described in chapter 7, there have been no problems at the floor of the orbit or in the periorbital area. This may be due to careful subperiosteal dissection of the anterior portion of the floor of the orbit and to the use of protected osteotomes with particular angulation (Fig 13-5). Furthermore, the authors have never had any episodes of postoperative diplopia.

The incidence of paresthesia of the infraorbital nerves in the immediate postoperative period is inevitably higher with maxillomalar osteotomy than with other types of maxillary osteotomy. However, this also regresses spontaneously within a few weeks, leaving no permanent damage.

Undoubtedly the risk of undesired fractures at the anterior wall of the maxilla is more serious. Such fractures are inversely proportional to the size of the bone fragment that is mobilized. We have had two cases with this type of complication. The first was resolved with fixation and stabilization using microplates, while the second required a small bone graft (taken from the mandibular cortex during the associated mandibular osteotomy).

Schuchardt lateroposterior segmental osteotomy

The complications linked to this type of osteotomy are the same as for the multiple-piece Le Fort I osteotomy (see the section above).

Early Postoperative Complications

The expression *early postoperative complications* may be taken to mean those occurring during the immediate postoperative period and those that arise within the first 3 or 4 weeks after surgery.

Complications in the immediate postoperative period are edema, vomiting, and bleeding. These complications may be caused by surgical and anesthesiologic techniques and maneuvers, and correct surgical and anesthesiologic management of the patient considerably reduces their incidence. Furthermore, adequate medical therapy with cortisone and antiemetic drugs makes a significant contribution to reducing edema and vomiting. It is equally clear that these complications may be managed very easily where internal rigid fixation has been used. In the increasingly rare cases in which maxillomandibular fixation is used, the patient must be kept under continual observation for at least 12 hours in an appropriate environment, which does not necessarily have to be an intensive care unit. Lastly, in no case does bleeding require additional surgery for hemostatic purposes. Slight bleeding from the nasal fossae or from oral incisions can be easily controlled and managed by gentle nasal tamponade (preferably only on the side of bleeding), aspiration in

the oral cavity, or, additionally, use of drainage at the level of the mandibular intraoral suture.

A dangerous complication in the first few days postsurgery consists of the occurrence of malocclusion with gross discrepancy with the planned occlusion, due to faulty realignment of the mandibular segments and/or condylar displacement (in cases of mandibular osteotomy). Normally, in the first 24 to 48 hours there is a very slight degree of mandibular retrusion due to the pain-avoiding adaptation in the posture of the internal pterygoid, masseter, mylohyoid, and geniohyoid muscles (see also chapter 11), which can easily be treated with light interocclusal guiding elastics. Slight deviation on opening and closing may be dealt with in the same way. However, the serious loss of occlusion that cannot be restored with elastics indicates either a faulty alignment of the osteotomy segments or a significant condylar dislocation (hence the importance of radiographic checkup in the immediate postoperative period through oblique transcranial radiographs of the temporomandibular joint [TMJ]). In these circumstances, it is obviously necessary to perform additional surgery as quickly as possible to set the segments in the correct position. The authors have had to perform additional surgery in two cases of condylar dislocation, to reposition the segments and reapply fixation.

An alternative to early additional surgery may, in some cases, be manipulation of the bone callus, according to the concepts of the floating bone technique (Hoffmeister et al 1999). In practice, in situations in which there is slight malocclusion with no evident or pronounced condylar dislocation, but that cannot be corrected under the guidance of the usual interocclusal elastic traction, the means of fixation may be removed at about 3 weeks postsurgery, and an interocclusal corrective elastic traction may be begun, exploiting the possibility of manipulating the bone callus. However, it is necessary that the fixation be removed no later than week 3; in any case, since the degree of calcification of the bone callus obviously varies by individual and is subject to numerous factors, the callus itself cannot always be manipulated sufficiently. This situation may produce an abnormal and dangerous degree of stress on the mandibular condyles and joint structures in general.

Diastasis of the sutures is not infrequent in orthognathic surgery; it occurs more frequently in the retromolar area than in superior buccal incisions and cannot truly be considered a complication, being very easily managed by lavage with antibiotic solution and/or low-volume hydrogen peroxide. Generally, healing is achieved within a few days. However, the situation is different if bone grafts or alloplastic material have been used. In these cases, diastasis becomes

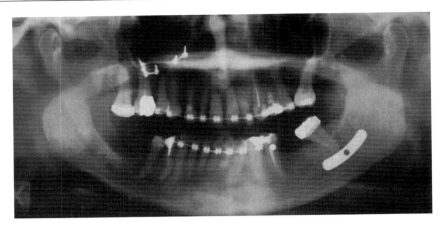

Fig 13-6 Severe osteitis consequent to a herpes infection with marked bone lysis in the subcondylar region.

a dangerous complication and requires immediate additional surgery for cleansing, curettage, and suture; otherwise, the graft or implanted material will be lost.

Osteitis at the osteotomy segments has been described in the literature usually for proximal mandibular segments, mainly due to reduced vascularization of the segments. This situation may be associated with defective consolidation of the segments. These cases of osteitis, if not properly treated medically and surgically (debridement of the bone and graft, if any), may also lead to the loss of the segment. The authors had one unfortunate case of serious unilateral osteitis in a 35-year-old patient who developed a severe diffuse herpes infection throughout the oral cavity and circumoral area immediately postsurgery, with bacterial superimposition at the bone of the right proximal mandibular segment. Despite all the treatment that was implemented, both medical and surgical (debridement and removal of the osteosynthesis plate), after healing the shape of the mandibular segment had changed significantly, with resorption at the neck of the condyle (Fig 13-6).

Another type of complication reported in the literature, and which the authors have observed in some cases, though rarely, is late nosebleed, appearing in the first few weeks postsurgery. This normally resolves without any particular difficulty by means of anterior nasal tamponade since it is due to bleeding of the peripheral blood vessels. More severe cases of late hemorrhage from the sphenopalatine artery or from the descending palatine artery have also been described, though with a very low incidence. Recently, Benech

and colleagues (1998) described a case of late hemorrhage consequent to the rupture of a pseudoaneurism of the sphenopalatine artery.

Delayed or defective consolidation of the maxilla, following osteotomy of the median third, may have varying etiology: marked advancement of the maxilla with little surface contact, very thin bone walls, compromised vascularization after particular surgical maneuvers, insufficient fixation of the segments, occlusal instability with premature contacts and occlusal overloading, general or local predisposing conditions (diabetes, poor nutrition, heavy smoking, lack of patient collaboration with regard to diet). In general, these complications are more frequent in osteotomy of the maxilla alone because the presence of an intact mandible enables greater pressure to be put on the maxilla. Furthermore, these patients usually pay less attention to their diet. When the failure to consolidate is recognized at an early stage, within the first 3 or 4 weeks, all possible etiologic factors must be removed, especially tooth premature contacts and occlusal overloading. It is also of fundamental importance to immediately cease the use of interocclusal elastics and put the patient on a liquid diet for several weeks. In cases in which the consolidation anomaly is recognized at a later stage, it is no longer susceptible to conservative treatment and additional surgery will be necessary. This will involve a further maxillary osteotomy: absolutely all intervening fibrous tissue must be removed, the bone margins cleanly recut, and fresh fixation applied with interposition of autologous bone graft, if necessary.

Neurosensory Disorders

As has already been said, this type of complication is undoubtedly the most frequent in the field of orthognathic surgery, especially surgery to the mandible. In this sense, the operations with the highest incidence of neurosensory disorders of the inferior alveolar nerve are Obwegeser–Dal Pont or Gotte osteotomy, genioplasty, and Kole anterior subapical osteotomy.

The literature contains many data concerning this problem, with incidences in different reports varying from 0% to 85%. This wide variability is due to a number of factors. First and foremost, subjective disorders of sensitivity must be clearly distinguished from objective alterations, which can be measured scientifically and compared. Hence, reports based exclusively on subjective perception or on patient questionnaires do not appear to be particularly reliable. Indeed, there is an enormous difference in percentage terms between alterations to the sensitivity that are objectively present and disorders actually perceived as such by the patient, such as painful paresthesia, tingling with pain spots, and complete anesthesia. The methods used in the various studies to measure these conditions also differ widely since some studies only consider qualitative alterations, while others consider both quantitative and qualitative ones. Tests of sensitivity, to be complete and scientifically valid, should be done with the correct equipment, such as the Von Frey monofilament device (Von Frey 1992) and suitably calibrated thermal probes; they should be performed in appropriate premises, properly prepared, with the patient relaxed, eyes closed, and fully collaborating. They should concern tactile sensitivity, capability to locate and discriminate between two points, and thermal sensitivity. Measurements should always be repeated and performed exclusively by a single person. In reality, not all studies reported in the literature provide this guarantee. Among the most complete reports from the scientific standpoint are those by Giannì et al (2002), Leira and Gilhuus-Moe (1991), Lindquist and Obeid (1988), and Van Sickels et al (2002).

Another aspect that, in our opinion, should be taken into consideration, but that is unfortunately neglected in most studies, is the correlation between traumatic lesions that effectively occurred and were noted at the time of surgery and long-term neurosensory disorders. Cases with true anatomic lesions should be distinguished from those that resulted from stretching and/or compression. From this standpoint, the reports by Leira and Gilhuus-Moe (1991) and Westermark et al (1998) appear to be well documented.

One last aspect that is no less important concerns whether surgical procedures are performed in isolation or in conjunction (Obwegeser–Dal Pont or Gotte osteotomy, genioplasty, Kole anterior subapical osteotomy). Although there is great variability in the data, some conclusions may be drawn from an analysis of the literature. First and foremost, neurosensory alterations should be evaluated at least 1 year after surgery. The incidence of intraoperative traumatic lesions (partial or total nerve interruption) varies from 0% to 12%. Damage consequent to manipulation, stretching, exposure, and compression reaches as much as 66%. Alterations in sensitivity that can be demonstrated objectively affect about 30% to 40% of cases of Obwegeser–Dal Pont osteotomy performed alone, and they increase markedly if this is associated with genioplasty (as high as 50% to 60%). These data relate to rigorously and scientifically valid tests, which are very sensitive. Moreover, there is some uniformity of opinion on the fact that neurosensory disorders are more accentuated in older patients. The type and extent of mandibular repositioning may also play a role. Advancement greater than 7 to 8 mm appears to bring a higher incidence of neurosensory disorders, probably because of the stretching that the vascular-nervous bundle usually undergoes.

Nevertheless, faced with the rather high percentage of alterations that can be measured objectively, one conclusion appears to be made by all studies. In very few cases, and in some reports in no case, do these alterations to sensitivity constitute a true disorder, from the patient's standpoint, of sufficient severity to compromise the results obtained or the quality of life. Furthermore, it generally happens in patients older than 40 years. The percentage of patients with disorders that are subjectively perceived as a severe disorder, and may even be partially invalidating, can be estimated at 3% or below. This is probably due to psychologic factors of various types, among which the quality of the final results achieved, from the esthetic and functional standpoints, is certainly of some importance.

The authors have almost never had any particular problem in this sense (except for two or three cases, in patients over 30 years of age), although obviously we have seen cases of intraoperative lesions and objective alterations in sensitivity, within the incidence range reported in the literature. It is interesting to note that there is a marked difference between the perception of neurosensory disorders by patients who underwent surgery for dentofacial anomalies and patients subjected to preprosthetic operations, including implant placement, or to removal of impacted third molars. In these patients, clearly for psychologic reasons of a different type, neurosensory disorders are reported as being much more serious and decreasing their quality of life.

Hence, disorders of inferior alveolar nerve sensitivity, although they occur in a relatively high percentage of cases from an objective standpoint, should not be a deterrent for surgical correction of dentofacial anomalies. However, this obviously does not affect the obligation to provide the patient with full and accurate information on this point. Indeed, the better the patient is informed in a clear and comprehensive fashion on all surgical problems linked to possible nerve damage, including the percentages of risk reported in the literature, the more he or she will have a positively predisposed approach and will therefore be more tolerant of any objective, or subjective, alterations in sensitivity.

Late Postoperative Complications

The so-called late complications have onset after 3 to 4 weeks from surgery and are undoubtedly those with greater clinical impact, both for the doctor and for the patient, because they may partially or wholly compromise the success of the orthodontic-surgical treatment. In particular this applies to disorders of the TMJ, resorption of the condyle, and long-term relapse.

Disorders of the temporomandibular joint

With regard to the influence of surgery on joint functionality, opinions in the literature are not in full agreement. Favorable effects of orthognathic surgery on TMJ disorders have been reported, due to improved occlusion (de Clercq et al 1995; White and Dolwick 1992). On the contrary, others report that this type of surgery may involve risks at the TMJ, both in terms of worsening any preexisting symptoms and, in some cases, even triggering the onset of new symptoms (Onizawa et al 1995; Sanders et al 1990).

We have already seen in chapters 1 and 3 that, in practice, the incidence of TMJ disorders in a healthy population and in a group of patients with facial anomalies is essentially the same. There are undoubtedly some types of dentoskeletal malocclusion in which these disorders are objectively more frequent, namely Class II deep bite or open bite and dentofacial asymmetries with dental interferences. Most studies on the influence of surgery on joint function consider groups of patients, some quite large, without distinguishing between underlying types of malocclusion in any detail, nor do they differentiate analytically between patients who are initially asymptomatic, those who are subjectively and/or objectively symptomatic, and those who have undergone specific concomitant gnathologic treatment.

Generally, the overall incidence of TMJ disorders is reported as being higher in patients before surgery than in the postoperative phase. However, this is too general an indication. Furthermore, the literature shows that, in general, the incidence of TMJ problems is higher in northern European (particularly Scandinavian) populations, in whom there is a higher incidence of collagen diseases and, above all, rheumatoid arthritis. Undoubtedly the role these factors play in the onset of joint symptoms is also far from negligible in patients with dentofacial anomalies. The overall improvement in joint function in these patients is, thus, undoubtedly an important statistic, but it is nonspecific and, all in all, logically predictable because of the improved occlusion and reduced stresses, both masticatory (occlusal and muscular) and psychologic.

Much more important in the discussion of possible complications is the onset of TMJ disorders in patients who are *surely asymptomatic* before surgery. We have already seen (see chapters 1 and 3) that in reality patients who are subjectively asymptomatic may, on careful clinical examination, show some signs of initial dysfunction, and thus highly accurate studies with greater precision in this respect would be of considerable interest. Nevertheless, from the data reported in the literature it is clear that the onset of postoperative disorders (or the aggravation of preexisting clinical signs) may have an incidence between 4% and 11%. The higher percentages relate to more exposed populations (as we have already seen) and to dentoskeletal malocclusions (likewise already mentioned) that predispose to joint dysfunction.

One of the most frequent signs in the initial phases is joint hypomobility. This is clearly much more frequent in patients who have undergone maxillomandibular fixation versus those treated with rigid fixation and early rehabilitation. In any case, adequate and timely physiotherapy, both active and passive, as described in chapter 11, can effectively resolve this problem.

The occurrence of acute locking with anterior disc dislocation is certainly less frequent, but also more worrisome. It may have onset at 3 to 4 weeks from surgery, or at the point in time when the patient is approaching maximum mouth opening. In these cases it is obviously necessary to recapture the disc through manual maneuvers or application of an anterior repositioning splint, if necessary with lateral guide walls. Once the acute event is resolved, though, it is imperative that the patient continue for some months with active and passive physiotherapy.

In cases in which marked hypomobility persists, and in which the procedure described has not had any success, joint lavage via arthrocentesis is indicated. This relatively simple procedure is not particularly invasive. In the great majority of cases it resolves even the most complex situations. In the authors' experience, use of this method was necessary in a fairly low percentage of patients, not more than 1% to 2% at most.

The onset in the postoperative period of the classic trio of symptoms that characterize TMJ disorders (pain, joint noises, functional limitation) is perhaps more difficult to treat, and its origin is undoubtedly multifactorial: slight condylar dislocation that is not visible radiographically, postsurgery tissue alterations affecting the condyle and/or disc, muscle spasms and contractions, premature tooth contacts or interferences, and persistent parafunctional and undesirable habits. These disorders are much more frequent in patients in whom the underlying malocclusion could be considered "at risk" with regard to joint function (Class II deep bite or open bite, dentofacial asymmetries with tooth interference and segmental deep bite). Treatment in these situations is multifaceted, employing drugs, physiotherapy, and gnathologic devices, which were examined in the discussion of patients with dysfunction (see chapters 1 and 3). Again, if the condition does not respond to this treatment, joint lavage via arthrocentesis may be indicated.

It is the authors' belief that the onset of TMJ problems, whether acute, subacute, or chronic, is inversely proportional to the care taken in initial diagnosis and monitoring of the patient's TMJ and muscle condition throughout all treatment phases. Monitoring the condition and equilibrium of the muscle and maintaining the correct condyle-fossa relationship and perfect postoperative occlusion are fundamental for all patients. The more precisely and rigorously this principle is observed, the lower the incidence of postoperative TMJ problems will be. However, this does not mean that the patient need not be scrupulously informed of the risk of this problem, and the therapeutic possibilities available to deal with it.

Condylar resorption

This is a dangerous and irreversible complication that occurs following split osteotomy of the mandible, whether or not this is associated with maxillary os-

teotomy, and that may present between 6 months and 2 years after surgery. Over the last 15 years, various reports in the literature have looked at this question; however, some points still remain obscure.

First and foremost, we must define what is meant by condylar resorption and, above all, differentiate resorption from remodeling. We have already said that adaptation and remodeling of the joint structures, above all of the condyle, always occur after surgery. This remodeling takes place at both histologic and morphologic levels. Condylar resorption is, on the contrary, a progressive process that leads to varying degrees of reduction in the size of the condyle, in terms of its vertical, sagittal, and lateral dimensions, with alteration of the condyle-fossa relationship, and which also affects the entire mandibular ramus. It is generally accepted in the literature that to speak of condylar resorption there must be at least a 2-mm shortening of the condyle or, more precisely, a reduction in the total height of the mandibular ramus, as measured on a panoramic radiograph, of 6% or more compared with the preoperative situation. In these conditions, the process inevitably leads to a loss of the occlusion achieved after surgery, with a tendency toward Class II malocclusion and/or open bite.

This alteration almost exclusively affects young women between the ages of 20 and 30 years, typically slim, with Class II open bite and an increased sella-nasion/gonion-menton (SN–Go-Me) angle. It occurs more frequently after double-jaw osteotomy than after mandibular osteotomy alone. The etiopathogenesis is multifactorial. Various factors have been indicated as being responsible: nonvascular necrosis secondary to surgery; dislocation of the condyle, especially if there is also posterior inclination; hormonal factors; and change in intensity and direction of the load to which the condyle is subjected. With regard to the latter two possible factors, a hormonal etiopathogenesis would explain why the disease affects almost exclusively young women, although there is no certain proof of such a cause-effect relationship. With regard to changes in the load to which the condyle is subjected, some studies (O'Ryan and Epker 1984) stress the different ultrastructural anatomy of the condyle in patients with deep bite or open bite, who also exhibit radiographic variations; the transition from a situation (open bite) in which the masticatory load is concentrated more on the molars and less on the condyles to a different situation (after surgery) in which the condyles are subjected to a load that is more normal, but in any case increased, would explain the onset of condylar resorption, especially in consideration of the particular anatomy of the condyles in patients with open bite. Other causes, such as the presence of preoperative joint disorders, the extent of surgical advancement, and the type of fixation (rigid or wire), do not at present appear to play significant roles in the etiogenesis.

As previously stated, the phenomenon appears in the postoperative period in particular categories of patients and tends to stabilize itself over time, generally within 2 years. Nevertheless, it may already be present at the start of treatment (see chapter 1) and, though rarely, may also appear postsurgery in patients who are typically not at risk. The incidence of this phenomenon ranges from 1.2% to 5% in a general group of patients with dentofacial anomalies, between 5.5% and 11% among northern European patients, who have a higher incidence of collagen diseases and rheumatoid arthritis, and reaches a peak at around 30% in the at-risk group, that is to say young women with Class II open bite and an increased SN–Go-Me angle.

Prevention of condylar resorption plays an important role in patients at risk. In these cases it is imperative to avoid any type of stress or compression on the condyle, both during preoperative orthodontic treatment (Class III interocclusal elastics should absolutely never be used) and especially during surgery. It is very important to avoid any movement of the jaws during surgery that might, for geometric reasons, lead to condylar compression. Furthermore, during the maneuvers to fix the mandibular segments, care must be taken to avoid putting excessive posterior or upward traction on the proximal segment, which must be manipulated and put into place in an absolutely passive and physiologic fashion.

Not many reports concerning treatment are available in the literature. Since condylar resorption inevitably leads to an alteration of the postoperative occlusion, with a tendency to Class II malocclusion and/or open bite and subjective symptoms that may vary from slight to severe at the TMJ, treatment is generally gnathologic (superior or anterior repositioning splints and selective grinding if necessary), orthodontic (orthodontic correction, when possible, of the Class II malocclusion and the open bite), and if necessary prosthetic. Additional surgery should only be considered with extreme care and only after the phenomenon has fully stabilized. In this regard, full-mouth radiographs must be taken over time, using panoramic radiography and TMJ scintigraphy. Furthermore, it is preferable to intervene only on the maxilla, or if necessary using a segmental dentoalveolar approach (Kole anterior subapical osteotomy).

Lastly, it is clear that patients, especially those at risk, must be fully provided with information on the possible outcome, as well as on the treatment available for this complication.

Long-term relapse

This is undoubtedly the most significant complication in the field of orthodontic-surgical treatment of dentofacial anomalies. It must not be confused with postoperative malocclusion (discussed above in the section on early postoperative complications), which is due to condylar malposition or to the segments' not having been abutted in the correct position. The etiopathogenesis of relapse is undoubtedly multifactorial; therefore, this section attempts to analyze all possible causes, how to prevent it, and how to treat it if it does occur.

Naturally, the concept of relapse goes hand in hand with that of stability, and it is therefore initially necessary to define what should be meant by *stability* and *relapse*. First and foremost, it must be considered that relapse never, or almost never, involves the complete return to the initial or postoperative situation.

Relapse is therefore defined as loss of the final result, in terms of occlusion, with a tendency to return toward the initial disease, without necessarily compromising the esthetic outcome.

With regard to the concept of stability, it is fundamental to distinguish absolute skeletal stability from overall clinical-functional stability in the widest sense.

Strictly speaking, absolute skeletal stability should be evaluated at intervals of time exclusively on cephalometric radiographs that are of optimal quality and precisely comparable and, if possible, taken with the same device.

Only under these conditions is it possible to speak of skeletal stability, and it must also be said that stability is almost never absolute since there is almost always some musculoskeletal adaptation that continues over time. This is true no matter which of the possible configurations of rigid fixation is used. In general, in the literature, a situation is considered stable if it involves a deviation or a displacement of the bony bases with regard to the control situation (normally the postoperative situation) that is not more than 2 mm.

However, the authors feel that global stability is perhaps more important, if this expression refers to the maintenance of the final occlusion that was achieved—in terms of molar and canine relationships, overjet and overbite, and coincidence of the dental midlines in association with a normal muscular equilibrium.

However, it is significant that this clinical occlusal stability can be maintained in some cases because the dentition adapts to the minimal and inevitable post-operative skeletal oscillations. Some like to define this process as *orthodontic relapse that compensates for surgical relapse*. In reality, it appears more appropriate to talk about the teeth and the occlusion adapting to the postoperative adaptation of the muscles and skeleton. The earlier these processes occur, and above all the nearer to simultaneous they are (as occurs with rigid fixation and immediate postoperative physiotherapy; see chapter 11), the better that stability will be in the widest sense. And it is just this stability in the widest sense that chiefly interests both clinician and patient.

Coming now to skeletal stability, two fundamental concepts stand out: *(1)* this stability is only in part proportional to the type of fixation used and *(2)* it varies with the type of surgery performed. With regard to the type of fixation (rigid or wire), the authors believe that rigid fixation, in itself, does not increase long-term stability (as we have already said, it is not, in fact, entirely rigid, but should more properly be called *semirigid*). However, rigid internal fixation may play an important role in immediate postsurgical stability and may be determinant in the later period because it favors immediate and physiologic postsurgical reeducation in conjunction with musculoskeletal adaptation, processes that underlie medium- and long-term stability.

The literature has much to say about the correlation between skeletal stability and type of surgery, although the most complete discussion is still the work by Proffit and coworkers (1996). The most stable surgical procedure appears to be superior repositioning of the maxilla, followed immediately by mandibular advancement in patients with normal or decreased facial height; the combination of these two operations (in patients with increased facial height) is significantly less stable. In Class III cases, advancement of the maxilla appears to be reasonably stable; mandibular setback is less stable (and depends on the extent of setback, the type of osteotomy, and the inclination of the mandibular ramus). Combination of the two methods has no effect on the stability of the individual bony bases involved. The surgical operation that is the least stable in absolute terms is segmental surgical expansion of the maxilla in two or three pieces: This is chiefly due to the fact that the palatine fibromucosa is inelastic and justifies the use of an alternative procedure, such as surgical-orthodontic expansion (see chapters 4 and 7). Inferior repositioning of the maxilla is also not very stable; nevertheless, interposition of autologous bone grafts and fixation with four miniplates (two anterior, two posterior) improves stability.

> In conclusion, the two fundamental principles on which satisfactory overall clinical stability rests are stable and valid occlusion and physiologic equilibrium of the musculature.

With regard to the occlusion, posterior premature tooth contacts, any crossbite, posterior lateral open bite, and occlusal imperfections may cause the mandible to slip or slide, and may produce a tendency toward open bite or deviation and, subsequently, may also cause surgical relapse.

With regard to the muscles, if these fail to accept the new spatial configuration of the skeleton and enter into spasm, the risk of relapse will increase. The masseter muscle and the internal pterygoid muscles (the so-called pterygomasseteric sling) appear to be particularly critical. Excessive stretching of this sling, caused by excessive or badly planned surgical displacement, will inevitably lead to relapse regardless of what type of fixation is used. Another critical group of muscles, though less so than the former, are the superhyoid muscles (in particular the geniohyoid and the digastric muscles). Studies have reported that these muscles can stretch and adapt, initially due to a lengthening of the connective and later the muscular structures (Reynolds et al 1988). Another indirect proof of this ability to adapt comes from the experiences that have been reported of treating patients with obstructive sleep apnea syndrome through double-jaw advancement. Tension is placed on the muscular and aponeurotic structures of the superhyoid muscles and the lateral walls of the pharynx in these patients, and is maintained over time; this constitutes the cornerstone for therapeutic success. However, in patients with dentofacial anomalies subjected to mandibular advancement, the mandibular lengthening and consequent stretching cannot go beyond a certain limit. In general, lengthening of the geniohyoid muscles not more than 15% or 20% of their initial length may be considered acceptable. Other possible causes of relapse may be condylar malposition, condylar resorption, or surgical operation at too early an age (especially in Class III cases).

All the means that are available to avoid and prevent condylar malposition, as well as methods to monitor the condyle-fossa relationship over time, are described in chapter 6. However, even with all these strategies and all due monitoring, condylar dislocation may still occur, sometimes over a span of several months; indeed, this is the only possible explanation for some otherwise inexplicable relapses. As discussed above, clearly condylar resorption may play a role in determining relapse in Class II patients, especially in those with a tendency for increased vertical dimension and open bite.

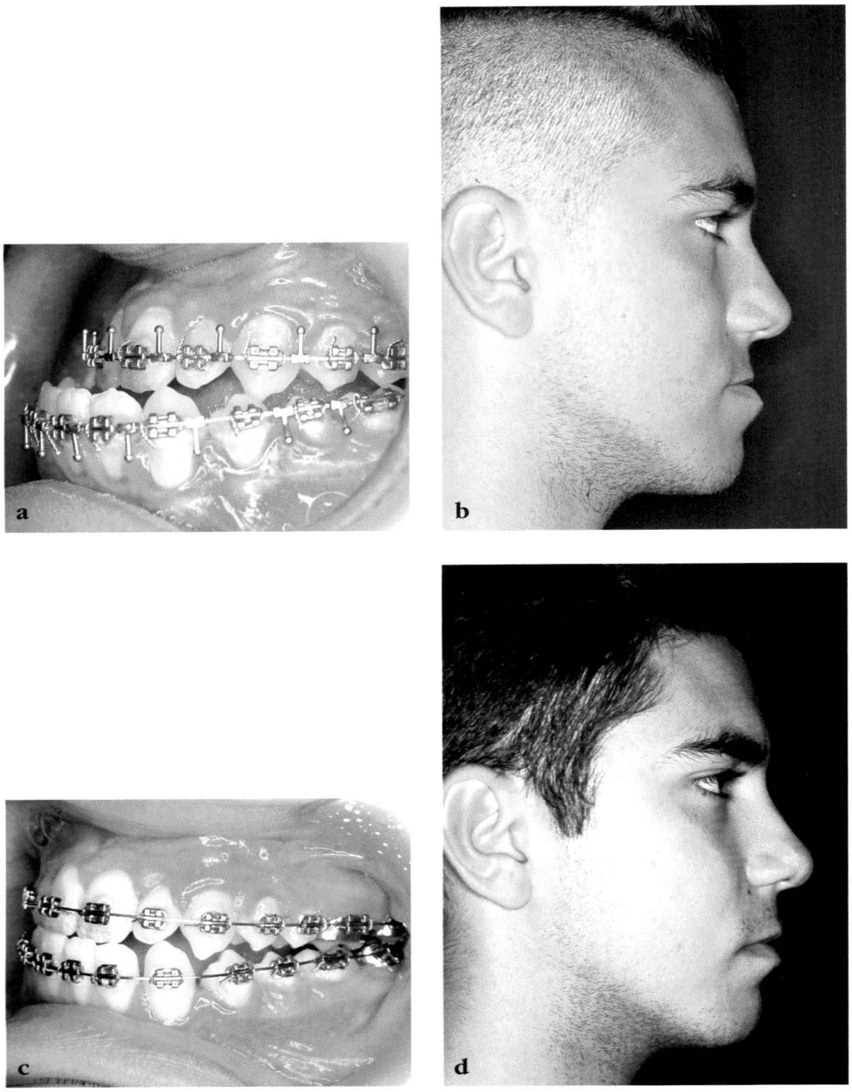

Fig 13-7 *(a and b)* Skeletal Class III case with a mixed maxillary-mandibular component. Occlusal relapse is evident after 6 months *(c)*, although the esthetic result does not appear compromised *(d)*.

In Class III patients, surgery must absolutely be delayed until completion of growth (see chapter 9) although in some cases this may involve disagreement with the patient, who is frequently in a hurry to correct the anomaly. The case presented in Fig 13-7 is exemplary from this standpoint. There is a clear relapse at 6 months after surgery (double-jaw osteotomy with rigid fixation) although the esthetic result was not significantly compromised. The relapse in this patient might to some extent depend on the stretching of the pterygomasseteric sling (there are no condylar problems), but the fact that surgery was performed too early (age 18 years, 9 months) may have been a factor in that there was residual mandibular growth.

In another patient, age 22 (Fig 13-8), who was likewise subjected to double-jaw osteotomy with rigid fixation for Class III malocclusion, the relapse presented 2 years after surgery and clearly had occlusal origin.

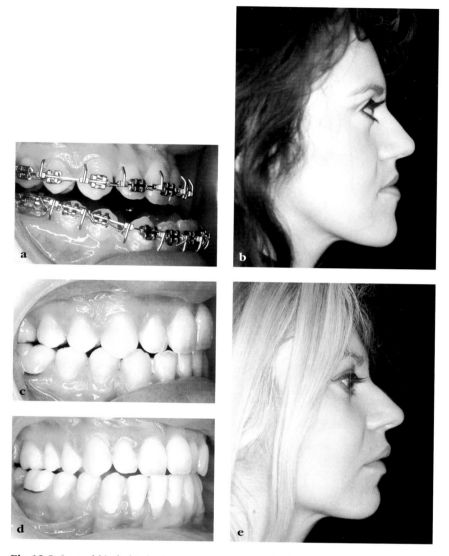

Fig 13-8 *(a and b)* Skeletal Class III case with a mixed maxillary-mandibular component. *(c)* The final occlusal result is not optimal with regard to overjet and overbite. There is an evident relapse at 2 years, resulting from occlusal causes *(d)*, although the esthetic result may be considered satisfactory *(e)*.

The final occlusion does not show a correct overjet and overbite (see chapters 3 and 10); in addition, a transverse contraction clearly contributed to the mandible sliding forward, even after considerable time. Although the esthetic result has been maintained over time, with unchanged patient satisfaction, this is clearly a relapse due to occlusal causes.

Occlusal causes may also be the reason for some relapses in dentofacial asymmetry cases. In these pa-

tients it is not always easy to achieve a valid and stable occlusion with perfect coincidence of the dental midlines because frequently some tooth anomalies (consisting of different mesiodistal diameters of some of the teeth) are responsible for alterations in the Bolton index, particularly in the segment from canine to canine. Furthermore, in these cases, there may be a transverse contraction of the maxillary arch over time, with a tendency of the mandible to slide later-

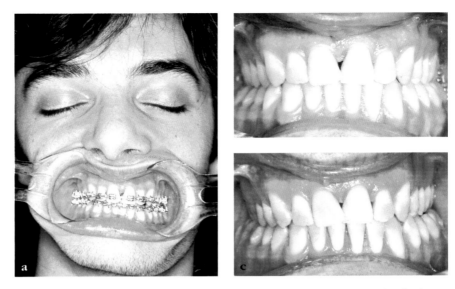

Fig 13-9 *(a)* Dentofacial asymmetry with mandibular hyperplasia. *(b)* The final occlusal result after double-jaw surgery with wire osteosynthesis and intermaxillary fixation. *(c)* Two years later the mandible shows a slight tendency to slide to the left (see dental midlines) due to occlusal reasons (dental interferences and narrowness of maxillary arch).

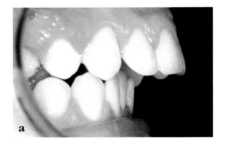
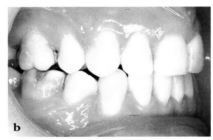
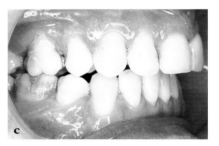

Fig 13-10 *(a)* Adult patient with moderate skeletal Class II malocclusion. *(b)* The final occlusal result after orthodontic-surgical treament and Obwegeser–Dal Pont osteotomy with rigid fixation. *(c)* Evident relapse 3 years later, most likely secondary to muscular problems.

ally, and thus the possibility of a slight occlusal relapse, although the general morphologic result remains substantially unvaried (Fig 13-9).

Where relapse is more frequent, both statistically and in the authors' experience, is undoubtedly in Class II cases with open bite. Although the concept of multifactorial etiopathogenesis remains valid, in these patients the muscular component is dominant, in association with condylar problems, particularly in relation to condylar resorption in patients who are at risk (see the above section). The case presented in Fig 13-10 is exemplary from this standpoint. This patient is a 20-year-old man with evident skeletal Class II malocclusion, subjected to mandibular advancement osteotomy, with rigid fixation, after orthodontic preparation with four extractions; the relapse occurred about 3 years after surgery, and, in the absence of certain condylar causes, may reasonably be considered to have a muscular etiology.

From the preceding text it is clear that the most dangerous and frequent complication in orthognathic surgery is the late relapse. It undoubtedly has multifactorial etiology (muscles, condyles, occlusion, age, initial disease), and all possible procedures and strategies must be brought into play to prevent it, particularly in patients and for types of malocclusion that are most at risk. Thus the orthodontic preparation must be rigorous, so as to reach all the planned preoperative goals in full, and to achieve a valid postsurgery occlusion and full surgical feasibility. It is essential to avoid being influenced by the patient, who is often in a hurry to have the operation, and not to be persuaded to advance the surgical time frame inappropriately. Surgical planning, especially for those malocclusions with high risk of relapse, must avoid excessive stretching of critical muscular groups, such as the pterygomasseteric sling and, to a lesser extent, the superhyoid musculature. Particular care must be paid during surgery to repositioning the condylar segment of the mandible, and the condyle-fossa relationship must be carefully observed during the postoperative period. Rigid fixation may help to prevent relapse, but it is not a panacea for all problems. The fight against relapse is won, above all, by paying careful attention to all the other details and the other strategies that have been mentioned repeatedly (occlusion, muscle, and joint equilibrium).

However, unfortunately, even putting into practice all of the above, some relapses may occur after a considerable time for which the etiopathogenesis cannot be identified. This is a risk that the orthodontist and surgeon must know and face, obviously providing proper information to the patient in a complete and understandable form. However, as we have said, such relapses never involve a return to the initial situation, and in general the esthetic result is substantially maintained. The patient, for whom this is the most important aspect, luckily tends to accept a slight occlusal relapse in a fairly positive frame of mind, provided that it does not involve functional problems.

Treatment in cases of relapse depends on the type of relapse presented. In slight cases, in which the cause is only or mainly occlusal, treatment may be limited to orthodontics with recovery of satisfactory occlusion, if necessary producing some slight dental compensation. Cases characterized by condylar resorption are discussed in the section above. In cases with muscular etiopathogenesis, or in which the relapse is quantitatively more significant and thus cannot be managed by orthodontics alone, the only possibility is to plan new orthodontic-surgical treatment, trying to understand in depth the etiopathogenic mechanism underlying the relapse and thus bring into play all possible therapeutic procedures aimed at avoiding it so as not to risk a further, and very unpleasant, failure.

Bibliography

Abeloos J, De Clercq C, Neyt L. Skeletal stability following miniplate fixation after bilateral sagittal split osteotomy for mandibular advancement. J Oral Maxillofac Surg 1993; 51:366-369.

Al-Kassab B, Barker GR. A computerized measurement of dental relapse following orthognathic surgery. Int J Adult Orthodon Orthognath Surg 1991;6:241-246.

Ayoub AF, Lalani Z, Moos KF, Wood GA. Complications following orthognathic surgery that required early surgical intervention: Fifteen years' experience. Int J Adult Orthodon Orthognath Surg 2001;16:138-144.

Bays RA, Greco JM. Surgically assisted rapid palatal expansion: An outpatient technique with long-term stability. J Oral Maxillofac Surg 1992;50:110-113.

Bell WH. Revascularization and bone healing after anterior maxillary osteotomy: A study using adult rhesus monkeys. J Oral Surg 1969;27:249-261.

Bell WH, Fonseca RJ, Kennedy JW, Levy BM. Bone healing and revascularization after total maxillary osteotomy. J Oral Surg 1975;33:253-260.

Bell WH, Proffit WR. Maxillary excess. In: Bell WH, Proffit WR, White RP Jr (eds). Surgical Correction of Dentofacial Deformities. Philadelphia: Saunders, 1980:341-343.

Benech A, Roccia F, Madaro E. Complicanza vascolare della chirurgia ortognatica: Rottura di uno pseudoaneurisma dell'arteria sfenopalatina a seguito di osteotomia secondo Le Fort I. Presentazione di un caso clinico e revisione della letteratura. Riv Ital Chir Maxillofac 1998;9:47-51.

Bouloux GF, Bays RA. Neurosensory recovery after ligation of the descending palatine neurovascular bundle during Le Fort I osteotomy. J Oral Maxillofac Surg 2000;58:841-845.

Bouwman JP, Kerstens HC, Tuinzing DB. Condylar resorption in orthognathic surgery: The role of intermaxillary fixation. Oral Surg Oral Med Oral Pathol 1994;78:138-141.

Brusati R, Fiamminghi L, Sesenna E, Gazzotti A. Functional disturbances of the inferior alveolar nerve after sagittal osteotomy of the mandibular ramus: Operating technique for prevention. J Maxillofac Surg 1981;9:123-125.

Busby BR, Bailey LJ, Proffit WR, Phillips C, White RP Jr. Long-term stability of surgical Class III treatment: A study of 5-year postsurgical results. Int J Adult Orthodon Orthognath Surg 2002;17:159-170.

Carlotti AE, Schendel SA. An analysis of factors influencing the stability of surgical advancement of the maxilla by the Le Fort I osteotomy. J Oral Maxillofac Surg 1987;45:924-930.

Carroll WJ, Haug RH, Bissada NF, Goldberg J, Hans M. The effects of the Le Fort I osteotomy on the periodontium. J Oral Maxillofac Surg 1992;50:128-132.

Coghlan KM, Irvine GH. Neurological damage after sagittal split osteotomy. Int J Oral Maxillofac Surg 1986;15:369-371.

Costa F, Robiony M, Politi M. Stability of Le Fort I osteotomy in maxillary advancement: Review of the literature. Int J Adult Orthodon Orthognath Surg 1999;14:207-213.

Costa F, Robiony M, Politi M. Stability of Le Fort I osteotomy in maxillary inferior repositioning: Review of the literature. Int J Adult Orthodon Orthognath Surg 2000;15:197-204.

Costa F, Robiony M, Politi M. Stability of sagittal split ramus osteotomy used to correct Class III malocclusion: Review of the literature. Int J Adult Orthodon Orthognath Surg 2001; 16:121-129.

Cutbirth M, Van Sickels JE, Thrash WJ. Condylar resorption after bicortical screw fixation of mandibular advancement. J Oral Maxillofac Surg 1998;56:178-182.

De Clercq CA, Neyt LF, Mommaerts MY, Abeloos JV, De Mot BM. Condylar resorption in orthognathic surgery: A retrospective study. Int J Adult Orthodon Orthognath Surg 1994;9:233-240.

De Clercq CA, Abeloos JV, Mommaerts MY, Neyt LF. Temporomandibular joint symptoms in an orthognathic surgery population. J Craniomaxillofac Surg 1995;23:195-199.

De Jongh M, Barnard D, Birnie D. Sensory nerve morbidity following Le Fort I osteotomy. J Maxillofac Surg 1986;14: 10–13.

De Mol van Otterloo JJ, Tuinzing DB, Greebe RB, van der Kwast WA. Intra- and early postoperative complications of the Le Fort I osteotomy. A retrospective study on 410 cases. J Craniomaxillofac Surg 1991;19:217–222.

De Mol van Otterloo JJ, Tuinzing DB, Kostense P. Inferior positioning of the maxilla by a Le Fort I osteotomy: A review of 25 patients with vertical maxillary deficiency. J Craniomaxillofac Surg 1996;24:69–77.

Dimitroulis G. A simple classification of orthognathic surgery complications. Int J Adult Orthodon Orthognath Surg 1998;13:79–87.

Dodson TB, Bays RA, Neuenschwander MC. Maxillary perfusion during Le Fort I osteotomy after ligation of the descending palatine artery. J Oral Maxillofac Surg 1997;55: 51–55.

Donoff RB. Surgical management of inferior alveolar nerve injuries (part I): The case for early repair. J Oral Maxillofac Surg 1995;53:1327–1329.

Dorfman HS, Turvey TA. Alterations in osseous crestal height following interdental osteotomies. Oral Surg 1979;48: 120–125.

Douma E, Kuftinec MM, Moshiri F. A comparative study of stability after mandibular advancement surgery. Am J Orthod Dentofacial Orthop 1992;6:21–34.

Fox ME, Stephens WF, Wolford LM, El Deeb M. Effects of interdental osteotomies on the periodontal and osseous supporting tissues. Int J Adult Orthodon Orthognath Surg 1991;6:39–46.

Franco JE, Van Sickels JE, Thrash WJ. Factors contributing to relapse in rigidly fixed mandibular setbacks. J Oral Maxillofac Surg 1989;47:451–456.

Fridrich KL, Holton TJ, Pansegrau KJ, Buckley MJ. Neurosensory recovery following the mandibular bilateral sagittal split osteotomy. J Oral Maxillofac Surg 1995;53:1300–1306.

Gallagher DM, Epker BN. Infection following intraoral surgical correction of dentofacial deformities: A review of 140 consecutive cases. J Oral Surg 1980;38:117–125.

Gassmann CJ, Van Sickels JE, Thrash WJ. Causes, location, and timing of relapse following rigid fixation after mandibular advancement. J Oral Maxillofac Surg 1990;48:450–454.

Giannì AB, D'Orto O, Biglioli F, Bozzetti A, Brusati R. Neurosensory alterations of the inferior alveolar and mental nerves after genioplasty alone or associated with sagittal osteotomy of the mandibular ramus. J Craniomaxillofac Surg 2002;30:295–303.

Gregg JM. Surgical management of inferior alveolar nerve injuries (part II): The case for delayed management. J Oral Maxillofac Surg 1995;53:1330–1333.

Hoffmeister B, Marks C, Wolff KD. Floating bone concept in mandibular distraction. Int J Oral Maxillofac Surg 1999; 28:90–97.

Hwang S, Haers PE, Sailer HF. The role of a posteriorly inclined condylar neck in condylar resorption after orthognathic surgery. J Craniomaxillofac Surg 2000;28:85–90.

Jones JK, Van Sickels JE. Facial nerve injuries associated with orthognathic surgery: A review of incidence and management. J Oral Maxillofac Surg 1991;49:740–744.

Karabouta I, Martis C. The TMJ dysfunction syndrome before and after sagittal split osteotomy of the rami. J Maxillofac Surg 1985;13:185–188.

Karas ND, Boyd SB, Sinn DP. Recovery of neurosensory function following orthognathic surgery. J Oral Maxillofac Surg 1990;48:124–127.

Kerstens HC, Tuinzing DB, Golding RP, van der Kwast WA. Condylar atrophy and osteoarthrosis after bimaxillary surgery. Oral Surg Oral Med Oral Pathol 1990;69:274–280.

Kobayashi T, Watanabe I, Ueda K, Nakajima T. Stability of the mandible after sagittal ramus osteotomy for correction of prognathism. J Oral Maxillofac Surg 1986;44:693–697.

Kwon H, Pihlstrom B, Waite DE. Effects on the periodontium of vertical bone cutting for segmental osteotomy. J Oral Maxillofac Surg 1985;43:952–955.

Lanigan DT, West RA. Management of postoperative hemorrhage following the Le Fort I maxillary osteotomy. J Oral Maxillofac Surg 1984;42:367–375.

Lanigan DT. Injuries to the internal carotid artery following orthognathic surgery. Int J Adult Orthodon Orthognath Surg 1988;3:215–220.

Lanigan DT, Hey JH, West RA. Aseptic necrosis of the maxilla. Report of 36 cases. J Oral Maxillofac Surg 1990a;48: 142–156.

Lanigan DT, Hey JH, West RA. Major vascular complications of orthognathic surgery: Hemorrhage associated with the Le Fort I osteotomies. J Oral Maxillofac Surg 1990b;48: 561–573.

Lanigan DT, Hey JH, West RA. Major complications of orthognathic surgery: False aneurysm and arteriovenous fistulas following orthognathic surgery. J Oral Maxillofac Surg 1991;49:571–577.

Leira JI, Gilhuus-Moe OT. Sensory impairment following sagittal split osteotomy for correction of mandibular retrognathism. Int J Adult Orthodon Orthognath Surg 1991;6: 161–167.

Levrini A, Lanteri C. Relapse and retention. Part I [in Italian]. Mondo Ortod 1988a;13(4):11–39.

Levrini A, Lanteri C. Relapse and retention. Part II [in Italian]. Mondo Ortod 1988b;13(5):29–69.

Lindquist CC, Obeid G. Complications of genioplasty done alone or in combination with sagittal split ramus osteotomy. Oral Surg Oral Med Oral Pathol 1988;66:13–16.

MacIntosh RB. Experience with the sagittal osteotomy of the mandibular ramus: A 13-year review. J Maxillofac Surg 1981;9:151–153.

Major PW, Philippson GE, Glover KE, Grace MG. Stability of maxilla downgrafting after rigid or wire fixation. J Oral Maxillofac Surg 1996;54:1287–1291.

Merkx MAW, Van Damme PA. Condylar resorption after orthognathic surgery. Evaluation of treatment in 8 patients. J Craniomaxillofac Surg 1994;22:53–58.

Michiwaki Y, Yoshida H, Ohno K, Michi K. Factors contributing to skeletal relapse after surgical correction of mandibular prognathism. J Craniomaxillofac Surg 1990; 18:195-200.

Moenning JE, Bussard DA, Lapp TH, Garrison BT. A comparison of relapse in bilateral sagittal split osteotomies for mandibular advancement: Rigid internal fixation (screw) versus inferior border wiring with anterior skeletal fixation. Int J Adult Orthodon Orthognath Surg 1990a;5: 175-182.

Moenning JE, Garrison BT, Lapp TH, Bussard DA. Early screw removal for correction of occlusion discrepancies following rigid internal fixation in orthognathic surgery. Int J Adult Orthodon Orthognath Surg 1990b;5:225-232.

Moldez MA, Sugawara J, Umemori M, Mitani H, Kawamura H. Long-term dentofacial stability after bimaxillary surgery in skeletal Class III open bite patients. Int J Adult Orthodon Orthognath Surg 2000;15:309-319.

Moore KE, Gooris PJJ, Stoelinga PJW. The contributing role of condylar resorption to skeletal relapse following mandibular advancement surgery: Report of five cases. J Oral Maxillofac Surg 1991;49:448-460.

Mordenfeld A, Andersson L. Periodontal and pulpal condition of the central incisors after midline osteotomy of the maxilla. J Oral Maxillofac Surg 1999;57:523-529.

Morgan TA, Fridrich KL. Effects of the multiple-piece maxillary osteotomy on the periodontium. Int J Adult Orthodon Orthognath Surg 2001;16:255-265.

Obwegeser JA, Wieselmann G. Can inferior alveolar nerve lesions be avoided during sagittal splitting? Anatomy, surgical technique and neurological aspects [in German]. Z Stomatol 1989;86:481-490.

Onizawa K, Schmelzeisen R, Vogt S. Alteration of temporomandibular joint symptoms after orthognathic surgery: Comparison with healthy volunteers. J Oral Maxillofac Surg 1995;53:117-121.

O'Ryan F, Epker BN. Temporomandibular joint function and morphology: Observation on the spectra of normalcy. Oral Surg Oral Med Oral Pathol 1984;58:272-279.

Panula K, Finne K, Oikarinen K. Incidence of complications and problems related to orthognathic surgery: A review of 655 patients. J Oral Maxillofac Surg 2001;59:1128-1136.

Perko M. Maxillary sinus and surgical movement of maxilla. Int J Oral Surg 1972;1:177-184.

Pogrel MA, Kaban LB, Vargervik K, Baumrind S. Surgically assisted rapid maxillary expansion in adults. Int J Adult Orthodon Orthognath Surg 1992;7:37-41.

Politi M, Costa F, Robiony M, Soldano F, Isola M, Soldano F. Stability of maxillary advancement for correction of skeletal Class III malocclusion after combined maxillary and mandibular procedures: Preliminary results of an active control equivalence trial for semirigid and rigid fixation of the maxilla. Int J Adult Orthodon Orthognath Surg 2002; 17:98-110.

Proffit WR, Phillips C. Adaptations in lip posture and pressure following orthognathic surgery. Am J Orthod Dentofacial Orthop 1988;93:294-304.

Proffit WR, Turvey TA, Phillips C. Orthognathic surgery: A hierarchy of stability. Int J Adult Orthodon Orthognath Surg 1996;11:191-204.

Quinn PD, Wedell D. Complications from intraoral vertical subsigmoid osteotomy: Review of literature and report of two cases. Int J Adult Orthodon Orthognath Surg 1988;3:189-196.

Reynolds ST, Ellis E 3rd, Carlson DS. Adaptation of the suprahyoid muscle complex to large mandibular advancements. J Oral Maxillofac Surg 1988;46:1077-1085.

Rosenquist B. Anterior segmental maxillary osteotomy: A 24-month follow-up. Int J Oral Maxillofac Surg 1993;22: 210-213.

Sanders B, Kaminishi R, Buoncristiani R, Davis C. Arthroscopic surgery for treatment of temporomandibular joint hypomobility after mandibular sagittal osteotomy. Oral Surg Oral Med Oral Pathol 1990;69:539-546.

Schultes G, Gaggl A, Karcher H. Periodontal disease associated with interdental osteotomies after orthognathic surgery. J Oral Maxillofac Surg 1998;56:414-417.

Schultze-Mosgau S, Reich RH. Assessment of inferior alveolar and lingual nerve disturbances after dentoalveolar surgery, and of recovery of sensitivity. Int J Oral Maxillofac Surg 1993;22:214-217.

Sesenna E, Raffaini M. Bilateral condylar atrophy after combined osteotomy for correction of mandibular retrusion. A case report. J Maxillofac Surg 1985;13:263-266.

Stajcic Z, Roncevic R. Facial nerve palsy following combined maxillary and mandibular osteotomy. J Craniomaxillofac Surg 1990;18:192-194.

Taglialatela F, Michelotti A, Farella M, Martina R. Neurosensory evaluation of orofacial region by Von Frey's monofilament device: A short and long term repeatability [in Italian]. Ortognatodonzia Ital 2002;11:51-57.

Taher AAY. Facial palsy: A complication of sagittal ramus osteotomy (Obwegeser–Dal Pont technique). Report of a case. Quintessence Int 1988;19:229-232.

Thuer U, Ingervall B, Vuillemin T. Functional and sensory impairment after sagittal split osteotomies. Int J Adult Orthodon Orthognath Surg 1997;12:263-272.

Turvey TA. Intraoperative complications of sagittal osteotomy of the mandibular ramus: Incidence and management. J Oral Maxillofac Surg 1985;43:504-509.

Van Merkesteyn JPR, Groot RH, Van Leeuwaarden R, Kroon FH. Intra-operative complications in sagittal and vertical ramus osteotomies. Int J Oral Maxillofac Surg 1987;16: 665-673.

Van Sickels JE, Jeter TS, Theriot BA. Management of an unfavorable lingual fracture during a sagittal split osteotomy. J Oral Maxillofac Surg 1985;43:808-809.

Van Sickels JE, Larsen AJ, Thrash WJ. Relapse after rigid fixation of mandibular advancement. J Oral Maxillofac Surg 1986;44:698-702.

Van Sickels JE, Tucker MR. Management of delayed union and nonunion of maxillary osteotomies. J Oral Maxillofac Surg 1990;48:1039-1044.

Van Sickels JE, Hatch JP, Dolce C, Bays RA, Rugh JD. Effects of age, amount of advancement, and genioplasty on neurosensory disturbance after a bilateral sagittal split osteotomy. J Oral Maxillofac Surg 2002;60:1012–1017.

Vedtofte P, Nattestad A. Pulp sensibility and pulp necrosis after Le Fort I osteotomy. J Craniomaxillofac Surg 1989;17:167–171.

Von Frey M. Verspatete Schmerzempfindungen. Z Gesamte Neurol Psychiatr 1992;79:324–333.

Walter JM, Gregg JM. Analysis of postsurgical neurologic alteration in the trigeminal nerve. J Oral Maxillofac Surg 1979;37:410–414.

Welch TB. Stability in the correction of dentofacial deformities: A comprehensive review. J Oral Maxillofac Surg 1989;47:1142–1151.

Westermark A, Bystedt H, von Konow L. Inferior alveolar nerve function after sagittal split osteotomy of the mandible: Correlation with degree of intraoperative nerve encounter and other variables in 496 operations. Br J Oral Maxillofac Surg 1998;36:429–437.

White CS, Dolwick MF. Prevalence and variance of temporomandibular dysfunction in orthognathic surgery patients. Int J Adult Orthodon Orthognath Surg 1992;7:7–14.

Will LA, Joondeph DR, Hohl TH, West RA. Condylar position following mandibular advancement: Its relationship to relapse. J Oral Maxillofac Surg 1984;42:578–588.

Wisth PJ. Mandibular function and dysfunction in patients with mandibular prognathism. Am J Orthod 1984;85:193–200.

Yamamoto R, Nakamura A, Ohno K, Michi K. Relationship of the mandibular canal to the lateral cortex of the mandibular ramus as a factor in the development of neurosensory disturbance after bilateral sagittal split osteotomy. J Oral Maxillofac Surg 2002;60:490–495.

Yeo JF, Loh FC, Egyedi P, Djeng SK. Serious circulatory disturbance after Le Fort I osteotomy: A case report. J Craniomaxillofac Surg 1989;17:222–225.

14

Clinical Cases

- Class III malocclusion
- Class II malocclusion
- Dentofacial asymmetry
- Open bite

This final chapter is a compendium of clinical cases, which are proposed as examples of the concepts presented in this book. The cases are subdivided into the different forms of dentofacial anomaly, and each case demonstrates both the diagnosis and the choice of the most appropriate therapeutic approach for the particular clinical situations specialists may be called upon to deal with.

Each case is presented with the same documentation: the essential clinical and radiographic records. On the left-hand page are, in order, the initial situation (face and occlusion), and the preoperative situation (occlusion). On the right-hand page are the medium-term final result and, in some cases, the long-term result (more than 7 years), together with some comments on the most significant clinical and therapeutic aspects. For the sake of brevity and simplicity, the radiographs are limited to those we believe to be essential for the clinician; ie, the initial and the preoperative views, which are set side by side for immediate comparison. On each radiograph the fundamental parameters as described in the book (incisal axes, mandibular plane,

palatal plane, cranial base) are indicated graphically. This layout echoes the clinical and esthetic principles that are the primary—if not the exclusive—guides to the surgical approach. Hence the emphasis in presenting the final result is fundamentally on occlusal balance, esthetic goals, and medium- and long-term stability, from both the esthetic and the functional standpoints.

Eighteen Class III cases are presented, together with six Class II cases, five dentofacial asymmetry cases, and four open bite cases. Four of these clinical cases (one in each group) also have severe temporomandibular joint (TMJ) disorders, which are discussed and commented upon in the individual cases. In these four cases, in addition to the standard documentation listed above, essential radiographs relevant to the TMJ are also provided and described.

For greater clarity and to focus the attention on the images, but also for reasons of space and to avoid reducing them in size, the photographs do not have individual legends. The reader will easily be able to reconstruct the diagnostic and therapeutic sequence from the comments accompanying each clinical case.

Class III Malocclusion

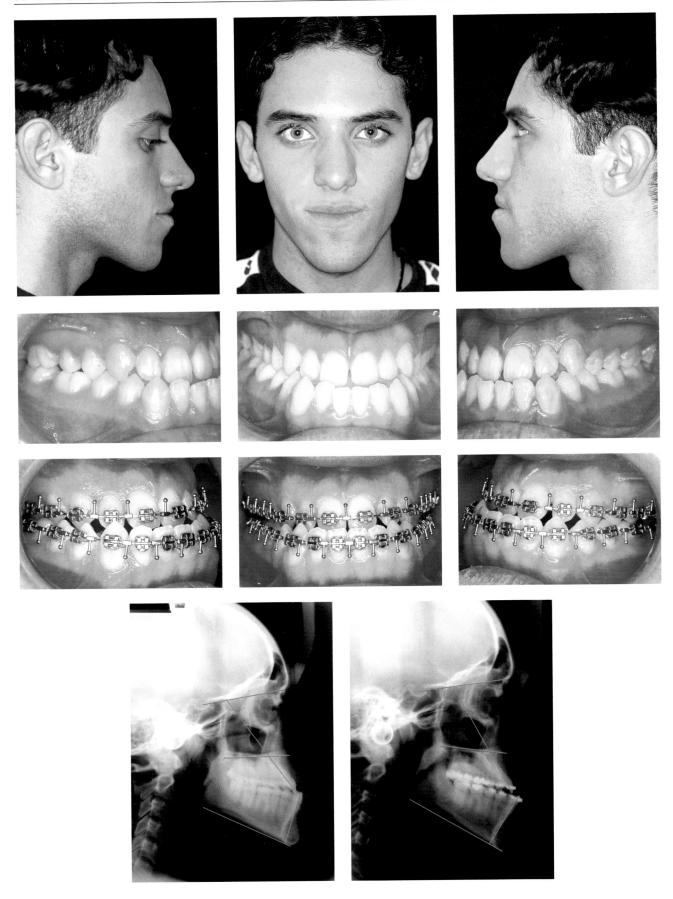

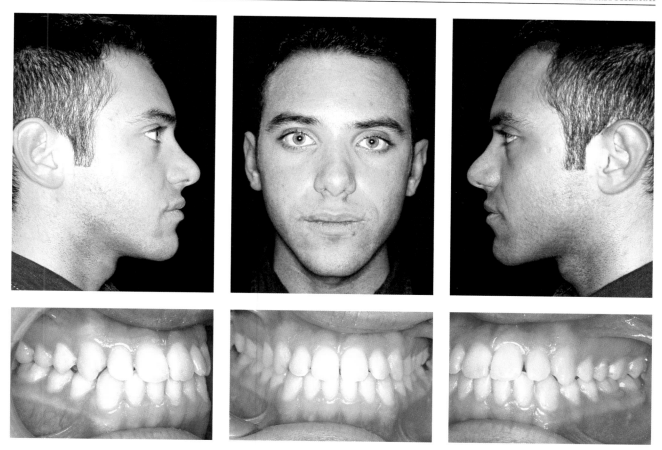

Case No. 1. Classic skeletal Class III case with pure mandibular component. Because the profile of the middle third is substantially acceptable, the choice is for a Gotte mandibular setback osteotomy (in all Class III cases presented, mandibular osteotomy is always performed with this technique, using rigid fixation). Presurgical orthodontic treatment, with alignment and decompensation following the rules given in the text, presented no particular problem. Rigid internal fixation (RIF) was adopted. The final result shown is at 3 years from the conclusion of active treatment. (Orthodontics: Dr A. Guariglia.)

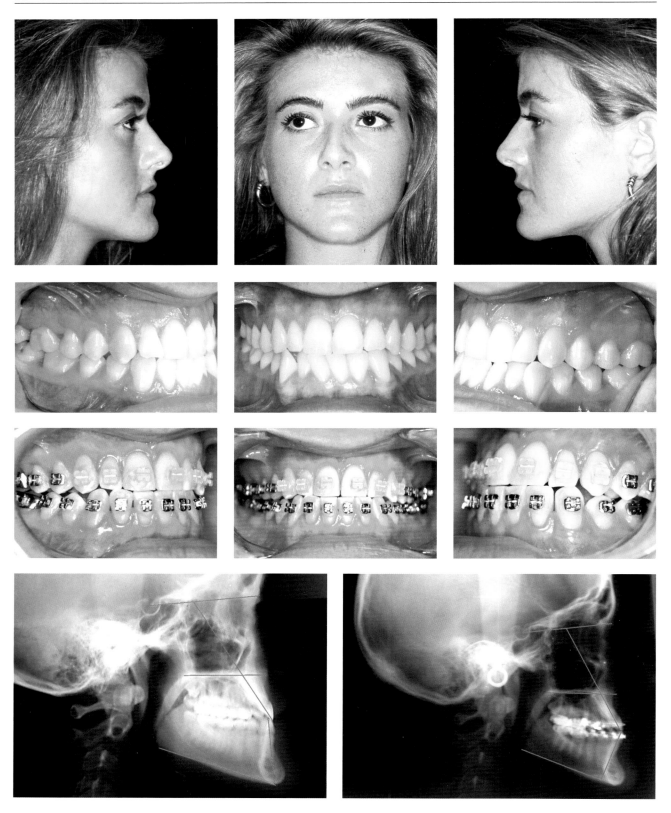

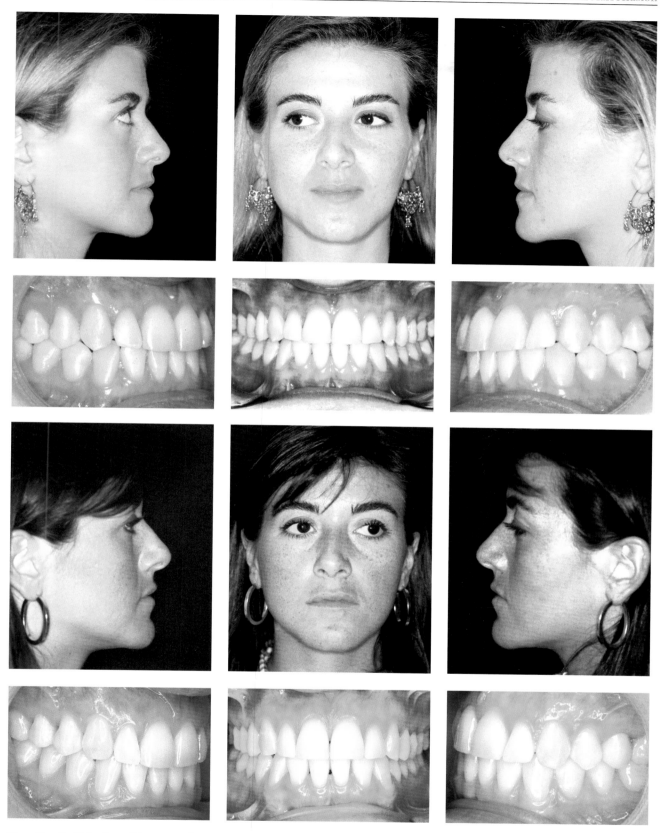

Case No. 2. This Class III case, with a pure mandibular component, may be considered a borderline case. The orthodontic and surgical choice was motivated by the patient's esthetic preferences and by the relatively quick preoperative orthodontic treatment. The orthodontic goals (leveling and perfecting the arches) were achieved in 8 months. A mandibular osteotomy with RIF was performed. The initial result *(above)* and that at 8 years *(below)* are shown; long-term stability is good. (Orthodontics: Dr A. Guariglia.)

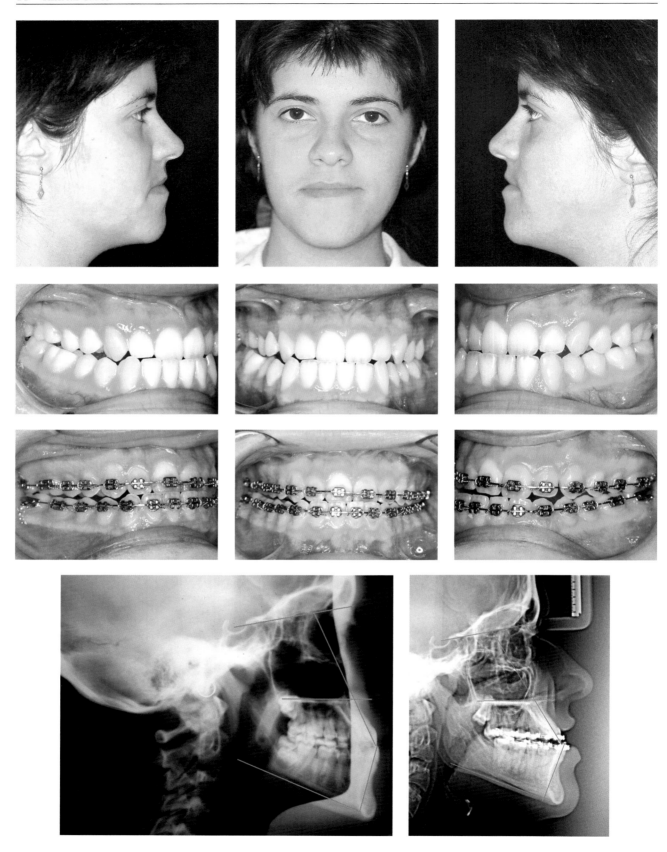

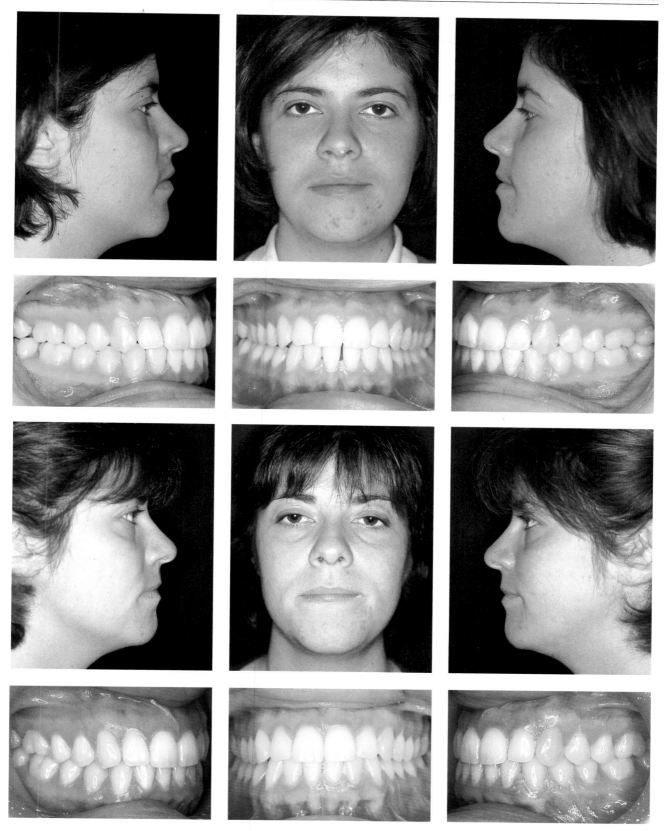

Case No. 3. The chief interest in this case, too, is the long-term result. Orthodontic treatment perfected the arches. This was followed by a mandibular setback osteotomy with RIF. Comparison between the initial result *(above)* and that at 10 years *(below)* shows the good stability of the result achieved. From the esthetic standpoint, the comparison between the final and long-term results shows that there has been some increase in the vertical dimension of the lower third over time. In this case, an associated genioplasty with vertical reduction would have been appropriate. (Orthodontics: Dr A. Guariglia.)

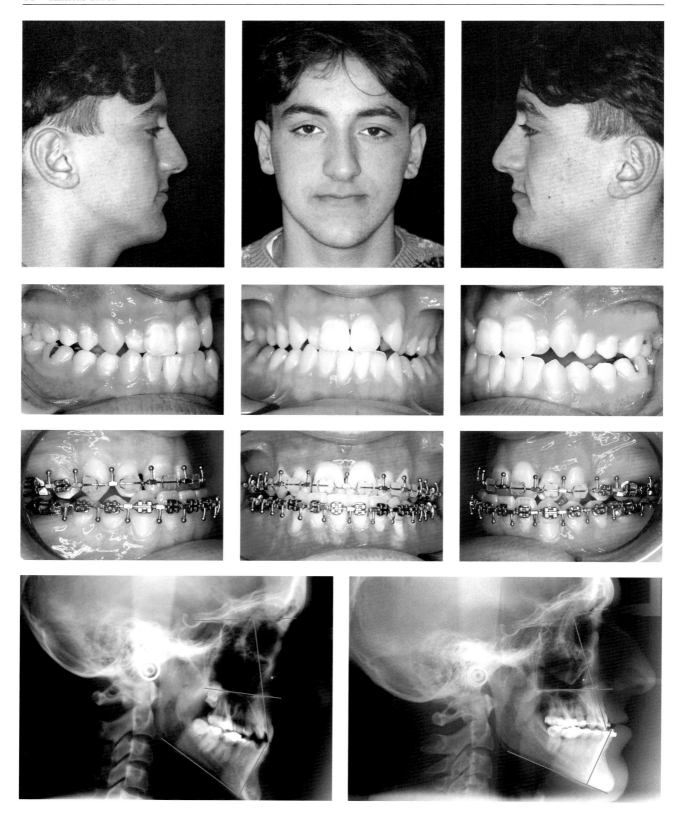

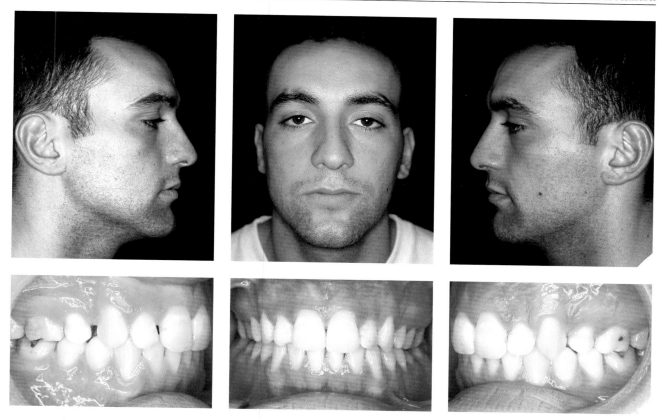

Case No. 4. This is a Class III case with a maxillary component, in which the choice of treatment (Le Fort I maxillary advancement osteotomy) was dictated by purely esthetic and profilometric considerations, independent of cephalometric values. To maintain the values of the maxillary incisal angle on the palatal plane within the ideal limits, and at the same time solve the maxillary crowding, it was necessary to extract two maxillary first premolars, with medial maximum anchorage at the first molars. The final result is at 3 years after completion of active treatment. (Orthodontics: Dr A. Guariglia.)

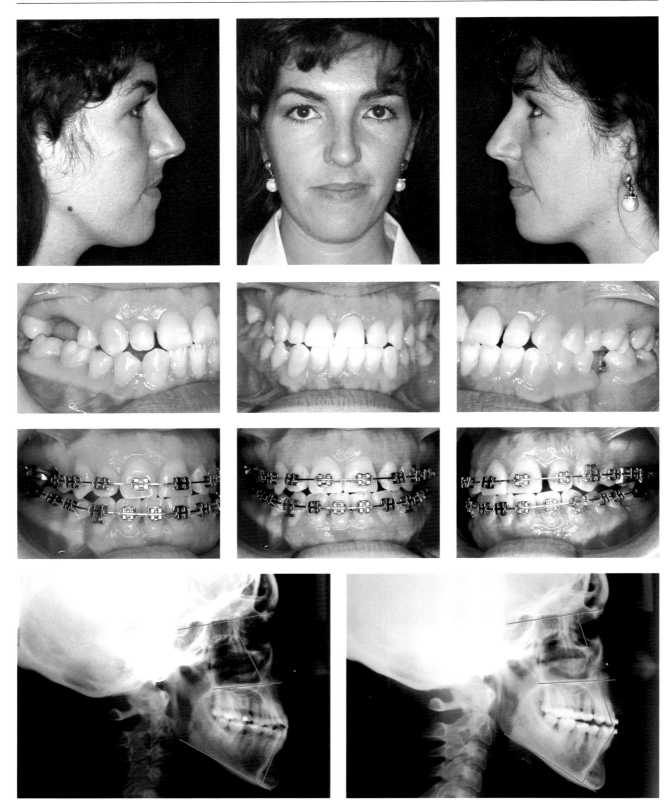

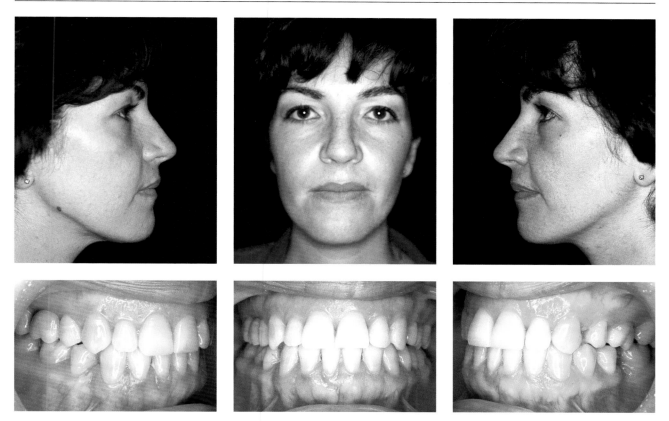

Case No. 5. The peculiarity of this Class III case consists in the choice of treatment, dictated by esthetic considerations, as always, but this time also by the age of the patient (35 years). Mandibular setback would have produced excessive relaxation of the soft tissue, with a risk of an aging effect. On the contrary, advancement of the maxilla, which was done with a Le Fort I osteotomy, not only resolved the occlusal problems, but undoubtedly produced an esthetic improvement and a lifting effect on the soft tissues. Note also the marked change in expression of the eyes. The presence of an edentulous space at the maxillary right posterior segment made favorable orthodontic decompensation possible, with the edgewise technique and maximum anchorage on the first molars. The final result shown is 4 years after completion of active treatment. Another characteristic of this case is that, because of a moderate alteration in the Bolton index at the incisor-canine level, which was due to a different mesiodistal diameter of the maxillary lateral incisors, a compromise was necessary: A slight difference (1 mm) between the two dental midlines had to be accepted, whereas the canine relationships are perfect Class I. (Orthodontics: Dr A. Guariglia.)

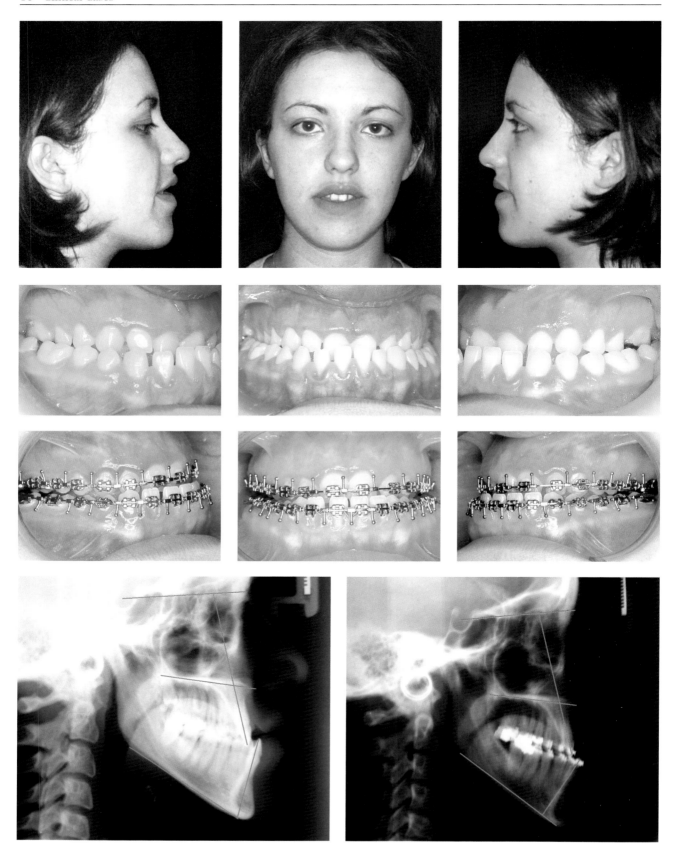

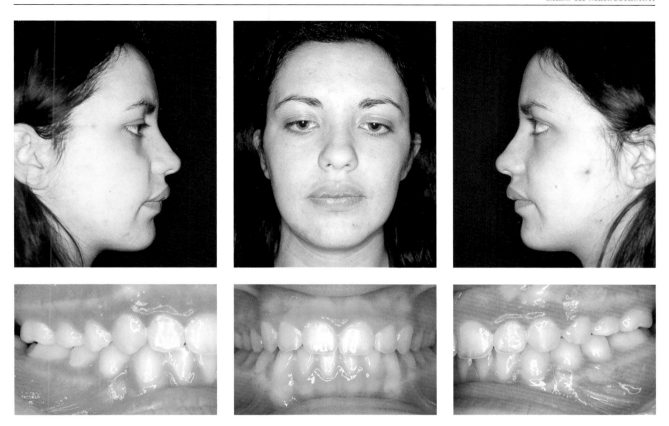

Case No. 6. This is a Class III case with mixed maxillary and mandibular components, with a slight vertical excess. The choice of treatment, Le Fort I osteotomy to advance and raise the maxilla with simultaneous mandibular setback osteotomy, was dictated by esthetic considerations. Furthermore, with some manipulation of the soft tissues when closing surgical access (V-Y suturing), the upper lip was deliberately given more fullness (perhaps excessively so). Orthodontic treatment, with the edgewise technique, above all produced a marked decompensation at the mandibular incisors, with marked accentuation of the negative overjet; this modification enabled the two jaws to be repositioned surgically to an adequate extent. RIF was used. The final result shown is at 1 year after completion of active treatment. (Orthodontics: Dr A. Guariglia.)

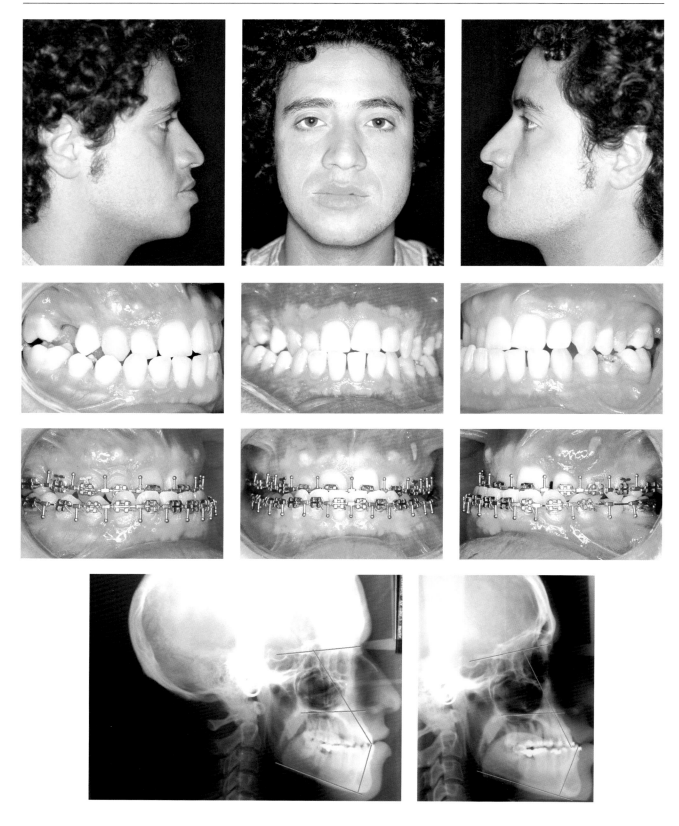

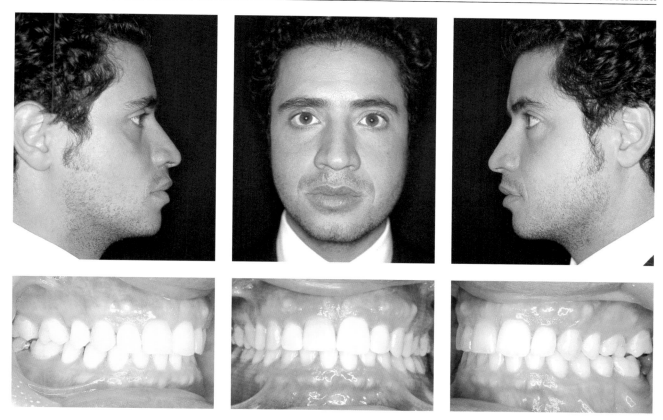

Case No. 7. This case is similar to the preceding one (Class III with mixed maxillary and mandibular components) and required effective decompensation during preoperative orthodontics, both at the mandibular arch and especially at the maxillary arch. In particular, because an edentulous space at the maxillary right second premolar tended to indicate extraction of the left second premolar, the anterior group was retruded with maximum anchorage on the first molars. The negative overjet achieved thus enabled the use of a double-jaw osteotomy (maxillary advancement plus mandibular setback) as indicated by clinical and esthetic analysis. As always in such Class III cases, RIF was adopted. In this patient, unlike the previous case, no particular treatment of the soft tissue of the lip (already rather prominent for a man) was employed and the difference over the preceding case is clear. The final result shown here is 3 years after the conclusion of active treatment. (Orthodontics: Dr A. Guariglia.)

223

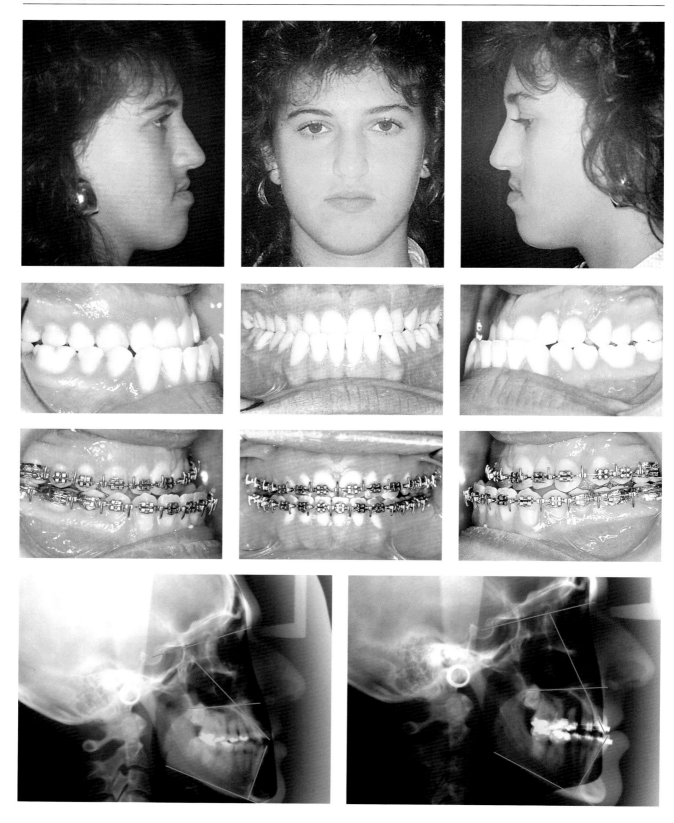

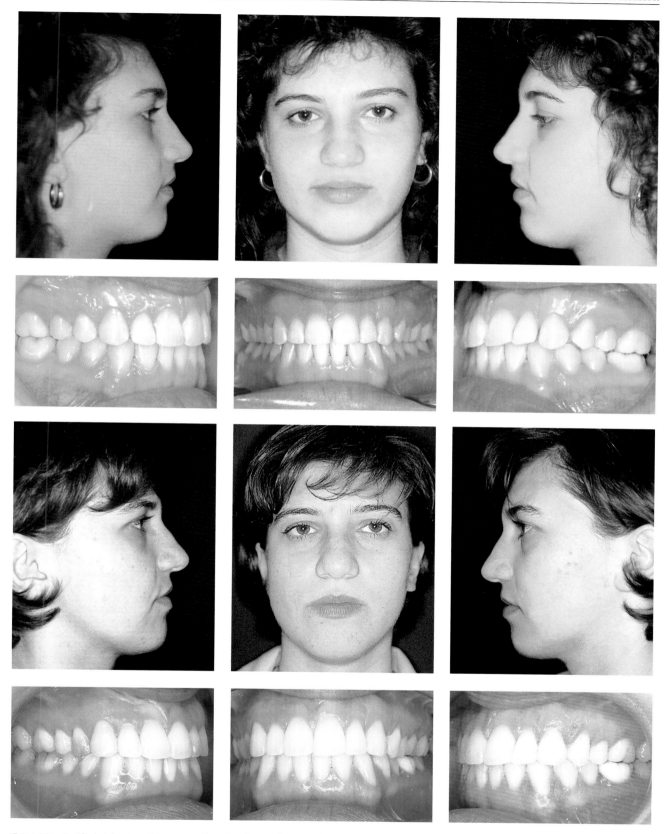

Case No. 8. Skeletal Class III case with mixed maxillary and mandibular components in which the interesting feature lies in the long-term outcome. Clinical and esthetic analysis suggested double-jaw osteotomy, with maxillary advancement and mandibular setback. Orthodontic treatment followed the classic principles (alignment, decompensation, perfecting the arches, no extractions). RIF was adopted. The results shown are at the end of active treatment *(above)* and at 13 years later *(below)*. From both the esthetic and the functional standpoints, stability may be considered optimal. (Orthodontics: Dr A. Guariglia.)

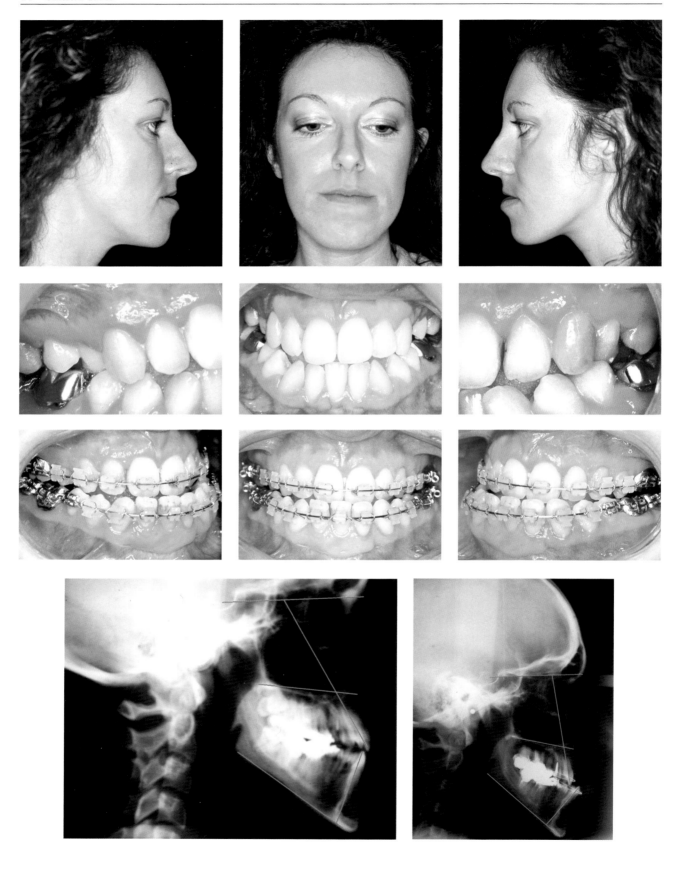

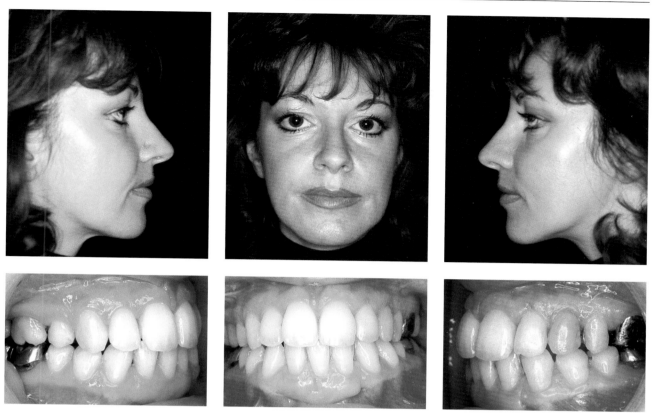

Case No. 9. This Class III case is exemplary of a particular situation: a frankly progenic profile, with slight vertical excess, accompanied by a Class III malocclusion that, at a superficial examination, might appear to be borderline. In reality, purely orthodontic correction of this malocclusion would produce an esthetic disaster. The treatment adopted consisted of extracting the first maxillary premolars, retruding the anterior group, again with maximum anchorage on the first molars, and mandibular decompensation with accentuated vestibularization of the incisors. (Note the absence of one incisor due to agenesis.) This made it possible to achieve a pronounced negative overjet, enabling the profile to be corrected to a greater extent through surgical advancement and superior repositioning of the maxilla, along with mandibular setback. This is exemplary of the concepts expressed throughout the book, that surgical operations can and should be modulated as a function of the orthodontic preparation achieved. RIF was adopted. Note also the spontaneous and marked improvement to the nose, consequent to maxillary osteotomy and appropriate manipulation of soft tissues during surgical closure, as well as the evident change in the expression of eyes and face. Given the lack of one mandibular incisor, the maxillary dental midline is centered on the axis of the one mandibular incisor. The results shown here are 2 years after completion of active treatment. (Orthodontics: Dr P. L. Botta.)

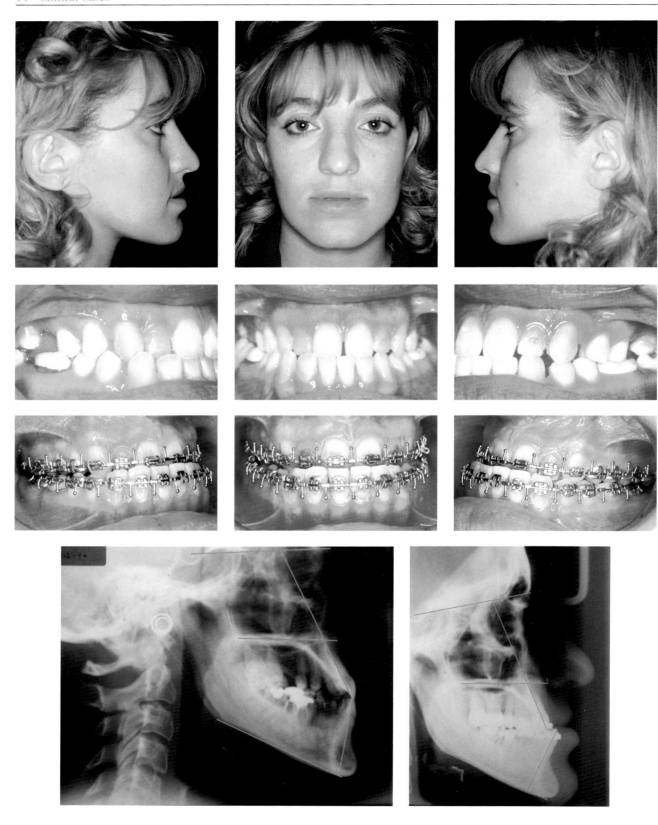

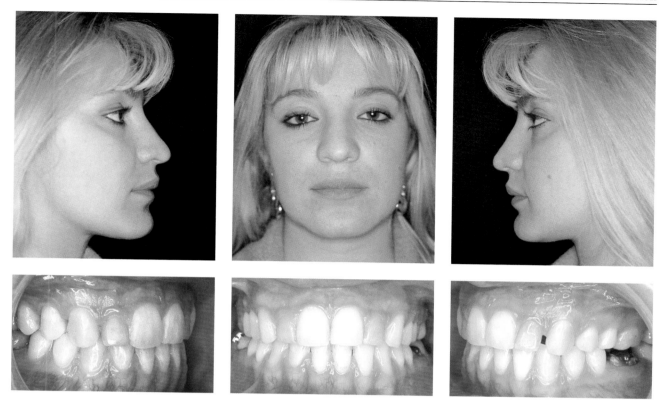

Case No. 10. The predominant factor in this case, which is skeletal Class III with mixed maxillary and mandibular components, is the lack of both maxillary first molars due to prior extraction. In this case, orthodontic preparation with lingualization of the maxillary incisors required longer and more elaborate treatment, starting with distalization of the premolars and canines, and subsequently of the incisors. Maximum anchorage was at the maxillary second molars. With regard to the mandibular arch, alignment and leveling with decompensation were performed. In this case, too, because a moderate negative overjet was achieved, it was possible to perform double-jaw osteotomy (maxillary advancement and mandibular setback) as esthetic considerations required. RIF was adopted. In this patient, too, greater prominence was given to the upper lip through appropriate manipulation of the soft tissues. The result shown is at 2 years after completion of active treatment. (Orthodontics: Dr M. Azzolina.)

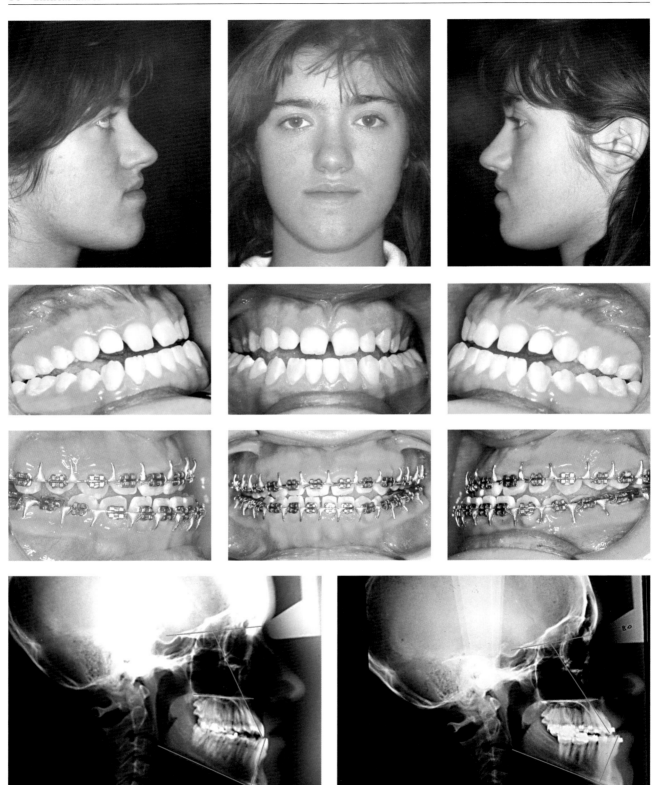

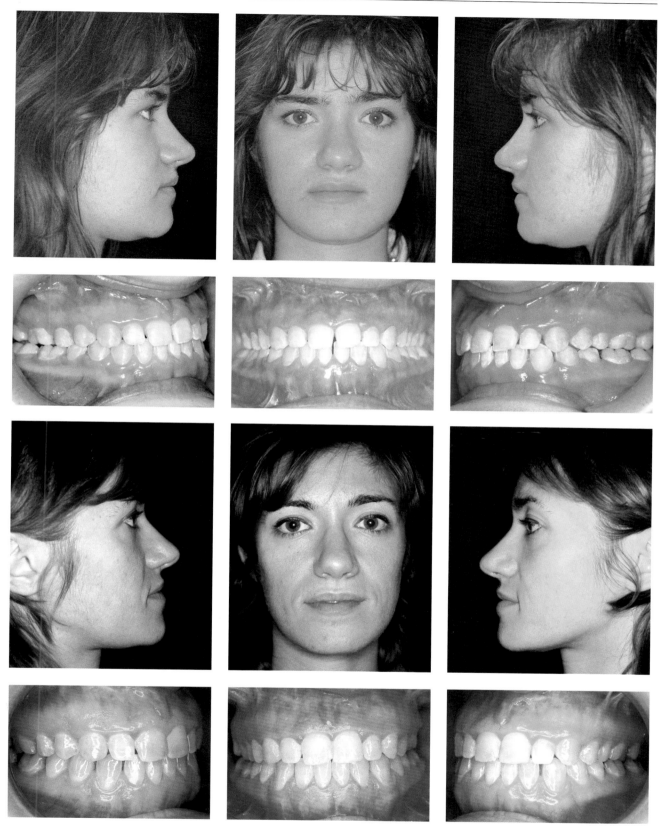

Case No. 11. The main features of this Class III case with mixed maxillary and mandibular components are the vertical excess at the lower third of the face and the long-term result. From the orthodontic standpoint, preparation followed the classic pattern as described, with no particular problems. From the surgical standpoint, the esthetic problem was resolved with advancement of the maxilla, mandibular setback, and vertical reduction genioplasty. RIF was adopted. The result shown is at completion of active treatment *(above)* and at 10 years *(below)*. (Orthodontics: Dr A. Guariglia.)

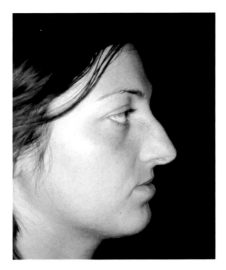
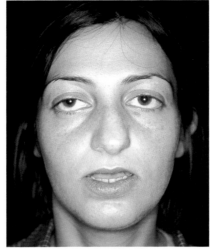
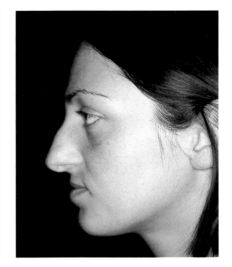

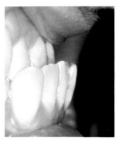
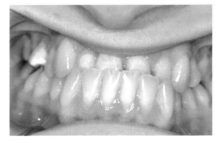
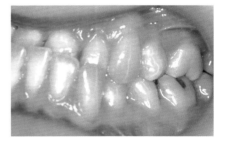

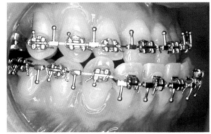
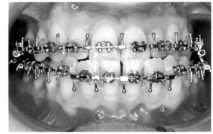
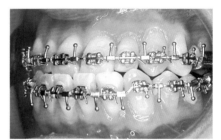

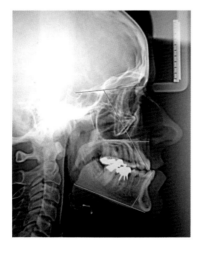
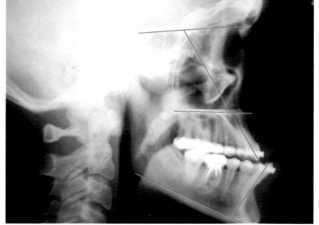

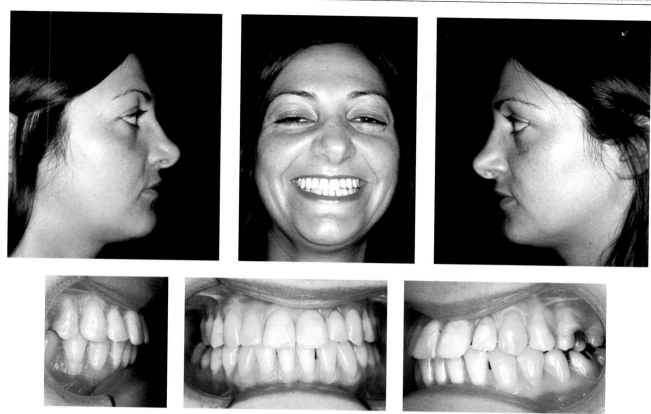

Case No. 12. This Class III case presents pure hypodevelopment of the maxilla (with no mandibular component) in both the sagittal and the vertical sense, with a complete lack of tooth exposure at rest and even when smiling. The nose is also significantly enlarged. The slight scleral exposure is not due to skeletal hypoplasia of the middle third, but to the hypotonic condition of the inferior orbicular muscles. Preoperative orthodontic treatment was complicated by gingival and periodontal problems present initially. Nevertheless, good coordination of the two arches was achieved, with satisfactory alignment of the incisal axes (note the absence of the maxillary left premolar due to prior extraction). Surgery consisted of advancement and inferior repositioning of the maxilla with interposition of bone graft harvested from the iliac crest and rigid fixation. Rhinoplasty was performed at the same time. The final result, 3 years after completion of active treatment, shows a satisfactory functional equilibrium and a good esthetic improvement, with normal tooth exposure when smiling. (Orthodontics: Dr G. Ambrosini.)

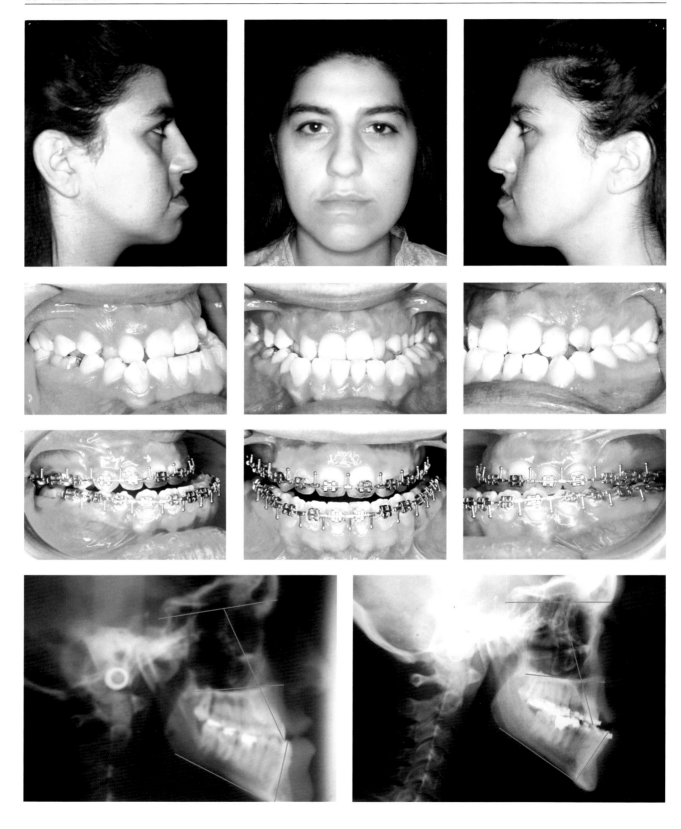

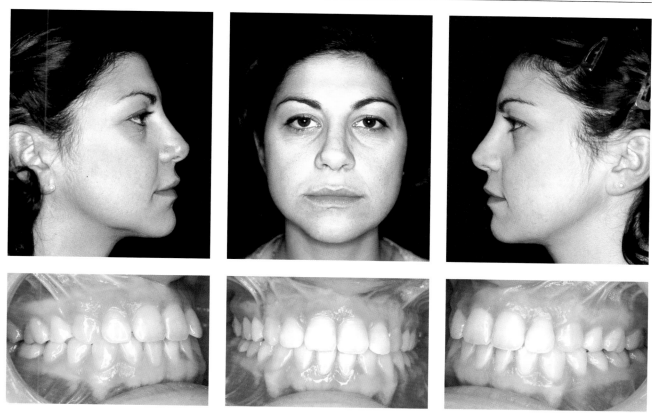

Case No. 13. This is an exemplary Class III case with mixed maxillary and mandibular components and an enlarged nose, in which rhinoplasty was associated with double-jaw osteotomy. This exploited the spontaneous favorable changes produced in the nose, together with small additional surgical corrections, and produced a satisfactory esthetic and functional result in a single operation. Orthodontic preparation followed the fundamental rules, with no extractions (decompensation, alignment, leveling and coordination of the two arches). RIF was adopted. The result shown is 5 years after completion of active treatment. (Orthodontics: Dr A. Guariglia.)

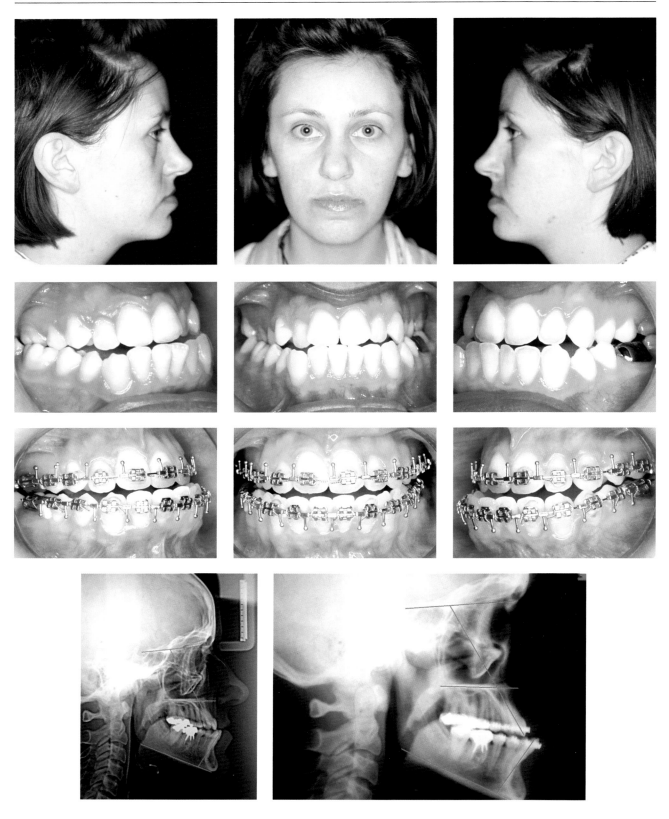

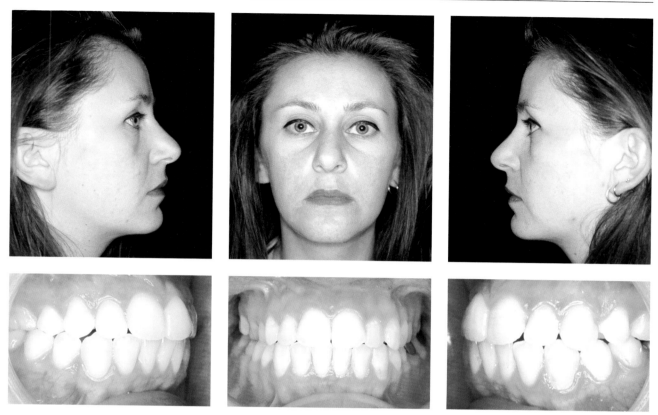

Case No. 14. This Class III case with mixed maxillary and mandibular components is exemplary because the situation is the opposite of the previous case. Clinical and esthetic analysis of the face suggested there was no doubt about the need for a double-jaw operation (advancement with Le Fort I osteotomy and mandibular setback) in consideration of the prominence of soft tissue pogonion and flattening of the paranasal areas. Furthermore, decompensation of the maxillary arch required extraction of both first premolars to enable the axis of the incisors to be normalized. The characteristics of the nose, with the tip already tilted upward and slight concavity in the supratip area, was nevertheless unsuited to maxillary osteotomy, which would certainly have worsened the situation by producing excessive tilting. In this patient, the associated rhinoplasty essentially consisted of contouring the alar cartilage and placing a cartilage graft above the tip (taken from the nasal septum after the downfracture). The goal was to eliminate the inevitable unfavorable effects and give greater support to the tip and dorsum of the nose. RIF was adopted. The final result shown here is at 2 years after completion of active treatment. (Orthodontics: Dr A. Guariglia.)

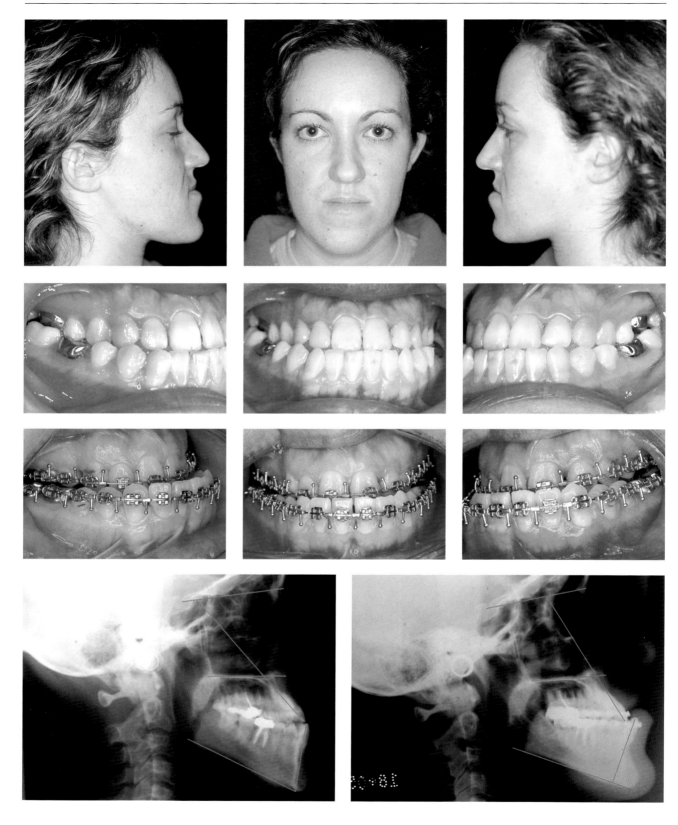

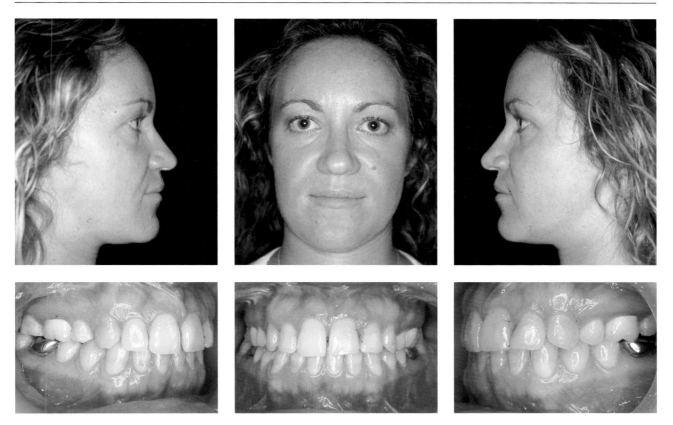

Case No. 15. This Class III case with mixed maxillary and mandibular components is characterized by marked hypoplasia of the middle third of the face at the level of the cheekbones. In this situation a Bell high maxillary osteotomy, described in chapter 7, is indicated, along with a Gotte mandibular setback osteotomy, as in all the Class III cases presented. In this case, too, the necessary decompensation at the maxillary arch required extraction of the first premolars; the maxillary anterior group was retruded, maximum anchorage being at the first and second molars. Mandibular alignment, here too with decompensation, did not require any extractions. RIF was adopted. The final result is shown 3 years after completion of active treatment. Note that in this case, too, there is a noticeable change in the expression of the eyes. (Orthodontics: Dr A. Guariglia.)

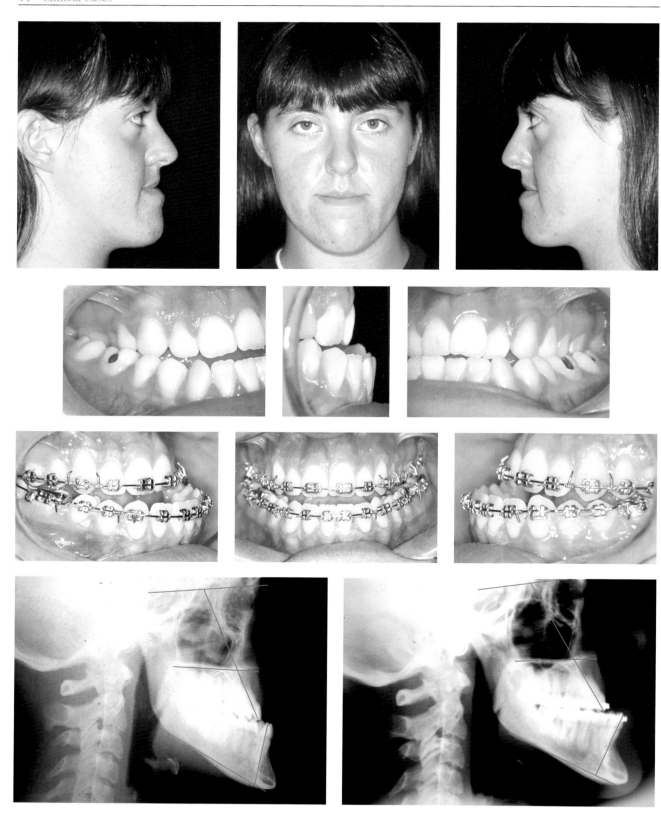

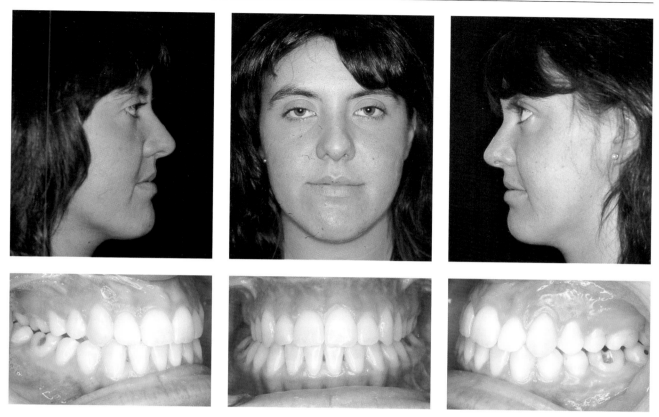

Case No. 16. This Class III case with mixed maxillary and mandibular components is characterized by an even more marked hypoplasia of the entire middle third, with flattening extending to the inferior orbital rim and marked scleral exposure. In these cases, a maxillomalar osteotomy performed intraorally is indicated (the technique is described in chapter 7), provided there are no particular contraindications (see chapter 9). Given the considerable negative overjet achieved during orthodontic preparation, mandibular osteotomy was associated. RIF was adopted. The final result is 4 years after completion of active treatment. Note the complete disappearance of scleral exposure. (Orthodontics: Dr C. Lanteri.)

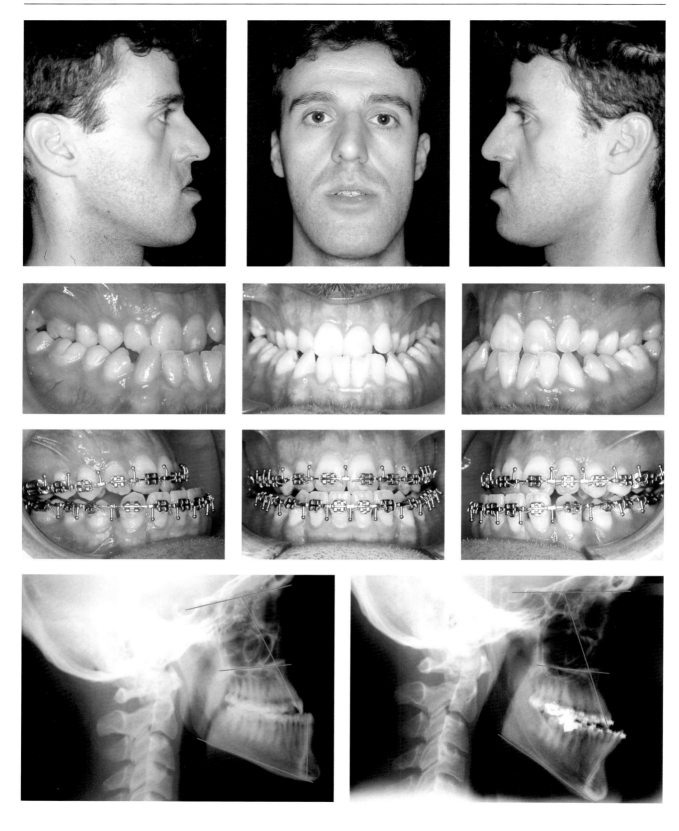

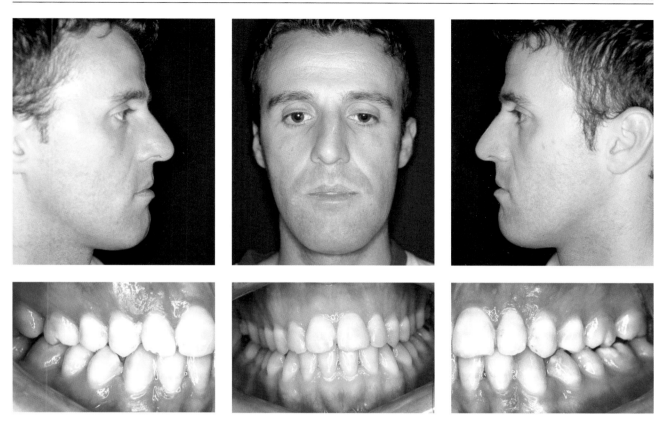

Case No. 17. This Class III case is similar to the previous one (mixed maxillary and mandibular components with severe hypoplasia of the entire middle third). Again the treatment preference was for maxillomalar osteotomy associated with mandibular setback. However, in this patient, to achieve effective decompensation and provide sufficient negative overjet, it was necessary to extract the maxillary first premolars and lingualize the maxillary incisors. In the mandibular arch, alignment and decompensation required no extractions. RIF was adopted. The final result is 2 years after completion of active treatment. Note that the hypoplasia of the middle third has been corrected. (Orthodontics: Dr A. Guariglia.)

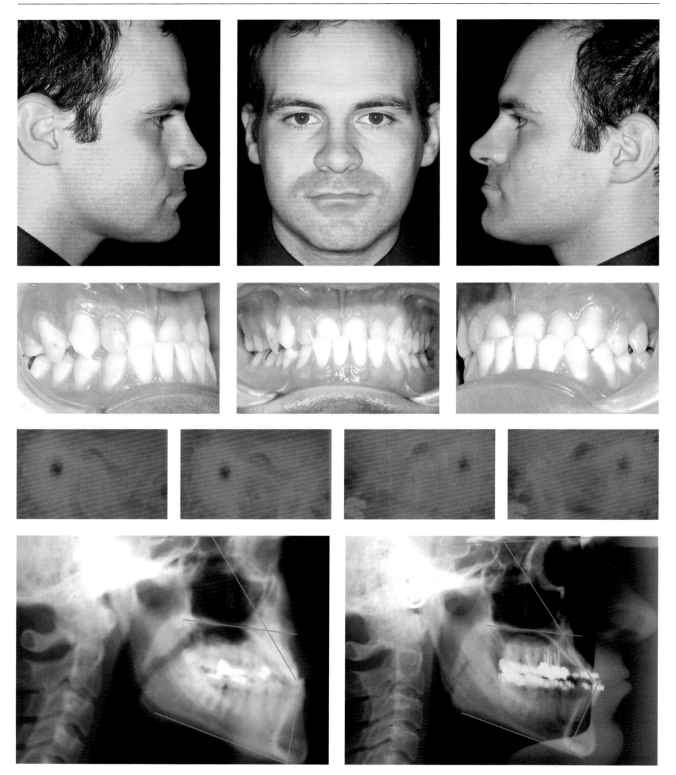

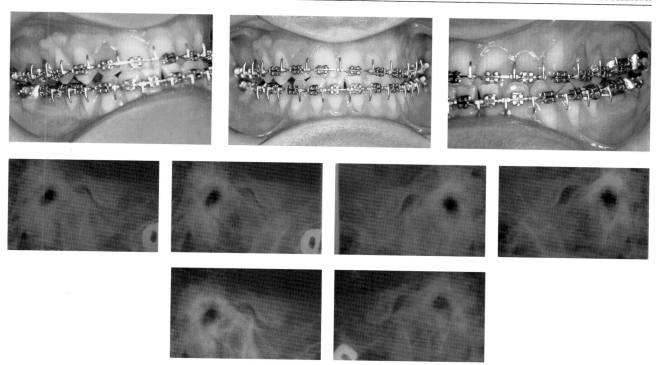

Case No. 18. This final Class III case, which may be diagnosed as progenic with a pure mandibular component and deep bite, also presented TMJ dysfunction, consisting of chronic relapsing partial dislocation of the mandibular condyles (see transcranial radiographs at open and closed mouth—first series on the left-hand page—where the condyles are clearly visible, markedly anterior to the articular tubercles). The patient presented to the office principally for this problem. Initial treatment with a repositioning splint resolved the relapsing partial dislocation, and preoperative orthodontic treatment was begun following the usual rules. After elimination of tooth interferences, the patient was able to discontinue use of the splint, although the condylar position was still monitored (see transcranial radiographs, second series, *above*). A Gotte mandibular osteotomy was performed, with fixation of the condylar position as described in chapter 6. The two transcranial radiographs presented above show the postoperative checkup on day 1, and the favorable maintenance of the condyle-fossa relationship achieved presurgically may be seen.

(continued on next page)

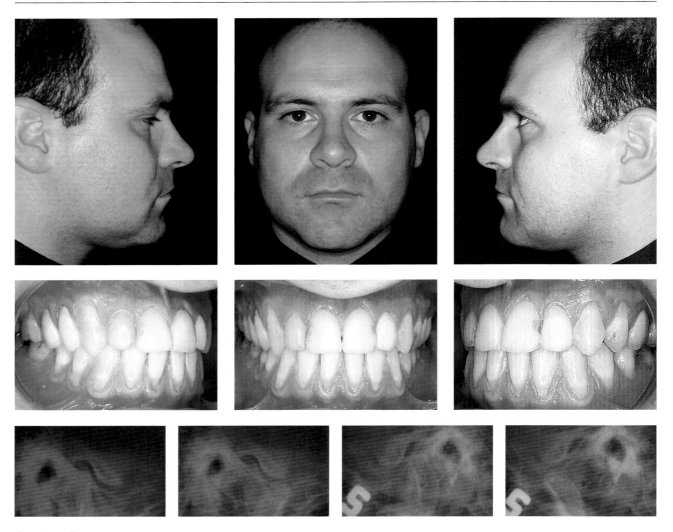

(continued)
The functional (more important in this case) and esthetic results are shown in the above photographs and the transcranial radiographs. These show the result 4 years after completion of active treatment. Note the favorable maintenance of the condyle-fossa relationship and the normalization of the condylar excursive movements. (Orthodontics: Drs L. Colombo and R. Moncada.)

Class II Malocclusion

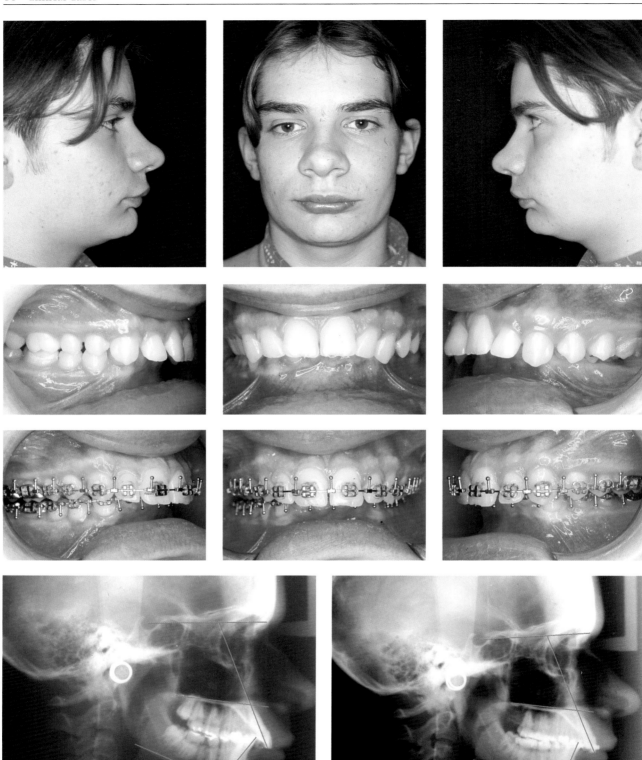

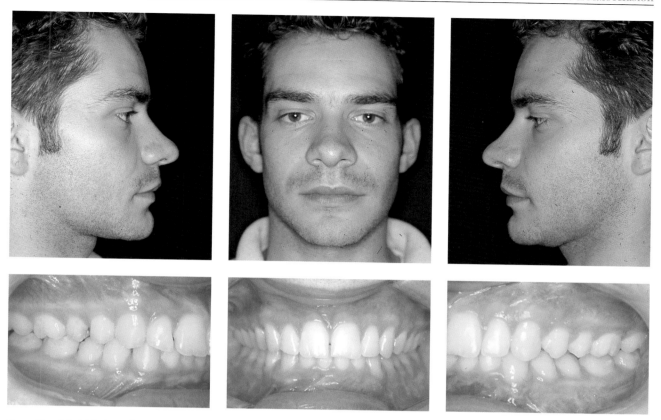

Case No. 19. This is a classic skeletal Class II case with a pure mandibular component and tendency to deep bite. The treatment selected was an Obwegeser–Dal Pont mandibular advancement osteotomy with RIF. Complete correction of the curve of Spee, which required leveling, was finalized and perfected in the postoperative phase, as described in chapter 11. The final result is at 4 years after completion of active treatment. (Orthodontics: Dr A. Guariglia.)

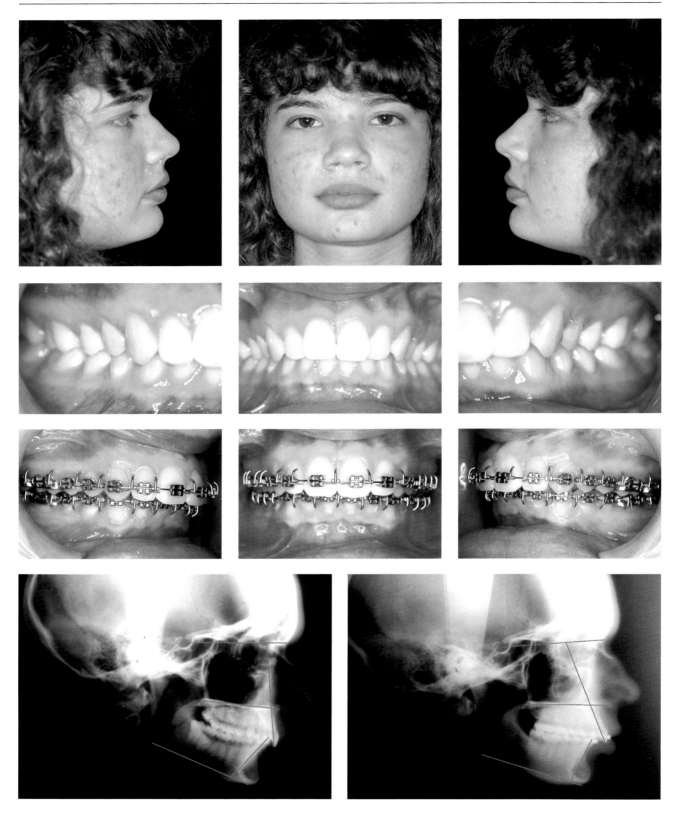

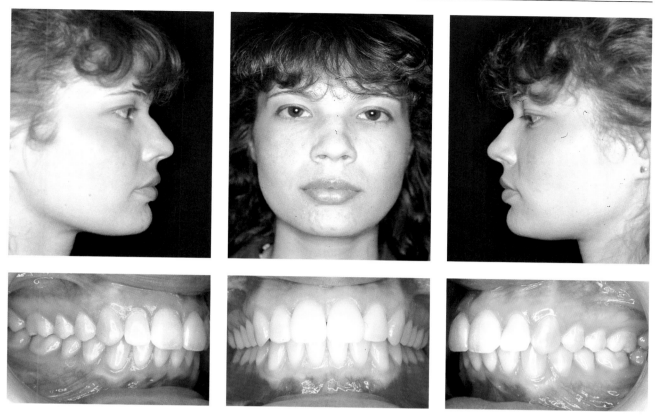

Case No. 20. This is a classic borderline case characterized by a slight Class II malocclusion with tendency to deep bite and an excessively square face. Orthodontic treatment alone would not have solved the esthetic and morphologic problems and would probably not have produced optimal medium- and long-term stability. The treatment selected was thus Obwegeser–Dal Pont mandibular advancement osteotomy with RIF. Preoperative orthodontic treatment was limited to aligning and perfecting the tooth arches. The result, at 5 years after completion of active treatment, shows satisfactory and stable esthetic and functional harmony. (Orthodontics: Dr A. Guariglia.)

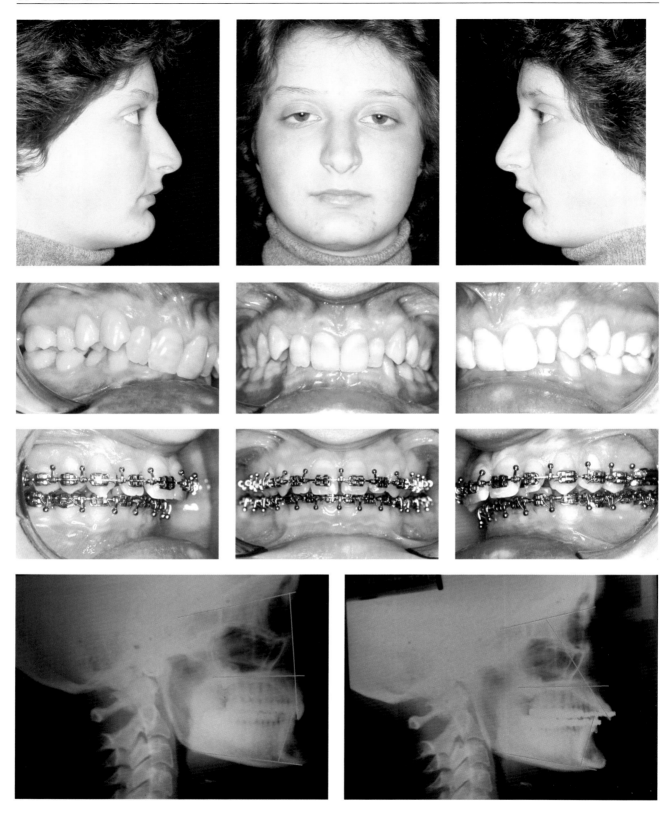

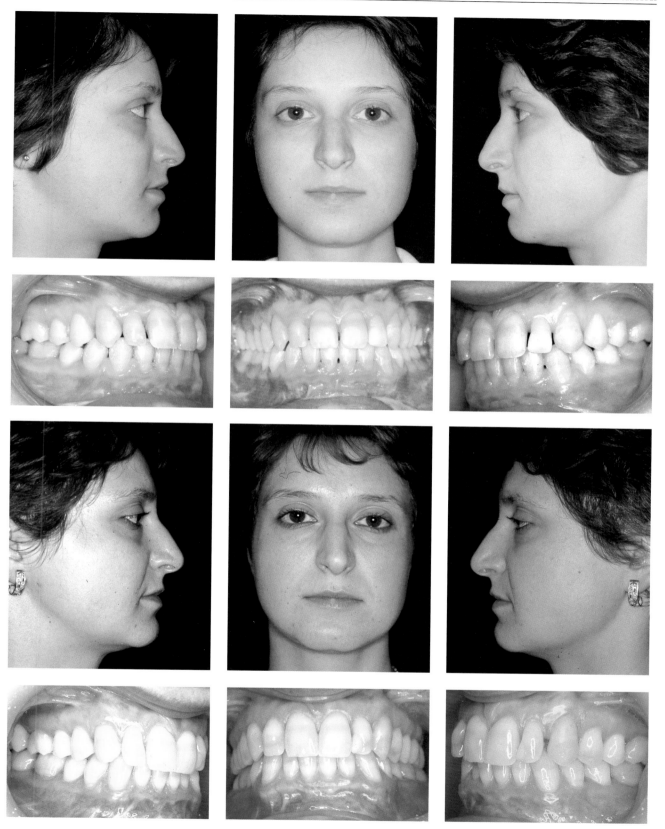

Case No. 21. What is notable about this classic Class II, division 2 case is the choice of treatment and the long-term stability achieved. Preoperative orthodontic treatment to perfect the arches and vestibularize the incisors transformed the malocclusion to Class I, division 1. With regard to surgery, an Obwegeser–Dal Pont osteotomy was performed with rigid fixation, accompanied by genioplasty for anteroposterior reduction. The initial result *(above)* and that at 13 years *(below)* show a harmonious esthetic and functional result. (Orthodontics: Dr A. Guariglia.)

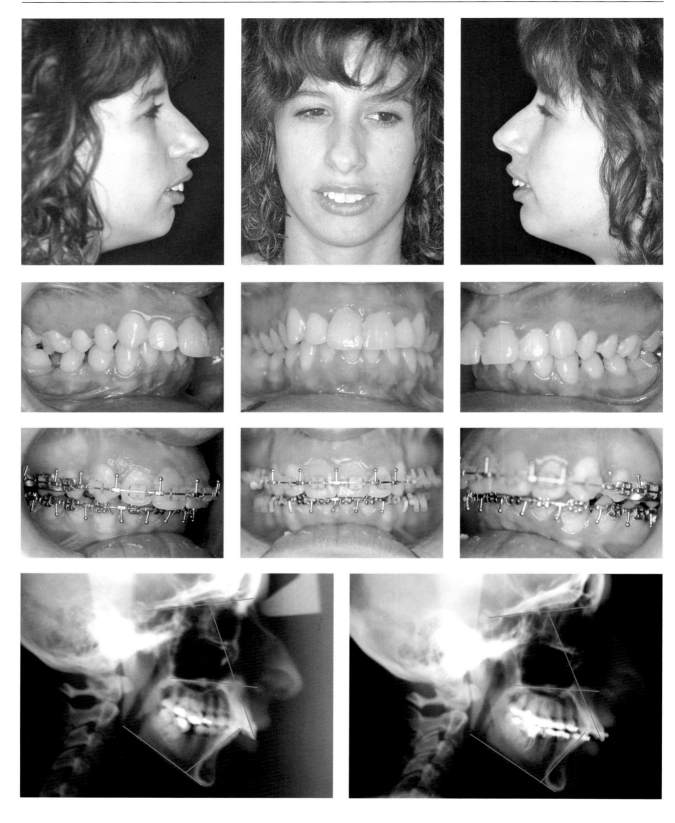

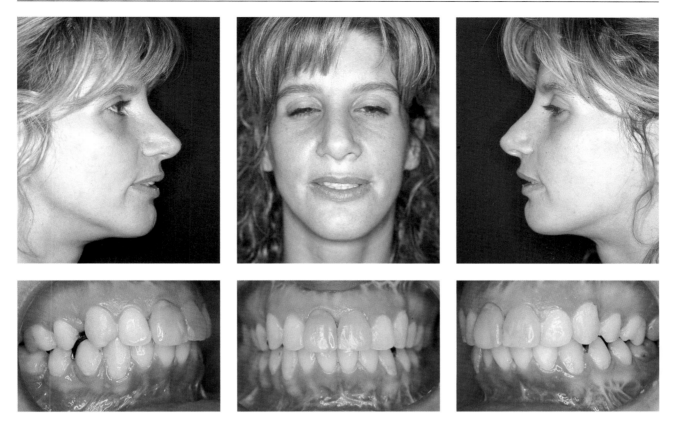

Case No. 22. This is an exemplary Class II case with vertical excess and transverse contraction of the maxilla. In agreement with measurements made following the school of McNamara, it also presented a vestibularization of the maxillary incisors, with no maxillary skeletal protrusion. The first step was to expand the maxillary arch surgically and orthodontically. This was followed by extraction of the maxillary first premolars and lingualization of the maxillary incisors. For the mandibular arch, simple alignment with leveling of the curve of Spee and modest lingualization of the mandibular incisors sufficed. From the surgical standpoint, double-jaw advancement with genioplasty was performed, based on exclusively esthetic rather than cephalometric considerations. This comprised Le Fort I osteotomy to advance and reposition the maxilla superiorly, Obwegeser–Dal Pont mandibular advancement, and advancement genioplasty. RIF was adopted. One year later, a slight corrective rhinoplasty was performed. (In this case it was decided to operate in two separate phases given the difficulty of predicting the spontaneous changes that would occur to the nose.) The final result is at 2 years after rhinoplasty. In this case, despite the evident morphologic and profilometric changes, the initial expression of the eyes has not improved significantly: A slight preexisting palpebral asymmetry is the cause. (Orthodontics: Dr A. Guariglia.)

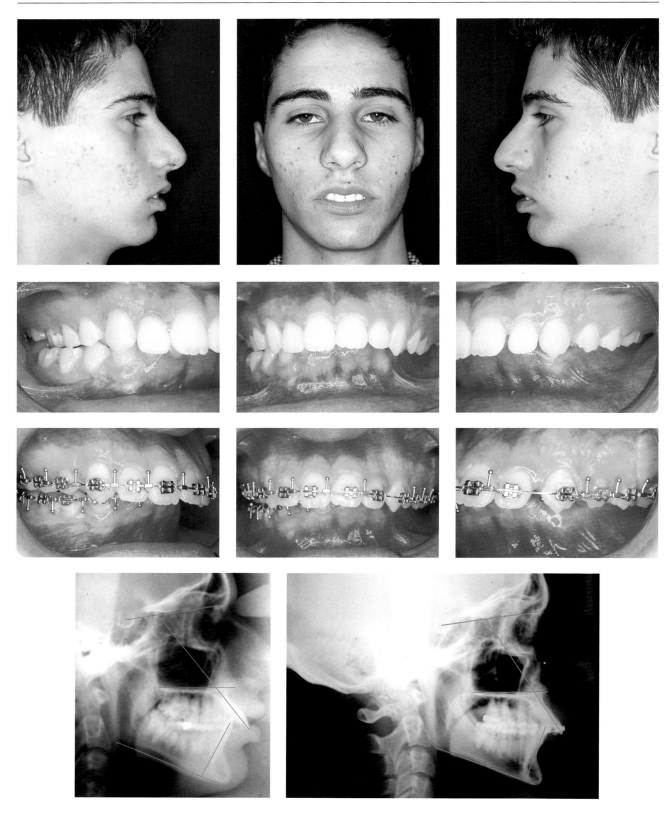

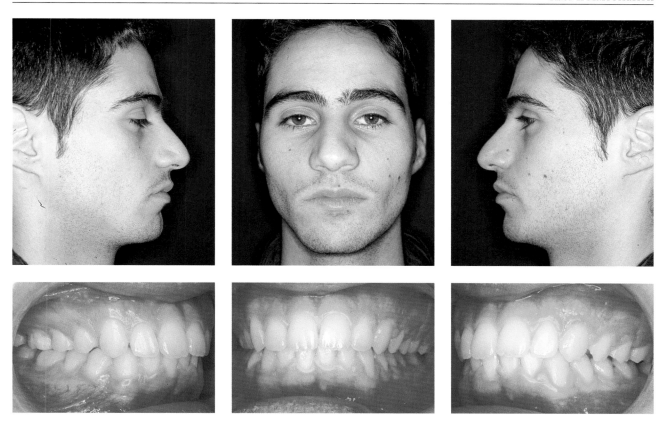

Case No. 23. This is an atypical case, but nevertheless an exemplary one, of Class II malocclusion with maxillary vertical excess and unilateral left Brodie syndrome. Furthermore, the maxillary occlusal plane is canted, being lower on the left, where a crossbite is present. Orthodontic preparation, given the impossibility of completely banding the mandibular arch due to the Brodie syndrome, was conducted partially by segments for the mandibular arch, whereas classic alignment of the maxillary arch to level and perfect it was performed. From the surgical standpoint, two-piece maxillary Le Fort I osteotomy was performed, with small palatal ostectomy and medialization of the left lateroposterior segment to correct the Brodie syndrome. This was associated with Obwegeser–Dal Pont mandibular advancement osteotomy and genioplasty to increase symmetry. RIF was adopted. Orthodontic treatment continued after surgery, with complete banding of the mandibular arch and the necessary orthodontic finishing treatment. The final result is at 3 years after completion of active treatment. (Orthodontics: Dr A. Guariglia.)

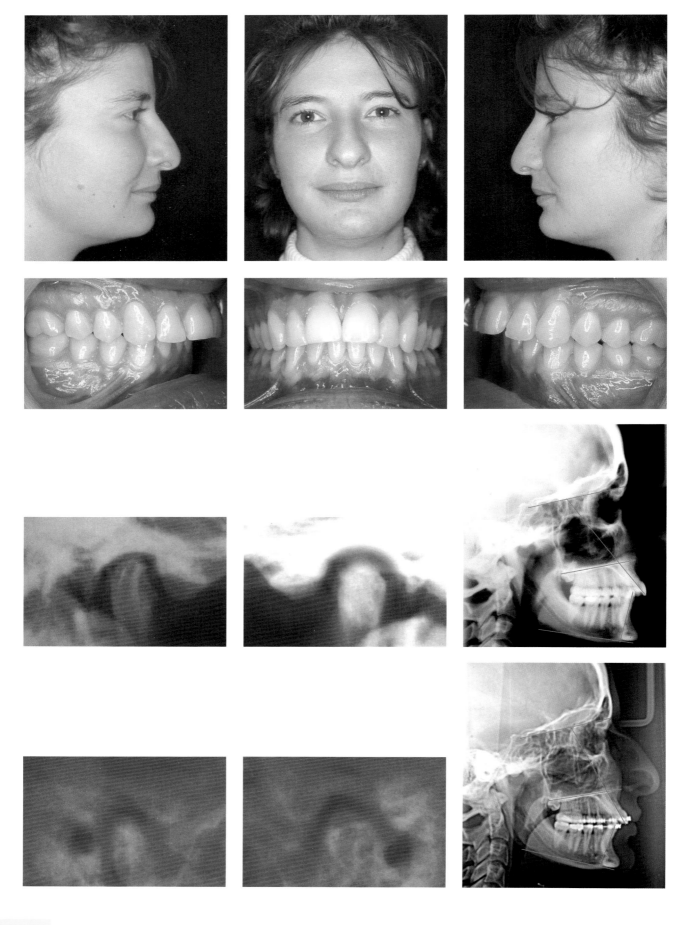

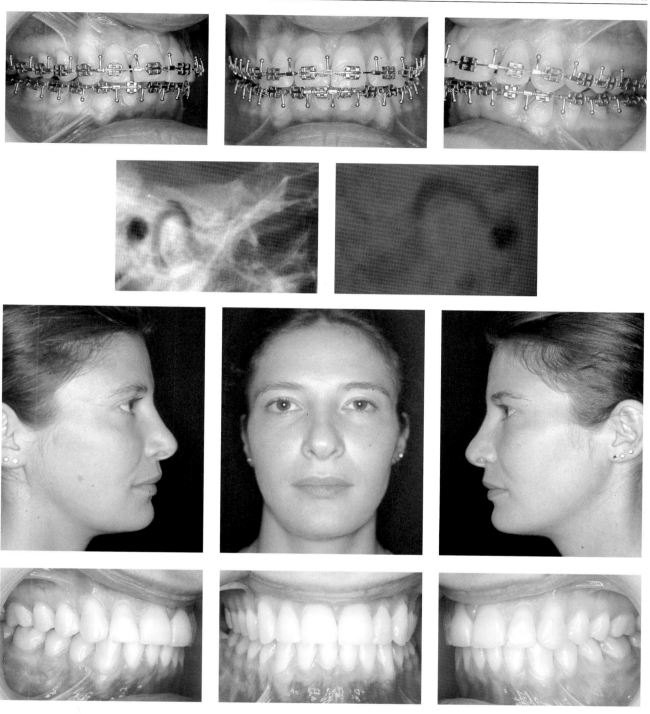

Case No. 24. This is a Class II case with a pure mandibular component, no vertical implications, and TMJ dysfunction. The subjective and objective TMJ disorders (pain and joint noises) were due to upward dislocation of the condyles with disk compression (see first series of TMJ radiographs on the left, in which the upward dislocation of the condyles is visible bilaterally). Initially, treatment was with an anterior repositioning splint; at disappearance of joint symptoms and elimination of some tooth interferences, this was followed by preoperative arch alignment. During this entire phase before the operation, the position of the condyles was monitored through transcranial radiographs (see second series of transcranial radiographs, bottom left). In this case, the required orthodontic decompensation was not marked (see radiographs). From the surgical standpoint, an Obwegeser–Dal Pont advancement osteotomy, with maintenance of the condylar position as described in chapter 6 and rigid fixation, was performed. This was accompanied by corrective rhinoplasty. The transcranial radiographs *(above)*, on day 1 postsurgery, show that the preoperative condyle position has been maintained. The final result, 2 years after the end of active treatment, shows that a satisfactory functional and esthetic equilibrium has been achieved. (Orthodontics: Dr A. Guariglia.)

Dentofacial Asymmetry

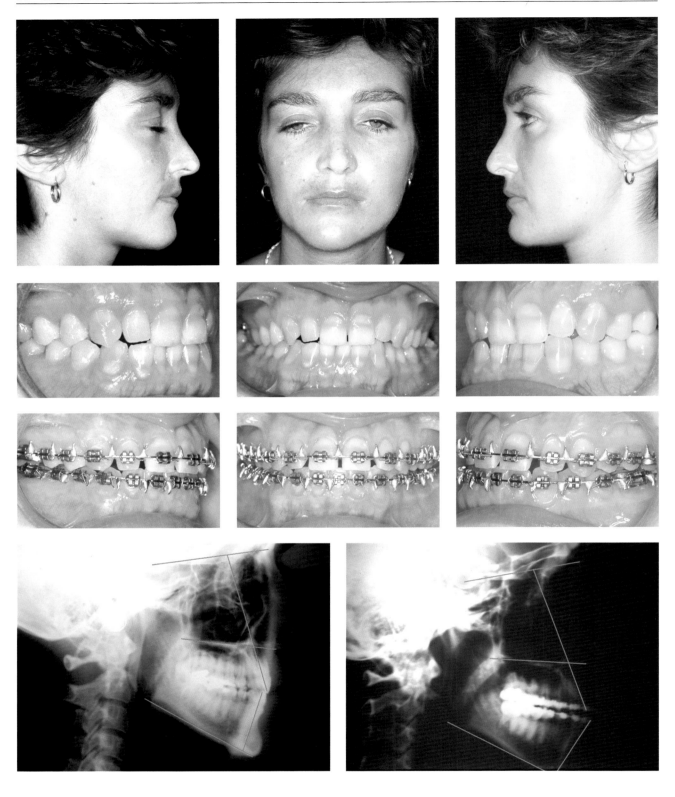

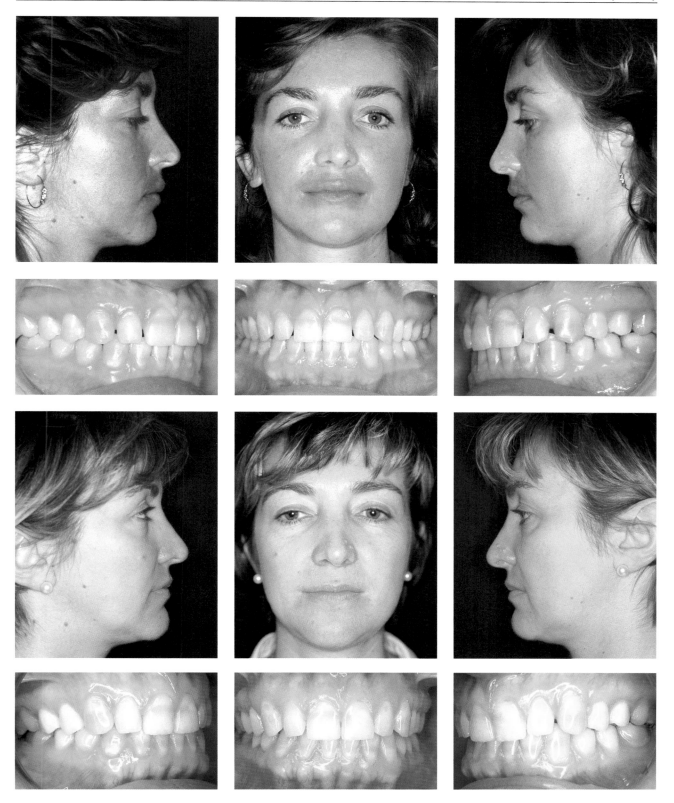

Case No. 25. This is an exemplary case of pure mandibular laterodeviation (hemimandibular elongation), with the maxilla perfectly centered, in a patient who has completed growth. Note the evident compensation of the mandibular incisors. Preoperative orthodontic treatment for perfection of the arches was relatively simple and quick. Gotte bilateral split osteotomy of the mandibular angle was performed with wiring and maxillomandibular fixation for 4 weeks. The initial result *(above)* and that at 14 years *(below)* are presented, showing good esthetic and functional stability. (Orthodontics: Dr A. Guariglia.)

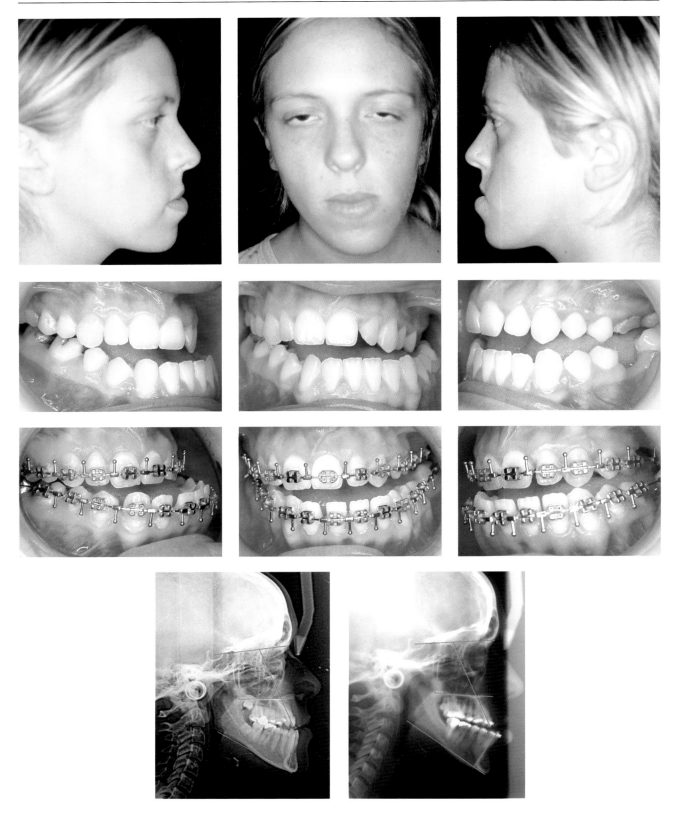

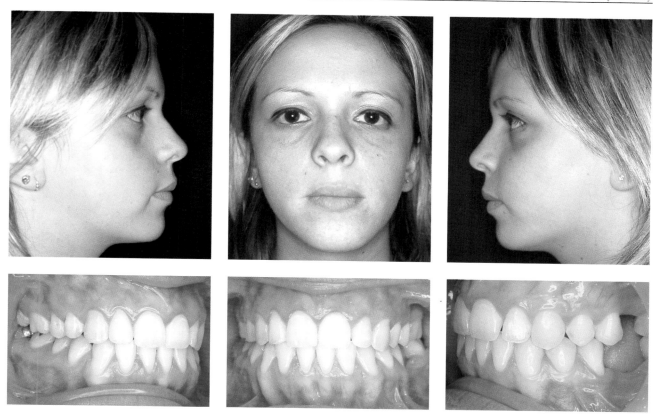

Case No. 26. This is a case of fairly severe dentofacial asymmetry with mixed maxillary and mandibular components and some Class III features. It may be considered a compound form of hemimandibular hyperplasia and hemimandibular elongation. Nevertheless, there is no evident condylar hyperplasia. Note the absence of the left mandibular first molar due to prior extraction and the need to extract the maxillary left first molar because of extensive caries. Preoperative orthodontics entailed no other particular problems. A double-jaw operation was performed (maxillary osteotomy of the Le Fort I type to increase symmetry and Gotte bilateral split osteotomy of the mandibular angle) with wire osteosynthesis and maxillomandibular fixation for 4 weeks. The result shown is 2 years after completion of active treatment. Note the overall marked improvement and the resulting lively expression of the eyes. (Orthodontics: Dr A. Guariglia.)

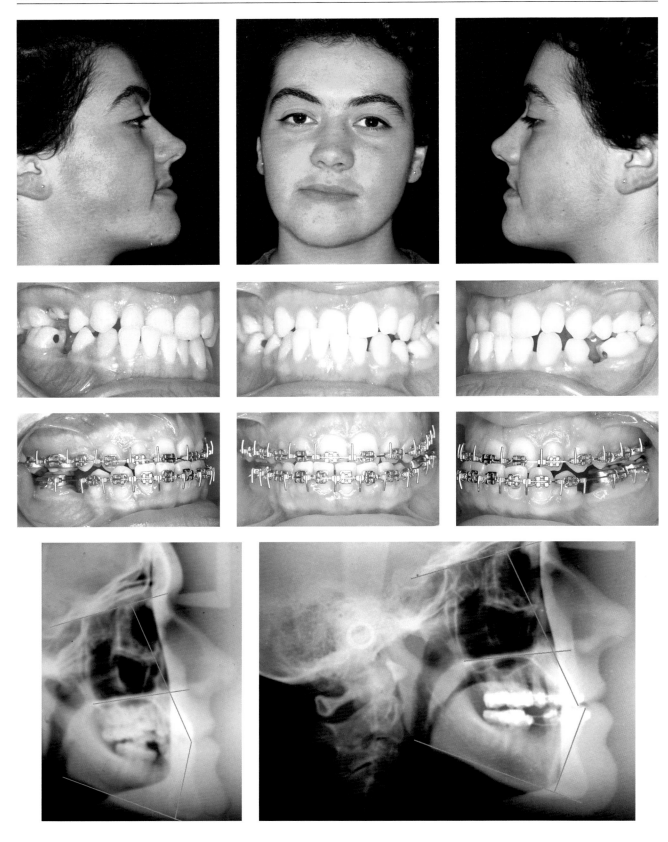

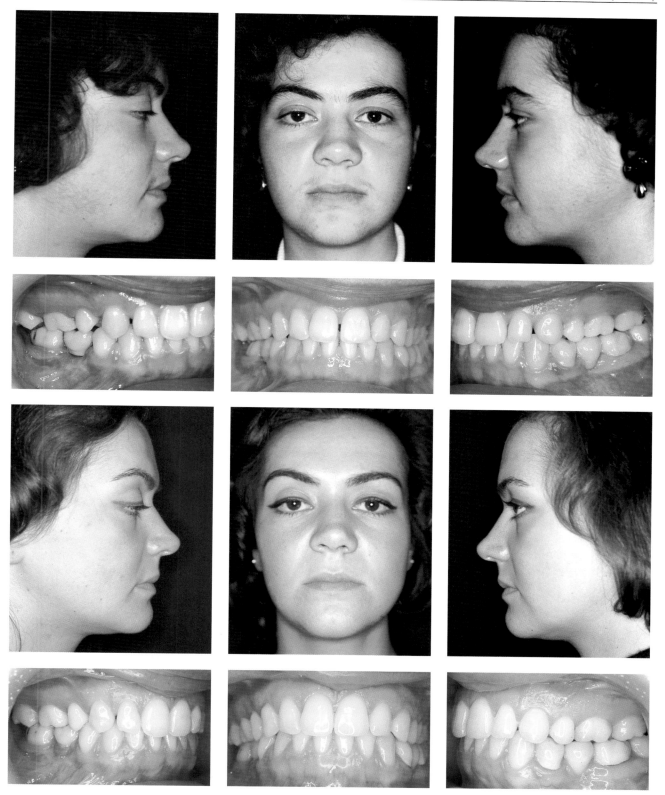

Case No. 27. This case is exemplary because of the long-term stability achieved. A double-jaw operation was performed, with wiring and maxillomandibular fixation. With regard to preoperative orthodontics, in consideration of the agenesis of all second premolars, it was decided to close the spaces in the maxillary arch and maintain the spaces in the mandibular arch for subsequent implant-supported prosthetic rehabilitation. This decision was motivated by the lack of sufficient bone support in the mandibular arch for mesialization of the first molars. The initial result is presented together with that at 9 years after completion of treatment. (Orthodontics: Dr A. Guariglia.)

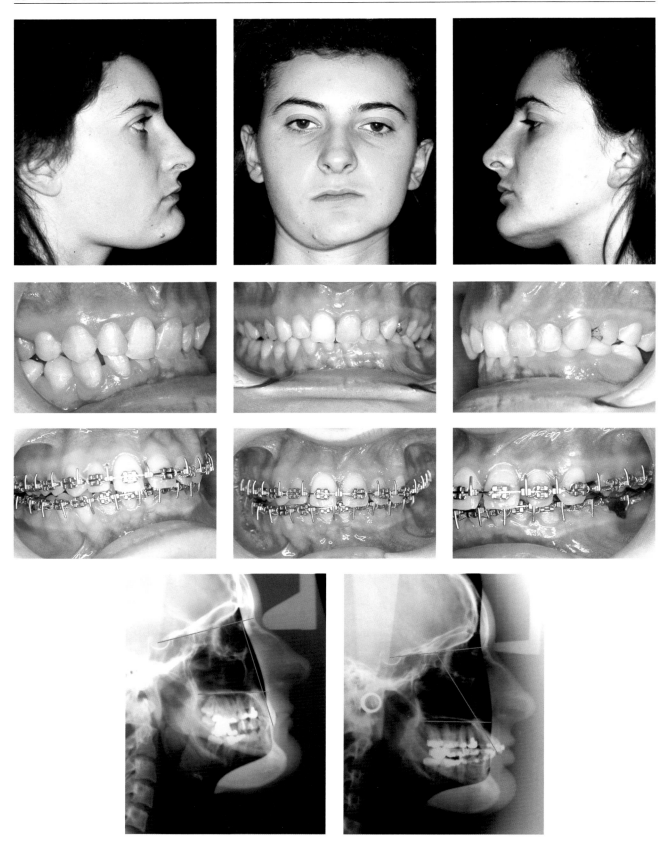

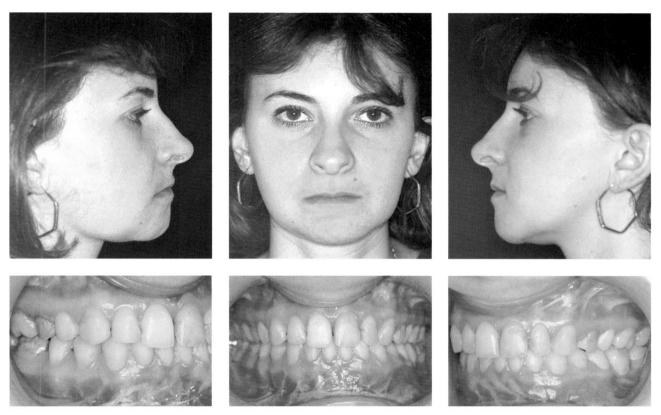

Case No. 28. This is a classic case of hemimandibular hyperplasia, with evident involvement of the maxilla. Scintigraphy did not reveal active condylar hyperplasia. After further scintigraphy at 6 months, it was decided to perform classic double-jaw osteotomy (Le Fort I osteotomy to increase symmetry plus Gotte mandibular osteotomy), with genioplasty and contouring of the mandibular margins postponed until 6 months later. Wiring and 4 weeks of maxillomandibular fixation were applied. Preoperative orthodontic treatment followed the fundamental and essential rules (note the lack of mandibular left first molar due to prior extraction). As shown in the lateral radiograph, the marked asymmetry of the mandibular margins made it impossible to identify the mandibular plane (gonion-menton) with confidence, so that in this case the axis of the mandibular incisors was not traced. The inclination of the mandibular incisors may also be evaluated clinically. The final result at 2 years is presented, after the ancillary surgical procedures were performed: genioplasty with cuneiform ostectomy and contouring of the body of the mandible at the right lower border. (Orthodontics: Dr A. Guariglia.)

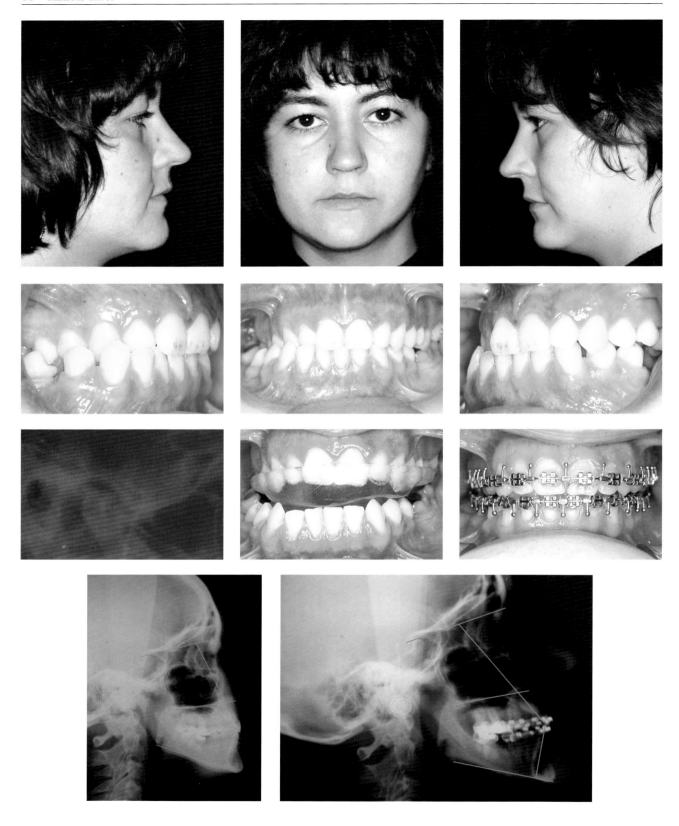

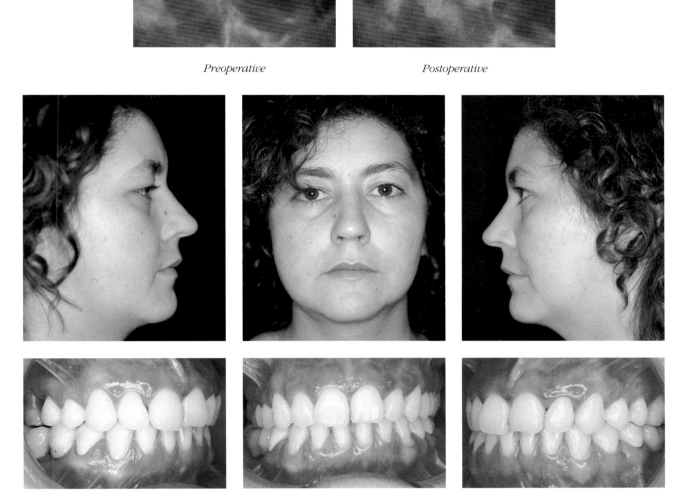

Preoperative   *Postoperative*

Case No. 29. A case of facial asymmetry with additional dysfunctional problems at the TMJ is presented. This patient had pure mandibular laterodeviation (hemimandibular elongation). Joint symptoms were present on the right in the form of pain and crepitation, resulting from an anterior position of the condyle (see transcranial radiograph on left-hand page). After application of an anterior repositioning splint, the condyle regained a central position within the glenoid fossa and the symptoms disappeared. This position was monitored throughout preoperative orthodontic treatment (see transcranial radiographs, *above left*). From the orthodontic standpoint, modest decompensation was obtained at the mandibular arch with vestibularization of the maxillary incisors. Laterodeviation only partially corrected itself, and thus a Gotte bilateral split osteotomy of the mandibular angle was performed with rigid fixation and maintenance of the position of the condyles, as described in chapter 6. The postoperative checkup on day 1 with transcranial radiograph *(above right)* shows maintenance of the preoperative position. The final result shown is 3 years after completion of active treatment. (Orthodontics: Dr A. Guariglia.)

271

Open Bite

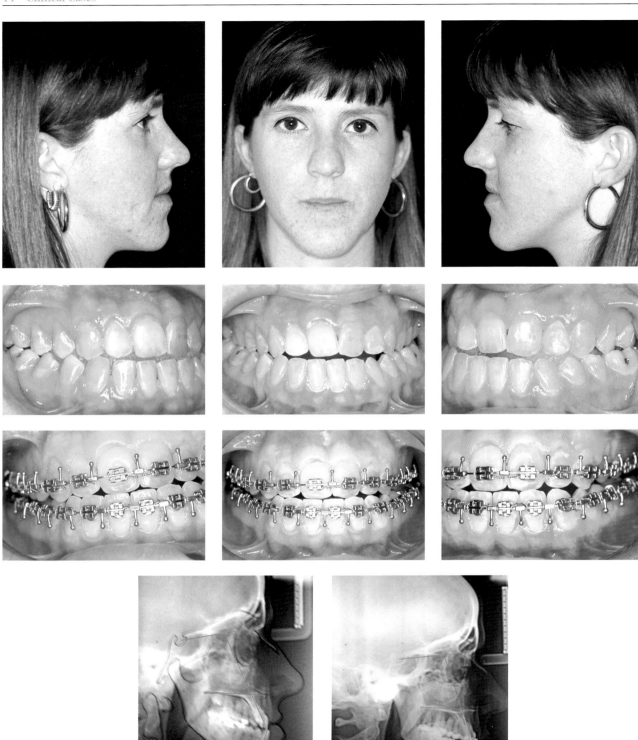

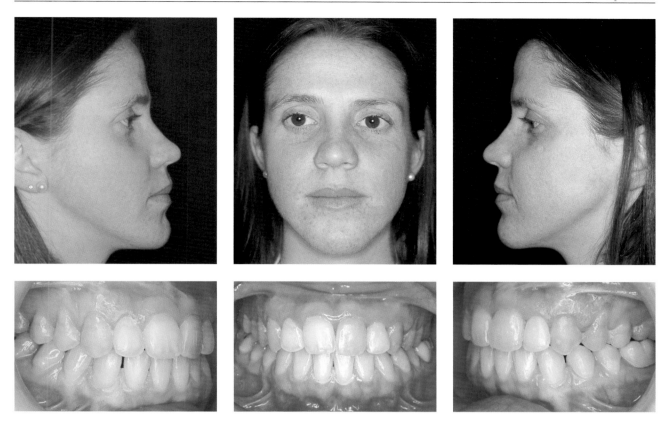

Case No. 30. This case is a slight open bite with a minimal Class III component. Preoperative orthodontic treatment was limited to alignment and coordination of the two arches. Le Fort I maxillary osteotomy was performed, with small posterior cuneiform ostectomy and rigid fixation. The final result shown is 6 months after completion of active treatment. (Orthodontics: Dr A. Guariglia.)

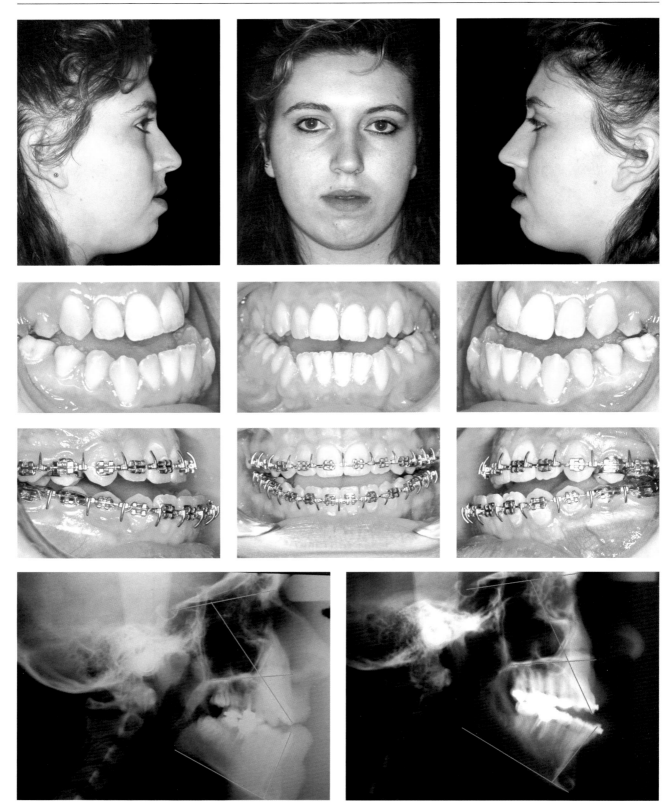

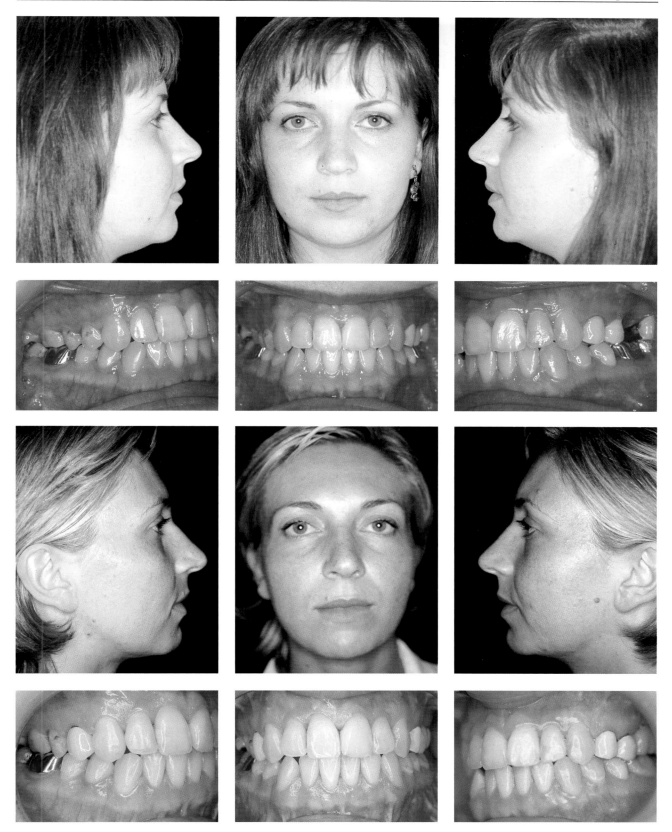

Case No. 31. This is a more severe total open bite with a moderate Class III component. In this case, surgery comprised osteotomy of the maxilla with posterior cuneiform ostectomy and Gotte bilateral split osteotomy of the mandibular angle, plus horizontal advancement genioplasty. RIF with maxillomandibular fixation for 7 days was adopted. Preoperative orthodontic treatment was simply a matter of aligning and perfecting the arches. The initial result and that at 9 years after completion of active treatment are shown, demonstrating good esthetic and functional equilibrium. (Orthodontics: Dr A. Guariglia.)

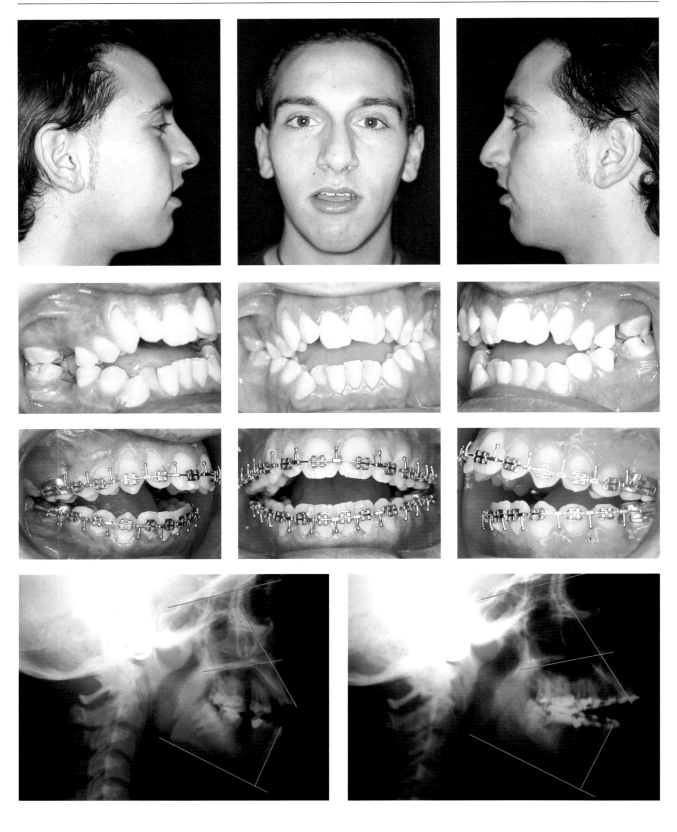

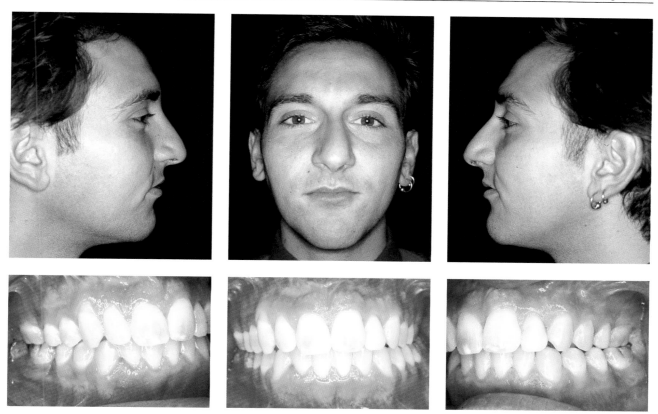

Case No. 32. This is an exemplary case of severe open bite, total and anterior, with some contraction of the maxilla. Orthodontic treatment was aimed at completely aligning the mandibular arch and normalizing the curve of Spee. For the maxillary arch, alignment was partial in preparation for three-piece Le Fort I osteotomy. This was associated with a Gotte bilateral split osteotomy of the mandibular angle. In this case, wiring with 4 weeks of maxillomandibular fixation was adopted. The final result shown is 2 years after completion of treatment. (Orthodontics: Drs L. Colombo and R. Moncado.)

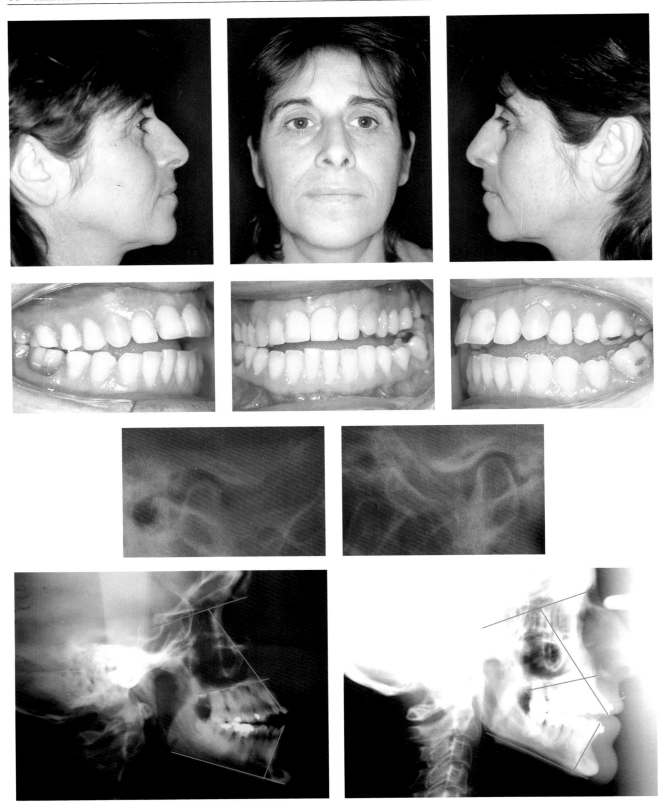

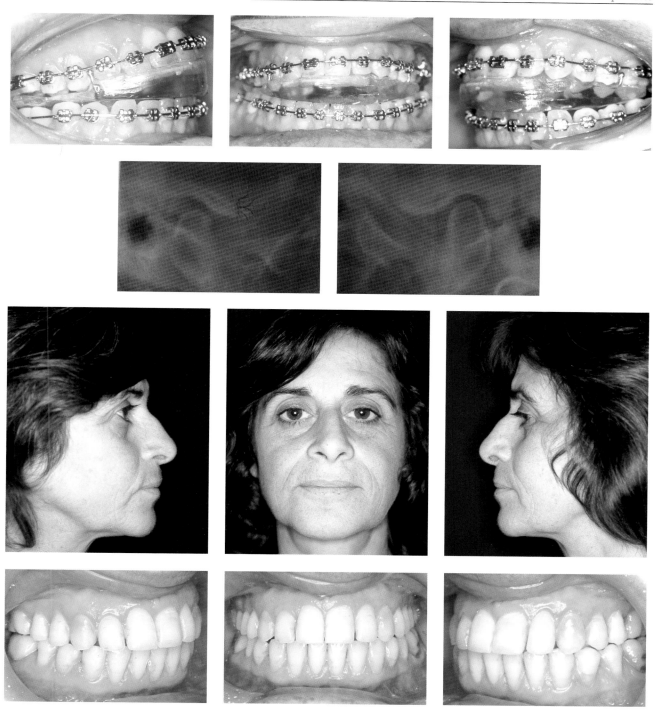

Case No. 33. The final case presented is a complex case of total open bite with significant pain and dysfunction at the TMJ. The patient's symptoms comprised pain, muscle spasm, and functional limitation, which were initially resolved with an anterior repositioning splint. However, maintenance of subjective and objective well-being was always and inevitably subordinated to the use of the splint, which the patient wore constantly throughout orthodontic preparation. The condylar position obtained with gnathologic and orthodontic treatment was monitored regularly by transcranial radiographs (see left-hand page). Orthodontic treatment included alignment and perfecting of the two arches with slight decompensation of the mandibular incisors. On completion of orthodontic preparation, double-jaw osteotomy was performed: at the maxilla, the Le Fort I type with posterior cuneiform ostectomy; at the mandible, Gotte bilateral split osteotomy of the mandibular angle. Rigid fixation was adopted with maintenance of the condylar position as described in chapter 6 and without maxillomandibular fixation. Postoperative transcranial radiographs *(above)* show perfect maintenance of the condylar position. The final result shown is at 1 year after surgery. (Orthodontics and craniomandibular orthopedics: Drs G. Cozzani and A. Modesti.)

INDEX